ESSENTIALS OF

Healthcare Management

ESSENTIALS OF Healthcare Management

SECOND EDITION

Cases, Concepts, and Skills

Leigh W. Cellucci | Michael R. Meacham | Tracy J. Farnsworth

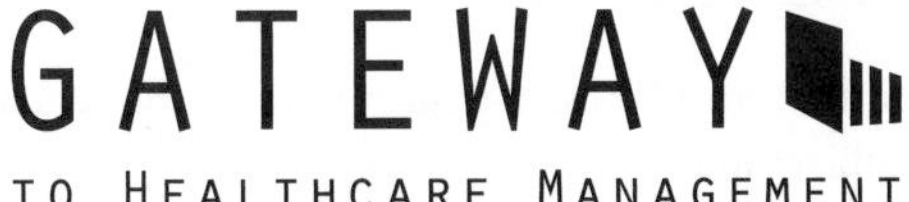

AUPHA

Health Administration Press, Chicago, Illinois
Association of University Programs in Health Administration, Washington, DC

Your board, staff, or clients may also benefit from this book's insight. For information on quantity discounts, contact the Health Administration Press Marketing Manager at (312) 424-9450.

23 22 21 20 19 5 4 3 2 1

Library of Congress Cataloging-in-Publication Data

Names: Cellucci, Leigh W., author. | Meacham, Michael R., author. | Farnsworth, Tracy J., author.
Title: Essentials of healthcare management : cases, concepts, and skills / Leigh W. Cellucci, Michael R. Meacham, Tracy J. Farnsworth.
Other titles: Essential techniques for healthcare managers
Description: Second edition. | Chicago, Illinois : Health Administration Press (HAP) ; Washington, DC : Association of University Programs in Health Administration (AUPHA), [2019] | Revision of: Essential techniques for healthcare managers / Leigh W. Cellucci and Carla Wiggins. 2010. | Includes bibliographical references and index.
Identifiers: LCCN 2018056290 (print) | LCCN 2018057913 (ebook) | ISBN 9781640550315 (ebook) | ISBN 9781640550322 (xml) | ISBN 9781640550339 (epub) | ISBN 9781640550346 (mobi) | ISBN 9781640550308 (print : alk. paper)
Subjects: LCSH: Health services administration.
Classification: LCC RA971 (ebook) | LCC RA971 .C43 2019 (print) | DDC 362.1068—dc23
LC record available at https://lccn.loc.gov/2018056290

The paper used in this publication meets the minimum requirements of American National Standard for Information Sciences—Permanence of Paper for Printed Library Materials, ANSI Z39.48-1984. ♾™

Acquisitions editor: Janet Davis; Manuscript editor: Adin Bookbinder; Project manager: Andrew Baumann; Cover designer: James Slate; Layout: Cepheus Edmondson

Found an error or a typo? We want to know! Please e-mail it to hapbooks@ache.org, mentioning the book's title and putting "Book Error" in the subject line.

Health Administration Press
A division of the Foundation of the
American College of Healthcare Executives
300 S. Riverside Plaza, Suite 1900
Chicago, IL 60606-6698
(312) 424-2800

Association of University Programs
in Health Administration
1730 M Street, NW
Suite 407
Washington, DC 20036
(202) 763-7283

In memory of a special mentor who possessed a genuine concern for the service of others,
Dr. Austin W. Bunch (1945–2017).
Courageous follower, celebrated leader, humorous colleague, and undaunted pirate.

To my husband Tony, who inspires me and is my best friend.
—L. W.C.

To Vicky Triponey, the love of my life and best friend.
—M.R.M.

To my sweetheart Michelle for her continuous support of my many endeavors.
—T.J.F.

BRIEF CONTENTS

DETAILED CONTENTS

FOREWORD

The fact that you are reading this means you are interested in working in healthcare. That interest is likely fueled by the desire to help others, to make a difference, and to have a meaningful career. Fundamentally, healthcare is about helping other people in need. It is a great way to spend your life's work.

Healthcare dominates the news cycle, political dialogue, and business agendas. There are many reasons why healthcare gets this attention. A major one is that the cost of healthcare in the United States is comparatively high, while the perceived quality of care is low. However, our healthcare system does great things for patients in their time of need and is vital to healthy communities. These varied issues and realities make healthcare a complex and sometimes confusing industry. It is undergoing rapid and transformational change. So, as a professional interested in healthcare management, the question you should ask is how you can address these varied and sometimes contradictory and complex dynamics while making individuals and communities healthier. In *Essentials of Health Care Management: Cases, Concepts and Skills*, Cellucci, Meacham, and Farnsworth help you begin to answer this overarching question.

Because management in healthcare is complex, professionals must possess a broad set of skills and a deep understanding of how healthcare works. The authors of this book introduce foundational concepts and skills that will position you for success. By equipping you with the needed management content and framing that content in practical vignettes, they provide you with a foundation of knowledge and practical applications. By learning important concepts such as professionalism, as well as technical principles and topics of business management, you will gain insights and skills that will help you drive performance and improvement in healthcare. By combining theory with practical application, this book will help you understand how healthcare works and gain knowledge and skills needed to manage in the real world.

After reading this book, you will be well on your way to a fulfilling and meaningful career in the complex, exciting, and meaningful profession of healthcare management.

Michael R. Waldrum, MD, MSc, MBA
CEO, Vidant Health
Distinguished Professor, Internal Medicine–Pulmonary and Critical Care
Brody School of Medicine at East Carolina University
Greenville, North Carolina

PREFACE

One of the benefits of authoring a book for Health Administration Press (HAP) is having a home base, so to speak, at the HAP exhibition table at all Association of University Programs in Health Administration (AUPHA) meetings. This home base enabled instructors who had adopted the first edition of this book to provide us with valuable feedback about it, including suggestions for improvement. We have enjoyed meeting our colleagues, and many of their comments inspired and informed this second edition, which we hope brings the best of teaching into the healthcare management classroom for students and professors alike.

We first met to plan this new edition during the 2015 AUPHA Undergraduate Workshop in Denver. We knew we wanted to retain the richness and detail that had been well received in the first edition. We also wanted to include substantial and comprehensive updates where appropriate and to provide a backdrop description of the current US healthcare system. Moreover, we wanted to keep the balance between theory and application to help the reader make the cognitive leap from passive reading to active understanding.

To this end, we have organized the book into three parts—(1) fundamental healthcare concepts, (2) interpersonal skills, and (3) business skills—to ensure that emerging and new healthcare professionals understand the foundation of effective management. We have added three in-depth, real-life case studies to introduce the parts. We have added six new chapters and thoroughly revised all chapters carried over from the first edition. We interwove cross-cultural learning and emphasized the significance of cultural diversity throughout the book.

The book examines health services management in the context that healthcare managers are more effective, in terms of decision-making and performance, if they possess a broad range of management skills as well as a thorough knowledge of how the US healthcare system works. This second edition begins with a case study titled "The Road to Accountable Care: Building Systems for Population Health Management." This case study introduces the first four chapters, all new to this edition:

- Chapter 1: A Brief History of the Development of Healthcare in America
- Chapter 2: Health Policy: Cost, Quality, and Access
- Chapter 3: The Healthcare System Today
- Chapter 4: Medical and Healthcare Environments

Part II, on interpersonal skills, begins with the case study "St. Luke's Health System: Transformational Leadership." Chapters 5–9 cover theory and practice in relation to leadership and managing change, professionalism and the significance of healthcare managers as members of the profession, communication and relationship management, teamwork and collaboration, and getting work done well and on time.

Finally, part III on business skills begins with "The Decision to Admit or Not to Admit," a case study describing one administrator's dilemma regarding whether to admit a potential patient to the state mental hospital. Chapters 10–12 in part III address healthcare ethics and law, finance and budgeting, and human resources. New to this edition are chapters 13 and 15 on strategic planning and marketing and health informatics, and chapter 14 on assessment of quality in health service delivery and management is an especially extensive revision.

In addition to the new chapters described above, this edition offers many features:

- True-life Case Studies translate theories to reality. The events described in the Case Studies are real; they actually occurred.

  Some of the cases are decision based—they place readers in a decision-making role and ask them to recommend how to handle or deal with the situation portrayed. Other cases are descriptive—they describe a real situation and then challenge readers to analyze, assess, and evaluate the situation and determine if the situation could have been handled more effectively. If informants asked to remain anonymous, modifications were made to disguise the people and sites involved. Otherwise, readers will know which organization faced which challenge and perhaps investigate further to discover what has happened in the time since this book was published.

  Each part of the book begins with a long, detailed Case Study that introduces the concepts covered in the upcoming chapters. Each chapter begins with a Case Study that sets the stage for particulars to be discussed, and each chapter ends with a Mini Case Study that highlights a topic covered in the chapter. The Mini Case Studies and part-opening Case Studies include discussion questions that prompt readers to make decisions about actions that should be taken or to assess actions that were taken.

- A list of Important Terms introduces every chapter to highlight the chapter's major topics.
- Learning Objectives list what the reader will be able to do after reading and studying each chapter's content.
- Points to Remember summarize the main concepts of every chapter.
- Challenge Yourself questions serve as a framework for student reflection on the material.
- For Your Consideration questions spur class discussion.
- Exercises (in select chapters) are class tested and provide individual or team-based opportunities to apply the chapter's concepts.
- Margin definitions accompany the first use of key terms, and all definitions are compiled into a convenient Glossary at the end of the book.
- Updated references, with classic references retained, help readers become familiar with the evolution of the field.

Writing this second edition was a collaborative team effort and a rewarding experience for us. We hope that you, too, find this book to be a valuable addition to your educational and career experiences.

Leigh W. Cellucci
East Carolina University
Greenville, North Carolina

Michael R. Meacham
Medical University of South Carolina
Charleston, South Carolina

Tracy J. Farnsworth
Idaho State University
Pocatello, Idaho

Instructor Resources

This book's Instructor Resources include a test bank, presentation PowerPoint slides, answer guides to the in-book Mini Case Study questions, teaching guides for the part-opener case studies, and a transition guide to the new edition.

For the most up-to-date information about this book and its Instructor Resources, go to ache.org/HAP and search for the book's order code (2375).

This book's Instructor Resources are available to instructors who adopt this book for use in their course. For access information, please e-mail hapbooks@ache.org.

ACKNOWLEDGMENTS

We thank our faculty colleagues and friends who let us endlessly discuss with them the healthcare management issues, challenges, and opportunities we encountered as we researched this book's case studies and end-of-chapter mini case studies. We have benefited greatly from the support of our colleagues at East Carolina University (ECU), the Medical University of South Carolina, and Idaho State University (ISU). Drs. Jami (DelliFraine) Jones, Xiaoming Zeng, and Dean Robert Orlikoff deserve special mention for their continued support.

Many of the case studies and end-of-chapter exercises were vetted in class or in roundtable discussions at conferences and workshops of the Association of University Programs in Health Administration. We benefited from the comments of numerous individuals there, particularly Drs. Macey Buker, Mark Diana, Christy Harris Lemak, Mary Helen McSweeney-Feld, and Carol Molinari. The undergraduate health services management students at ECU assessed (through in-class participation and feedback) which cases and exercises were worthy of print. Moreover, we greatly appreciate the work of Jenyqua Young, undergraduate assistant to the Department of Health Services and Information Management at ECU, whose unwavering enthusiasm regarding all things healthcare management was inspiring.

We thank the librarians of ECU's Laupus Health Sciences Library. Specifically, we are grateful to Carrie Forbes, interlibrary loan supervisor and distance education coordinator, for her careful attention to reference details.

We thank those who took time from their busy careers to speak with us about their work. In particular, we thank Jim Trounson, founder and CEO of Medical Management (MedMan) for his willingness to provide, review, and approve material for use in chapter 8. We thank Drew Burke, human resources director at Portneuf Medical Center, for supplying the job description and evaluation forms used in chapter 12. And we thank Dr. David Pate for sharing the story of St. Luke's transformation journey for the benefit of students and others.

Finally, we acknowledge the publishing professionals at Health Administration Press. Janet Davis served as our acquisitions editor, and her steadfast support is greatly appreciated. She championed our work on this second edition, and we value her calm leadership, good humor, and friendship. Adin Bookbinder served as our manuscript editor, and we appreciate her expert attention to detail and careful read of our drafts. We also thank Drew Baumann, editorial production manager, who handled the cover design and project management for the book, and Nancy Vitucci, marketing manager, who is leading marketing efforts.

On a personal note, Leigh Cellucci thanks her husband Tony, who showed faith in the work and her and did so with love. She also thanks her friends Louise Hudak, Mike Kennedy, Aurelia Monk, and Cara Peters, who regularly asked how the work was coming along, and Wanda Bunch, who graciously allowed the book to be dedicated to the memory of her husband Austin.

Mike Meacham thanks his wife, Vicky Triponey, who provided expert commentary for chapter 5 and careful proofreading of his portion of the book, as well as the love and support that made this effort possible.

Tracy Farnsworth thanks his friends and colleagues at ISU and at the Association of University Programs in Health Administration for their examples of scholarship and support.

PART I

CONCEPTS

CASE STUDY

The Road to Accountable Care: Building Systems for Population Health Management

Introduction

This book addresses many of the conceptual, interpersonal, and business skills associated with healthcare management, and part I covers an industry overview; health system organization; matters related to healthcare access, cost, and quality; industry issues and trends; and policy reforms that are radically reshaping the organization, financing, and delivery of healthcare. This opening case study, which describes the issues and strategies pursued by three institutions, illustrates many of these concepts and concerns. The discussion questions at the end provide additional insight and learning.

Background

A key reform goal of the 2010 Affordable Care Act was creating a healthcare system that rewards providers for achieving optimal care outcomes at a sustainable cost. As part of the law, the federal government has tested and implemented several new payment models designed to achieve this goal for the Medicare program; many of the models are built on academic blueprints (Fisher et al. 2007) and prior demonstrations (Colla et al. 2012). Likewise, several states are redesigning their Medicaid programs in pursuit of accountable care (Kocot et al. 2013; Silow-Carroll, Edwards, and Rodin 2013). Accountable care organizations (ACOs) are provider-based organizations that take responsibility for the healthcare needs of a defined population, with the goal of simultaneously improving health, improving patient experiences, and reducing per capita costs. Commercial insurers also are partnering with healthcare providers in various arrangements that strive to reward value rather than volume of services (Damore et al. 2013; Silow-Carroll and Edwards 2013; Van Citters et al. 2012).

These efforts stem from a consensus that payment reform is necessary to achieve what the Institute for Healthcare Improvement calls the "Triple Aim": improved care, healthier populations, and reduced costs. The early experiences of organizations participating in public and private payment reform programs may help policymakers gauge whether the programs are likely to achieve policy goals as well as how the programs may need to evolve to do so. Lessons learned also may help healthcare leaders decide whether to enter into such arrangements and, if so, how to increase the likelihood of success.

The following case studies describe how diverse delivery systems have responded to accountable care initiatives (see exhibit 1).[1] These organizations (or their founders) were the subject of prior research by the Commonwealth Fund, which investigated the attributes of high-performing, organized delivery systems (Shih et al. 2008). They were selected to illustrate a range of mature efforts, early successes, and ambitious aims for the accountable care model under different payment and local contexts.

Exhibit 1
Case Study Sites

Organization	Location	Type of Organization	ACO Participation	ACO Population
Health Share of Oregon*	Greater Portland, Oregon	Not-for-profit collaboration of medical and dental health plans, county mental health agencies, and community and social service agencies	Medicaid coordinated care organization	227,000 Medicaid beneficiaries residing in three Oregon counties
Hill Physicians Medical Group**	Northern California	Independent practice association of 3,800 private-practice physicians serving 300,000 patients	Several commercial ACOs, including a partnership with Dignity Health and Blue Shield of California in the Sacramento market	41,000 CalPERS members in the Sacramento market
Marshfield Clinic***	Central Wisconsin	Not-for-profit multispecialty medical group practice with 700 employed physicians serving 383,380 patients across 41 clinical sites	Medicare Shared Savings Program (following participation in Medicare's Physician Group Practice Demonstration)	30,000 traditional (fee-for-service) Medicare beneficiaries

Notes: ACO = accountable care organization; CalPERS = California Public Employees' Retirement System.
*CareOregon, a health plan that is one of Health Share's founders, was the subject of a previous Commonwealth Fund case study (Klein and McCarthy 2010).
**See Emswiler and Nichols (2009).
***See McCarthy, Mueller, and Klein (2009).

Impetus for ACO Formation and Development

The case study focuses on three organizations: Health Share of Oregon, Hill Physicians Medical Group, and the Marshfield Clinic. (See the box on page 4 for a detailed description of each entity.) All three groups shared the same main motivation for forming ACOs: The model was a natural progression of long-standing efforts to enhance primary care services and a means for extending quality improvement and care management initiatives. Other motives were unique to each site.

The creation of Health Share of Oregon, a regional Medicaid coordinated care organization, was prompted by Oregon governor John Kitzhaber's vision for transforming healthcare amid a Medicaid budget shortfall, which led the state to consolidate its vendor contracts to achieve greater efficiency and community service integration.

Market forces motivated Hill Physicians Medical Group to partner with hospitals and health plans to regain market share lost to Kaiser Permanente, an integrated delivery system that was underpricing its competitors. Meeting this challenge required the ACO partners to jointly reduce spending to bring their premiums below Kaiser's.

For the Marshfield Clinic, the Medicare Shared Savings Program offered a potential revenue source to support the continued evolution of mission-driven population health management for its patients. These physician-led efforts had begun seven years earlier through the clinic's participation in Medicare's Physician Group Practice (PGP) Demonstration, which tested the ACO concept.

Building a System for Population Health Management

The study sites adopted a variety of approaches and interventions to optimize care and identify opportunities to achieve performance and savings targets and goals. Exhibit 2 summarizes select examples of capabilities for population health management from the study sites.

Care redesign to improve the delivery and coordination of care

All three organizations were building on past efforts to redesign and strengthen primary care. Typically, this involved establishing the infrastructure and support needed for physician practices to function as patient-centered medical homes, a concept that will be discussed in chapter 4. Care coordination was key, and Hill Physicians Medical Group and its ACO partners aligned incentives to promote coordination across settings and collaborated as a cross-continuum team to successfully reduce hospital readmissions. Health Share sought to ensure that all members seeking behavioral health services received the same level of care from mental health agencies in three different counties; it created a single provider network

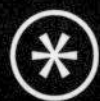

OVERVIEW OF THE CASE STUDY SITES

Health Share of Oregon is a nonprofit founded in 2012 by four competing health plans, three county-run mental health agencies, and several healthcare provider organizations to improve the care of Medicaid beneficiaries in a tricounty region encompassing Portland. As one of 16 coordinated care organizations designated by the state to oversee and integrate the delivery of medical, dental, and mental health care for a geographically defined population, Health Share receives a global budget, which it distributes in per capita payments to providers known as risk-accepting entities (RAEs). Each RAE determines how it will meet collective cost and quality goals. Through their participation in the governance of Health Share, the RAEs collaborate in adopting common practices for improving care for high-need, high-cost patients; achieving efficiencies by centralizing certain administrative functions; and creating accountability for performance. Health Share also facilitates partnerships of providers, community-based organizations, and social service agencies working to help high-need patients achieve better health.

Hill Physicians Medical Group—Northern California's largest independent practice association—joined local hospitals and commercial health plans in forming four separate ACOs aimed at improving quality, reducing fragmentation, and lowering the cost of care as a means of retaining business. The case study focused on the first and largest ACO, which was established in January 2010 to reduce premiums for 41,000 public sector employees and retirees covered by the California Public Employees' Retirement System (CalPERS). The ACO decreased hospital use and per-member per-month spending in its first three years, resulting in $59 million in savings to CalPERS, or $480 per member per year. Leaders credit their success to developing a mutual understanding of one another's strengths and challenges, which was a prerequisite for improving care coordination, increasing patient education, and reducing unwarranted variation in care.

Marshfield Clinic, a nonprofit multispecialty group practice in central Wisconsin, joined Medicare's Shared Savings Program in 2013, following its success in Medicare's Physician Group Practice Demonstration—the program's forerunner. The clinic's Medicare ACO benefits from the organization's past investment in advanced primary care infrastructure and disease-specific care management capabilities, which have yielded reductions in hospitalization and readmission rates. The clinic has an advanced, internally developed electronic health record system and enterprise data warehouse, which has enabled the internal performance reporting and identification of best practices that have galvanized physician support for quality improvement efforts. Marshfield Clinic's track record of achieving cost savings and quality targets set by Medicare suggests the importance of combining mission-driven performance improvement initiatives with a commitment to mutual accountability among providers in group practice.

Exhibit 2

Key Capabilities for Population Health Management: Examples from Study Sites*

Capability	Implementation Examples
Care redesign to improve the delivery and coordination of care	Delivery of behavioral health services was integrated across three counties and enhanced through colocation of services, improved transitions from psychiatric inpatient units to community mental health programs, and streamlining of administrative processes (Health Share).
	A standard hospital discharge practice was established to connect inpatient and outpatient care managers, arrange follow-up primary care appointments, enhance patient education, and create stronger links between skilled nursing facilities and in-home management services (Hill).
	Midlevel practitioners were employed to increase timely access to care, medical assistants were assigned to help physicians meet patients' care needs, and nurses staffing a 24-hour call line were given access to electronic records and care protocols to help route patients to appropriate care sites (Marshfield).
Care management of patients with complex, costly needs	Health resilience specialists engage, mentor, and help meet medical and nonmedical needs of at-risk patients (Health Share).
	An integrated referral process ensures patients needing case management services (e.g., for heart failure, diabetes, cancer) receive them from the most appropriate partner in the ACO, thus avoiding duplication of services (Hill).
	Virtual care teams comprising pharmacists, social workers, and case managers help primary care physicians manage the clinical and psychosocial needs of primary care patients with chronic conditions; physicians are deployed to Sacramento-area skilled nursing facilities to monitor patients and intervene when necessary to avoid admissions (Hill).
	Nurses embedded in primary care sites coordinate care and provide individualized care management to patients at risk of hospitalization; nurses receive electronic alerts when patients visit an ED or are hospitalized or discharged; patients with some chronic conditions are referred to specialized care management programs (Marshfield).
Patient/family engagement and activation	A community advisory council performs a community health assessment and develops a health improvement plan to guide care transformation (Health Share).
	A patient activation measure is used to assess patients' self-management capacities and determine appropriate support levels to achieve treatment goals (Marshfield).
Integrated data and analytics	Medical group monitors physician performance and provides coaching when there are signs of unnecessary use of services or inappropriate specialty referral patterns; physician, pharmacy, and hospital claims data identify high-cost patients needing care management (Hill).
	Risk-stratification data from Medicare are combined with in-house data on billed charges, numbers of specialists seen, medications prescribed, gender, and age to predict patients requiring care management (Marshfield).

Notes: ACO = accountable care organization; ED = emergency department.

*Findings are organized according to an evolving framework for population health management developed by John W. Whittington and the Institute for Healthcare Improvement in collaboration with healthcare organizations working toward the Triple Aim. See Institute for Healthcare Improvement (2018).

and streamlined the process for authorizing services and determining service levels to meet patient needs, an integration that enhanced the ACO's ability to measure and monitor the network's performance. Another common area of focus was improving transitions for patients moving from hospitals to post-acute or community settings, or from skilled nursing facilities to in-home care.

Care management of patients with costly, complex needs

All study sites invested resources to deploy care managers, outreach workers, or virtual care teams to engage with and help improve outcomes for patients with complex healthcare needs or at risk of incurring high costs. All three organizations provide in-person or telephone visits to provide an individualized approach to help identify and address unmet patient needs. For example, multidisciplinary care teams that included experts such as social workers, pharmacists, and case managers were deployed by urban safety-net clinics affiliated with Health Share and by the Hill Physicians Medical Group to help address the psychosocial and clinical factors that play a role in improving patients' health and treatment adherence. Marshfield Clinic embedded nurse care coordinators in its primary care clinics to help patients avoid unnecessary hospital use. (It later discontinued the program because it was partially duplicating a service offered by its health plan and because the program's cost was not sustainable without support from other payers.) The clinic retains a care management program serving heart failure patients and is reconfiguring its primary care teams to take over the care coordination responsibilities.

Patient and family engagement and patient activation initiatives

All the study sites recognized the value of engaging patients in their care management to identify personal goals for lifestyle change or treatment and educating them about their treatment options, though all felt they could do more in this regard. Health Share has had a unique opportunity to partner with community-based organizations and social service agencies to address nonmedical determinants of health within the practical constraints of its budget. However, Medicare ACOs face particular challenges when engaging patients because Medicare beneficiaries are not formally enrolled in an ACO and cannot be offered incentives to change their behavior. Therefore, Medicare ACOs must rely on their physicians' rapport with patients to encourage voluntary compliance with referrals within the ACO network and other recommendations.

Integrated data and analytics

Every site developed capabilities to identify patients who could benefit from more intensive care management, and several created systems to alert physicians or care managers when patients use or transition from the hospital. For example, through its partnership with Dignity Health in the Sacramento ACO, the Hill Physicians Medical Group was able to combine professional and hospital claims data to more accurately identify and intervene with patients at risk of hospital admission. Marshfield Clinic developed customized systems to study outcomes, identify variations and best practices in care, and report performance to physicians—a capability its leaders consider key to its success. All sites stressed the importance of achieving what is possible with available data and resources and noted that even when data are not yet electronically integrated, sharing timely information (e.g., daily hospital inpatient counts, known as "census") across ACO partners can provide insights into improving care coordination.

Supportive payment models and financial incentives

Capitation is a payment arrangement for healthcare providers such as physicians or nurse practitioners. It pays a physician or group of physicians a set amount for each enrolled person assigned to them, per period of time, whether or not that person seeks care. Capitation provides the greatest flexibility for creating a global budget to make strategic investments or to engage providers in novel ways. Yet, as exhibit 3 shows, it is perhaps easier and more feasible to add a shared-savings, or shared-risk model, on an existing reimbursement arrangement, at least initially. The Medicare Shared Savings Programs gives providers and suppliers (e.g., physicians, hospitals, others involved in patient care) an opportunity to create an ACO, which agrees to be held accountable for the quality, cost, and care experience of a Medicare population.

Results

While it is too early to tell if Health Share's bold experiment will prove successful in the Portland area, the Hill–Dignity–Blue Shield ACO and the Marshfield Clinic have established a record of savings (exhibit 3) that suggests the potential of the accountable care approach in two different contexts. Results for the Hill–Dignity–Blue Shield commercial ACO may be indicative of the kinds of savings that can be achieved when purchasers and marketplaces give consumers incentives to choose among competing value-based networks of providers.

In the Medicare arena, Marshfield Clinic was much more successful in reaping savings than other participants in the PGP demonstration, the forerunner to the Medicare Shared

EXHIBIT 3
ACO Payment Models and Results

Payment Model	Results
The state Medicaid agency allots Health Share a global per capita budget, which it apportions to RAEs that pay contracted providers on a capitated or fee-for-service basis. The state withholds 2% of Health Share's overall budget, contingent on the organization and its RAEs' cost and quality targets. Future increases in per capita payments to Health Share will be reduced by 1 percentage point in the first year and a cumulative 2 percentage points the second year.	Health Share has an ambitious plan to improve care and outcomes for Medicaid beneficiaries through the alignment of physical, capital, and human resources, with the expectation that its efforts will reduce avoidable hospitalizations and ED use and produce savings of $32.5 million in the first three years. In 2013, its first full year of operation, Health Share earned 100% of its performance incentive pool for meeting state benchmark or improvement targets on 12 of 16 measures, such as an 18% reduction in ED visits, and for enrolling more than 80% of its members in primary care medical homes.
Hill Physicians Medical Group and its partners in the Sacramento ACO (Dignity Health and Blue Shield of California) aimed to reduce spending by $15.5 million in the ACO's first year to bring premiums for Blue Shield's HMO product in line with or below those of its competitor, Kaiser Permanente. Risk and savings are shared among the medical group, hospital system, and health plan, proportional to each partner's ability to bear risk and influence spending.	The Sacramento ACO reduced spending by $20 million its first year, of which nearly $5 million in savings were shared among the three partners. Cost savings reflected reduced unit cost of services as well as reduced use of services, including a 15% reduction in 30-day readmissions; a 15% reduction in inpatient days per 1,000 members; and a 13% decline in the average length of a hospital stay for ACO patients. In total, the three-year pilot ACO reduced Blue Shield premiums for CalPERS beneficiaries by $59 million, or $480 per member per year.
Marshfield Clinic opted to participate in the Medicare Shared Savings Program's one-sided risk model,* which permits the organization to share up to 50% of the savings it produces for Medicare, provided it meets or exceeds a minimum savings rate and prescribed quality performance standards. Savings payments are capped at 10% of total benchmark expenditures each year.	During the five-year Medicare Physician Group Practice Demonstration, a forerunner of the Medicare Shared Savings Program, the clinic saved Medicare $118 million, of which it earned $56 million in shared savings for meeting quality and financial targets. The clinic reports reductions in hospitalization and readmission rates among patients engaged in its heart failure management program.

Notes: ACO = accountable care organization; CalPERS = California Public Employees' Retirement System; ED = emergency department; HMO = health maintenance organization; RAE = risk-accepting entity.
*Under one-sided risk-sharing, an ACO receives bonus payments for meeting quality and cost targets, but no direct penalty for not doing so. Under two-sided (upside and downside) risk-sharing, an ACO earns savings for meeting cost and quality targets and faces a financial penalty for failing to do so.

Savings Program. Many contemporary ACOs are expanding strategies for cost containment to include making better use of post-acute care, which was not a significant source of savings in the PGP demonstration (RTI International 2012). Such efforts take time to bear fruit. Hence, early results from the Medicare Shared Savings Program may not be indicative of the full potential of the model (CMS 2014).

Insights and Lessons Learned

Across the three study sites, gaining buy-in from providers and building systems for performance reporting and feedback were essential for fostering an environment of accountability. Each of these organizations had prior experience with managed care or shared-savings arrangements and, as a result, had developed internally managed reporting systems and feedback mechanisms that have been accepted by providers as a credible way of identifying opportunities for improvement. The organizations were also working toward explicit cost-reduction targets, whether set by federal or state governments or self-imposed based on market conditions. These targets helped them identify and prioritize programs that could lead to reductions in costs or improvements in quality.

Marshfield Clinic benefited from its dominant position and existing close working relationships with hospitals in its local, rural markets. As the sole sponsor of its ACO, the clinic did not share savings with hospitals, nor was it at risk for lost revenue from reductions in inpatient stays. This obviated the need for the trust-building exercises that were essential to Health Share and the Hill–Dignity–Blue Shield ACO, which sought to transform competitive relationships among partners. These trust-building exercises required time, patience, and perseverance. Moreover, the commercial ACO partners found that joint success required a shared willingness to reveal not only how each partner makes and loses money, but also how they underperform. The ACO's success also occurred in a mature managed care market with a dominant purchaser (CalPERS) that structured its benefit offerings to encourage cost-consciousness in its beneficiaries when they chose among competing health plan offerings. In effect, price-sensitive consumers and the market competition they fostered led the ACO partners to realize mutual benefit by acting together like a virtually integrated delivery system.

The ACOs also faced challenges. Chief among these was the difficulty of changing patient and provider behavior. The sites that produced early results had an infrastructure for robust data analytics to monitor performance and identify opportunities for improvement. The Marshfield Clinic had an enterprise-level integrated health information system—including telehealth capability—that connected its geographically dispersed ambulatory care sites and physicians. None of the sites had access to a functional regional health information exchange. This capability would likely have accelerated ACO development efforts among partners in Health Share and the Hill–Dignity–Blue Shield ACOs, which improvised in sharing information.

The method Medicare uses to determine whether ACOs qualify for shared savings presents another challenge for ACOs that need to invest in staff and technology to manage care. Some of the ACO's expenses (e.g., for case managers who oversee the care of patients with chronic and complex conditions) may recur each year, while Medicare's savings expectations will increase over time to ensure total spending for ACO patients continues to decrease relative to fee-for-service spending. In Marshfield Clinic's case, the benchmark savings target for its ACO reflected in part the reduced spending levels the clinic had previously achieved in the Physician Group Practice Demonstration, which made it more challenging for the clinic to finance intensified care management programs that could benefit its patients. The clinic's experience offers a cautionary lesson about the challenges Medicare ACOs may face when Medicare resets their shared savings benchmarks at the end of their initial participation in the program. From a policy perspective, the shared savings model may be only a halfway point on the road to more durable and comprehensive risk-sharing arrangements.

The leaders of the ACOs stress it is important to do the following:

1. Develop a portfolio of initiatives that take aim at several challenging problems (e.g., care coordination, patient engagement) because discrete quality improvement programs will not achieve the returns needed to qualify for shared savings or other payment incentives.
2. Create a system to ensure decisions made by the leaders of partner organizations and their staff are operating in lockstep. For Health Share, this meant establishing a medical directors' group that met regularly to discuss how they were carrying out the organization's mission.
3. Carefully consider each organization's willingness, readiness, and competency (including physician leadership capability) before engaging in an ACO or partnering with other organizations in an ACO relationship.

To promote successful engagement in accountable care arrangements among provider organizations that are less experienced than these case study sites, it will be important to continue to research how ACOs of many kinds are performing under a variety of circumstances. As these case studies suggest, some approaches are likely to require refinement and adaptation to address the challenges facing organizations and providers in diverse geographic markets that differ in spending levels, savings potential, and capacity for the partnerships necessary to achieve savings and quality goals. However, the progress that the case study sites have made to date suggests that payment and delivery system reforms are producing the willingness and accountability necessary to transform care and that these efforts are worthy of continued investment.

Discussion Questions

1. Define and explain the purpose of a value-based network of providers.
2. Explain why all three organizations discussed in the case study are building on past efforts to redesign and strengthen primary care. Give examples and comment on the effectiveness of their efforts.
3. All study sites have invested resources to deploy care managers, outreach workers, or virtual care teams to engage with and help improve outcomes for patients with complex needs or at risk of incurring high costs. Describe some examples and evaluate the effectiveness of their work.
4. The three sites recognized the value of engaging patients and families in care management to identify personal goals for lifestyle change or treatment and educating them about treatment options. Give examples and comment on the effectiveness of their efforts.
5. Identify and describe at least two major challenges the organizations faced in realizing benefit from their ACOs.
6. All study sites employed a combination of shared-savings or shared-risk payment models to incentivize provider behaviors. Identify these payment models and evaluate their results.
7. Explain why data integration and analytics are needed to achieve the Triple Aim. Give examples from the case study sites.
8. Explain why gaining buy-in from ACO providers and building systems for performance reporting and feedback appear essential for fostering an environment of accountability.

Note

1. The research team conducted a qualitative cross-case analysis of interview transcripts and secondary documents using case-ordered displays to identify commonalities and differences between study sites. See Miles, M., and A. Huberman. 1994. *Quantitative Data Analysis: An Expanded Sourcebook*, 2nd ed. Thousand Oaks, CA: Sage Publications.

References

Centers for Medicare & Medicaid Services (CMS). 2014. "Medicare's Delivery System Reform Initiatives Achieve Significant Savings and Quality Improvements." Accessed July 24, 2018. https://blog.cms.gov/2014/01/30/medicares-delivery-system-reform-initiatives-achieve-significant-savings-and-quality-improvements-off-to-a-strong-start/.

Colla, C. H., D. E. Wennberg, E. Meara, J. S. Skinner, D. Gottlieb, V. A. Lewis, C. M. Snyder, and E. S. Fisher. 2012. "Spending Differences Associated with the Medicare Physician Group Practice Demonstration." *Journal of the American Medical Association* 308 (10): 1015–23.

Damore, J. F., S. D. DeVore, R. W. Champion, E. A. Kroch, D. A. Lloyd, and D. W. Shannon. 2013. *The Many Journeys to Accountable Care: 4 Case Studies.* Charlotte, NC: Premier Research Institute.

Emswiler, T., and L. Nichols. 2009. *Hill Physicians Medical Group: Independent Physicians Working to Improve Quality and Reduce Costs.* New York: The Commonwealth Fund.

Fisher, E. S., D. O. Staiger, J. P. Bynum, and D. J. Gottlieb. 2007. "Creating Accountable Care Organizations: The Extended Hospital Medical Staff." *Health Affairs* 26 (1): w44–w57.

Institute for Healthcare Improvement. 2018. "Triple Aim for Populations." Accessed May 28. www.ihi.org/explore/tripleaim/pages/default.aspx.

Klein, S., and D. McCarthy. 2010. *CareOregon: Transforming the Role of a Medicaid Health Plan from Payer to Partner.* New York: The Commonwealth Fund.

Kocot, S. L., C. Dang-Vu, R. White, and M. McClellan. 2013. "Early Experiences with Accountable Care in Medicaid: Special Challenges, Big Opportunities." *Population Health Management* 16 (Suppl. 1): S4–S11.

McCarthy, D., K. Mueller, and S. Klein. 2009. *Marshfield Clinic: Health Information Technology Paves the Way for Population Health Management.* New York: The Commonwealth Fund.

RTI International. 2012. *Evaluation of the Medicare Physician Group Practice Demonstration: Final Report.* Published September. www.cms.gov/Medicare/Demonstration-Projects/DemoProjectsEvalRpts/Downloads/PhysicianGroupPracticeFinalReport.pdf.

Shih, A., K. Davis, S. C. Schoenbaum, A. Gauthier, R. Nuzum, and D. McCarthy. 2008. *Organizing the U.S. Health Care Delivery System for High Performance.* New York: The Commonwealth Fund.

Silow-Carroll, S., and J. N. Edwards. 2013. *Early Adopters of the Accountable Care Model: A Field Report on Improvements in Health Care Delivery.* New York: The Commonwealth Fund.

Silow-Carroll, S., J. N. Edwards, and D. Rodin. 2013. *Aligning Incentives in Medicaid: How Colorado, Minnesota, and Vermont Are Reforming Care Delivery and Payment to Improve Health and Lower Costs.* New York: The Commonwealth Fund.

Van Citters, A. D., B. K. Larson, K. L. Carluzzo, J. N. Gbemudu, S. A. Kreindler, F. M. Wu, S. M. Shortell, E. C. Nelson, and E. S. Fisher. 2012. *Four Health Care Organizations' Efforts to Improve Patient Care and Reduce Costs.* New York: The Commonwealth Fund.

Acknowledgment

The case studies were developed by Douglas McCarthy, Sarah Klein, and Alexander Cohen as part of a grant from the Commonwealth Fund to the Institute for Healthcare Improvement.

CHAPTER 1

A BRIEF HISTORY OF THE DEVELOPMENT OF HEALTHCARE IN AMERICA

Important Terms

- Adverse selection
- Affordable Care Act (ACA)
- Clinical integration
- Community rating
- Electronic health record (EHR)
- Employer-sponsored insurance (ESI)
- Germ theory
- Health maintenance organization (HMO)
- Hill-Burton Act
- Iron triangle
- Managed care organization (MCO)
- Medicaid
- Medicare
- National health expenditures (NHE)
- Social insurance
- Social Security Act of 1935

Learning Objectives

After reading this chapter, you will be able to do the following:

- ➤ Understand that the US healthcare system has evolved over time
- ➤ Understand the relationship between cost, quality, and access
- ➤ Understand the importance of germ theory to the development of the US healthcare system
- ➤ Understand the historical development of health insurance
- ➤ Understand that public policy decisions affect the healthcare system

Case Study: The Hill-Burton Act: A Major Landmark

One of the monumental legacies in American healthcare is a little-known piece of legislation popularly referred to as "Hill-Burton." Formally named the Hospital Survey and Construction Act, this bill was signed into law by President Truman on August 13, 1946. The Hill-Burton Act provided federal funding to states to build hospitals. The government distributed funds based on relative state wealth, such that poorer states received more money while wealthier states received less. Although construction of hospitals was part of Truman's broader national health agenda, some members of Congress, on both sides of the aisle, saw this bill as an opportunity to "do something" about healthcare while cooling the ardor of those who espoused the provision of national health insurance coverage.

The significance of Hill-Burton, however, goes well beyond its model of bipartisanship; it also provided funding for the backbone of American healthcare. When Hill-Burton appropriations ended and some of the law's provisions were folded into the Public Health Services Act in 1975, it had provided funding for more than 4,200 new hospitals and long-term care facilities. Most of these hospitals were located in poor communities or those with fewer than 10,000 people. For a hospital to receive the federal funds, the only stipulation was that it had to provide a certain amount of free care to those who could not otherwise afford it. Thus, Hill-Burton not only was a major impetus in building the infrastructure of American healthcare but also extended medical care to those who could not otherwise access it. The Hospital Survey and Construction Act of 1946 occupies a position in the pantheon of American healthcare policy initiatives similar to that of Medicare and Medicaid.

Introduction

People routinely describe the American health system as the best in the world. However, a number of questions should come to mind when we hear this declarative comment. First, does the United States really have a "health system"? Second, how does one define "the best in the world"? Does it have the best technology? Does it provide universal access to care? Does it provide the lowest-cost care? Is the access to and quality of care evenly distributed among all classes of our society? Finally, does the US health system provide high-quality care to the patient?

The answers to these questions are complex and compel us to ponder many variables. For now, a broad review of the US health system may be useful. What kind of "system" does the United States really have? And how did that healthcare system develop?

No one sat down and said, "Let's design a health system." The US healthcare system is the result of many economic and public policy outcomes sewn together like patchwork over roughly the past 240 years. Events of specific eras created certain economic or social conditions, to which the market and public policymakers responded. During one era, additional government involvement might have seemed appropriate, while conditions in other eras may have evoked a greater embrace of private markets and traditional capitalism. Indeed, even within eras of waxing or waning government engagement, some elements of the health system were more appropriately left in the hands of the free market while other elements required scrutiny by public authorities. Looking at the US health system through the prism of history will help explain how the system developed and will provide a foundation to answer questions about how well it really works.

Before the 1860s

The provision of care today—the medicine and the venues—bears no resemblance to the delivery of care before the 1860s.

Almshouses and Charlatans

Before the 1860s, hospitals were largely almshouses or places where people went because they could not get care at home. During this time, when a person fell ill, a family member or neighbor most frequently administered care in the home. Hospitals were enterprises established by a community's elite to provide charity care in the community for those who could not afford anything else. Most patients were residents of urban areas who could not pay for services and who suffered a wide variety of maladies. This era predates Louis Pasteur's germ theory and Joseph Lister's development of antiseptic procedures. Thus, hospitals were often not clean; it was common for patients to share beds, and a stench frequently permeated every corner. There were no "unit" or "ward" distinctions: A person with typhus might be in the bed next to a person with an unstable compound fracture (Rosenberg 1995).

Physicians during this era were little more than snake oil vendors and charlatans. There was no real scientific foundation nor were there academic standards on which to claim the title of "medical doctor." It was an "open market," meaning that virtually anyone could get into the business of "healing." Barbers frequently provided something akin to medical services, using leeches sometimes in the belief that "leeching" blood from a patient would alleviate the illness. No licensure standards prevented people from rendering all manner of care from leeching to selling potent elixirs designed to "cure" a wide range of ailments (Starr 1983).

Absence of Standards

One poignant example of "care" in this tradition comes from the July 2, 1881, assassination of President James Garfield. The assassin shot Garfield in the Washington, DC, train station, and the first doctor on the scene inserted his ungloved, unwashed finger into the bullet hole in search of the bullet, without success. Later, another physician used an unwashed probe for the same purpose (and with the same result). As the president lay suffering in the White House—because Garfield could receive care at his home, avoiding the hospital was imperative—he received brandy and morphine intermittently. His condition gradually worsened until he died two and a half months later, on September 19. Commentators have observed that Garfield likely would have survived the gunshot wound alone, as it did not involve any vital organs. The infection he contracted from his treatment is, ultimately, what killed him (Millard 2012).

During this era, medical schools were proprietary institutions with no uniform standards. There was no public investment in medical education, no authoritative governing bodies mandating curriculum standards, and, certainly, no experts who could be trusted to decide what topics should be taught.

In short, the delivery of care and the places in which that care took place were vastly different from one facility to the next. No agency or institution assured the public that such services would be effective. Patients turned to medicine out of personal belief amped up by the siren call of a panacea from the purveyor of an elixir on the town square. Healthcare was a crude combination of charity and chicanery with limited basis in science, often providing the illusion of hope rather than efficacious treatment.

Germ Theory to the Great War

From the middle of the nineteenth century to the beginning of the twentieth, several events combined to revolutionize medicine, thereby dramatically improving the delivery of healthcare in the United States.

Germs and Epidemiology

During the 1800s, medical science increased its understanding of the etiology of diseases—that is, their causes—and how diseases worked. Perhaps the best example is the story of Dr. John Snow, a London physician, who in 1854 uncovered the origins of cholera and, in the process, became the unofficial father of epidemiology.

Panic was widespread in mid-nineteenth-century London due to a series of seemingly random deaths throughout the capital. While London was quickly becoming a modern, industrialized metropolis, it still lacked the infrastructure needed to support its growing population. The accumulation of garbage in the streets and in the sewers that drained into the Thames River provided a perfect breeding ground for disease. Indeed, that is precisely what happened.

Because London did not provide a central water system, people obtained their drinking water from different companies throughout the city. One of the companies on the south side provided water to customers through what residents called the Broad Street pump. Snow observed that a population of people living in the same area all suffered from this strange and fatal disease at a disproportionately high frequency. He investigated by going door to door to learn where residents obtained their water and concluded that residents using the Broad Street pump had intercepted a bacterium that caused cholera, later known as *vibrio cholera*. Residents were dumping sewage and other materials into the Thames, thus exposing people who used water downstream from that location to the toxic bacterium (Johnson 2006).

The prevailing theory before Snow's discovery was that the great foggy mist that frequently enveloped the city, referred to as a miasma, caused the disease. Such was the context for medicine at the time: It was an emerging science with relatively few believers. Snow's breakthrough, however, demonstrated that the science of medicine could provide answers to questions left unanswered by the chorus of faith-based adherents of the miasma theory.

Early "Germ"-Related Science

A decade after Snow's discovery, the work of the great French chemist Louis Pasteur, centering on microbes and fermentation, contributed to the growing **germ theory** of disease. Pasteur's eponymous method to eliminate contamination in milk—pasteurization—added to the body of thought about diseases and their origins. While Pasteur is not responsible for germ theory itself, his work provided a scientific foundation to disprove the notion of "spontaneous generation": the impression that disease somehow spontaneously develops and spreads through the air. Pasteurization works by applying a mild heat to eliminate pathogens. Having thus shown how to eliminate germs, it was possible to prove that the existence of germs caused disease. Snow had already disproved the spontaneous generation theory regarding cholera; Pasteur's work made it possible to develop a more generalized theory on the way disease spread (Rosenberg 1995).

Germ theory
The theory stating that invisible microorganisms invade the body to cause disease.

In 1867, a few years after Pasteur's findings were published, Joseph Lister, a Scottish surgeon, used the Frenchman's work as the foundation for developing methods to sterilize surgical instruments and patient wounds. As his technique became more widely adopted, it dramatically reduced hospital-based infections (Rutkow 2010). President Garfield certainly would have benefited from this technique had American physicians of the day not been so reluctant to embrace it (Millard 2012).

Application of Science and Improvement in Medical Education

Contemporaneously in the United States, both "public health" (it was not called by that name at the time) and medical science advanced, though not at the same pace.

During the Civil War, the Union created the Sanitary Commission to help its army understand the nexus between disease and cure. The commission opened hospitals, encouraged the use of antiseptic techniques, and provided its active soldiers and veterans other forms of support focused on health and hygiene (Stille 1866).

Meanwhile, the number of American medical schools and students grew. This development, combined with an increasing number of legitimate practitioners and the enactment of licensure laws to keep unwanted pretenders on the sidelines, helped medicine slowly but inexorably assume a position of moral authority across the healthcare landscape (Starr 1983). The growing use of effective antiseptic techniques further helped the medical profession improve its reputation and standing. Science became the core of medical education, and students undertook internships and residencies to hone their classroom knowledge into a workable, salable set of skills. Doctors became more available and gained a greater degree of respect and acceptance. Licensure requirements erected barriers to the profession, making the proverbial "snake oil" charlatan a relic. No longer could one sell their cornucopia of potions and elixirs by simply purporting to lead unsuspecting citizens to healthier conditions.

In 1904, the American Medical Association called for minimum standards in education. That inspired further debate and review about what constituted the appropriate training of a "doctor." In 1910, the Flexner Report—published after a five-year study of medicine in the United States—concluded that medical education should include two years of science and two years of clinical training in hospitals. Further, the report recommended that medical schools affiliate with universities to advance the intellectual underpinnings of the science. As those developments continued, the proprietary schools began to vanish from the landscape because they could not afford the laboratories to support the science component of the curriculum (Flexner 1910).

All these developments combined to improve the quality of healthcare offered to and obtained by Americans. Providers were learning about the science of the human body, and medicine was thwarting the spread of disease or working to eliminate it based on scientific understanding. This gave rise to expanding access to more qualified and competent care.

Beginnings of Institutionalized Healthcare: From WWI to WWII

While science led to advancements in medicine and hospital care during the late nineteenth century, the early twentieth century saw significant developments in the process of delivering care and in the way providers were paid.

The Beginning and Proliferation of Health Insurance

Health insurance took a significant step forward in 1929 when Baylor University Hospital provided Dallas school district teachers 21 days of hospital coverage for 50 cents per month. The teachers were prepaying for care they might or might not need at some point in the future. This was the birth of Blue Cross plans, in which hospitals provided coverage for the insured (Buchmueller and Monheit 2009). (Blue Shield, the counterpart insurance covering physician care, came a decade later in mining and lumber camps in the northwest United States [Lichtenstein 2012].)

Still, commercial insurance companies at that time maintained their focus on life, property, and casualty and avoided health as a subject for coverage because they feared **adverse selection**, which occurs when healthy people do not purchase coverage. The commercial insurers worried that if only people who were sick bought insurance, rates would skyrocket because the costs of care would also be quite high. With no (or relatively few) healthy people in the pool to balance the risk, commercial insurers were reluctant to enter the market (Starr 1983).

Adverse selection
The phenomenon that occurs when there is a disproportionate percentage of patients with greater-than-average need for medical and hospital care enrolling in an insurance plan.

The Baylor plan, however, was strictly not-for-profit and included *all* teachers, healthy and sick alike. In addition, everyone paid the same "premium," 50 cents per month. That this occurred in 1929, the year the Great Depression began, is not a coincidence. As individuals started to avoid healthcare to save money, hospitals found they had vacant beds and declining revenue. By enrolling large numbers of teachers, the 50 cents per month per teacher provided Baylor University Hospital with much-needed cash and protected the teachers from at least some of the costs associated with a potentially catastrophic illness or injury, thereby spreading the cost over a larger group of people with varying health statuses.

As this idea caught on, 25 states enacted laws permitting Blue Cross to operate as a charitable foundation and waived the normally significant financial reserve required of insurance companies. Other organizations across the United States emulated the plan, and ultimately sister organizations known as Blue Shield provided similar coverage for physician services. "The Blues" continued to insure millions of Americans using **community rating** through late in the twentieth century.

Community rating
The process of establishing insurance premiums based on the average healthcare demands of an entire community or population without regard to any risk factors, resulting in identical premiums for every plan member regardless of age, gender, or other health risk.

Community rating is the practice of providing health coverage for a group of individuals where everyone pays the same amount for the insurance regardless of age, health risk, gender, or source of employment. This concept lost some of its appeal as commercial insurers became more active in the market in the post-Depression period. Employers, anxious to manage costs, engaged commercial insurers as they began to adjust for risk among various groups. "Risk adjustment" means that insurance companies adjust the premiums based on the relative risk of illness striking members of the insured group. Thus, for example, insurance for coal miners is likely to cost more, because of their exposure to coal dust and pollution-filled air, than insurance for office workers, who do not engage in any potentially hazardous activity associated with their employment.

The Impact of World War II

World War II also became a major impetus that forever changed the landscape in financing healthcare services in the United States. Not only did the federal government become more directly involved in providing and financing healthcare, but its wartime policies inexorably set in motion a trend to expand health insurance coverage for Americans.

Insurance became an attractive and popular negotiated benefit during World War II. The federal government imposed wage and price controls to avoid, for example, the makers of airplanes from raiding the employees of those companies making armaments. Thus, as wages were frozen, employers searched for alternative mechanisms to recruit and retain their labor force. Health insurance became that recruitment tool. This led to significant growth in **employer-sponsored insurance (ESI)**, which became the primary mechanism by which individual employees acquired insurance to cover the costs of their care.

Employer-sponsored insurance (ESI)
Insurance plans for which the employer pays part of the premium for the benefit of the employee and sometimes their family members. The primary way Americans obtain health insurance.

World War II also was a time when the federal government became more directly involved in providing health insurance. Congress enacted medical coverage for women and children dependent on members of the armed services and expanded coverage for all military personnel (Starr 1983).

As the first half of the twentieth century ended, the stage was set for a new era in American society, and a new era for healthcare. The Social Security Act (see box) provided

THE IMPORTANCE OF THE SOCIAL SECURITY ACT

The federal government's role also dramatically changed during the time between the two world wars. As the malaise of the Great Depression gripped the US economy, people looked to government policymakers for solutions. One piece of legislation that forever changed the nature of the contract the American people had with their government was the **Social Security Act of 1935.**

Social Security Act of 1935
Massive legislation that created direct federal benefits for American citizens in the form of cash payments to the elderly. The act also provided for unemployment insurance and worker's compensation for injured workers.

As the Roosevelt administration prepared the legislation, drafters considered including provisions for national health insurance. Advisers close to Roosevelt, specifically Dr. Harvey Cushing, voiced opposition to that concept, parroting the American Medical Association. Thus, national health insurance never made it into even the draft of the Social Security legislation (Blumenthal and Morone 2010).

The importance of the Social Security Act, however, rests in its sweeping scope of old-age benefits for workers, benefits for victims of industrial accidents, unemployment insurance, aid for dependent children, and aid for the blind and the physically disabled. Implementation of some of these programs came through the states with federal financial support. Some, such as the direct benefits for retired workers, came directly from the federal government. For the first time, the federal government would provide benefits directly to individual citizens, in the form of Social Security payments.

The act in its entirety, especially the direct payments to retired workers, established a broad precedent for the federal government's direct involvement in the lives of individuals, most particularly for the enactment of both Medicare and Medicaid some 30 years later. (Medicare and Medicaid will be discussed in depth later.) The Social Security Act provided the bedrock for what would become the pantheon of federal social programs, including healthcare, that directly affect the lives and well-being of individual citizens.

direct benefits for the American people. The concept of health insurance was born. War forced employers to embrace the concept of health insurance as an additional benefit for employees, and the federal government took an active role in providing insurance for a particular class of citizens. Combined, these developments served as the foundation for an era of unprecedented growth in all elements that together form what we today call the American healthcare system.

The Postwar Era to the Early 1970s

The post-World War II era was a period of profound growth in most aspects of American life, including healthcare. While many think of the 1950s as a relatively tranquil time in American history, often using the phrase "peace and prosperity in our time," it was in fact an era of unprecedented growth and the injection of new dynamics into American life (Halberstam 1993). With respect to health services delivery, this growth manifested itself in multiple ways.

Hospitals and Hill-Burton

When President Harry Truman proposed a universal healthcare plan in early 1945 (see box), Republicans in Congress found an alternative in legislation to expand the availability of hospitals. Authored by Senators Lister Hill, a Democrat from Alabama, and Harold Burton, a Republican from Ohio, the plan rested in a Senate committee until it became a watered-down substitute to the Truman plan (Perlstadt 1995). The heart of the act authorized $75 million annually for five years to build new hospitals or expand existing facilities. The legislation's funding distribution formula especially helped rural and poorer states where hospitals were rare or nonexistent. It also set a policy goal of creating 4.5 beds per 1,000 people. Hospitals that accepted **Hill-Burton** funding were then obligated to provide a "reasonable" amount of care for indigent patients who could not afford to pay the full cost of care. Because of this provision, Hill-Burton became the first federal legislation aimed at providing healthcare services for the uninsured (Perlstadt 1995). Hill-Burton was also significant in that it relied on the concept of federal–state cost sharing, a concept that would be used in subsequent health-related initiatives.

Hill-Burton Act
Bipartisan legislation aimed at funding the growth of community hospitals in the United States.

The Hill-Burton Act had a long run, beginning in 1946, including significant amendments to include long-term care facilities, rehabilitation centers, and certain outpatient facilities. When funding for the act was terminated in 1975, Hill-Burton had underwritten the bulwark of modern US healthcare infrastructure. It had provided $3.7 billion in federal funding, with $9.1 billion in matched funding from state and local governments. During that time, state and local governments added more than 410,000 hospital beds to the system in more than 10,000 projects. Since 1980, Hill-Burton hospitals and other facilities have provided more than $6 billion in uncompensated care for eligible patients (HRSA 2016).

Investing in Science

The postwar era also was a time when the United States invested billions in health-related science, significantly increasing funding to the National Institutes of Health (NIH). During the 1950s and 1960s, appropriations to the NIH grew from $52.7 million in 1950 to $291.8 million in 1959 to more than $1.1 billion a decade later (NIH 2018). As a result, scientists and public health providers all but eradicated smallpox; introduced and widely disseminated an effective vaccine for polio; discovered new diseases; deployed new methods of imaging and diagnosis; and deployed new therapies. A small sample of discovery during this period includes the use of diagnostic ultrasound (1953); kidney transplant (1953); the antibiotic tetracycline (1955); the cardiac pacemaker (1958); hip replacement (1962); the first oral vaccine for polio (1962); and liver and lung transplants (1963). Science was advancing knowledge about human anatomy and physiology at an astounding rate, finding new ways to diagnose "new" diseases and developing new methods of treatment and prevention (Stevens 1999).

Expansion of Medical Education

During this same time, the number of medical schools, medical students, and related research also exploded. Much of the NIH funding mentioned previously was allocated to medical schools for advanced research related to disease causation and treatment. Likewise, the federal government invested in health education facilities. Opposition by the American Medical Association, attempting to protect the markets for existing medical practitioners, stalled federal engagement in the issue of direct aid for the expansion of medical education throughout the 1950s. In 1963, however, Congress passed the Health Education Facilities Act that started a stream of funding to open 54 more medical schools (44 allopathic and 10 osteopathic), before federal appropriations ended in 1980 (Cooper 2003). To further address the perceived shortage of doctors, in addition to new students enrolling in the new medical schools, enrollments in existing schools went from an average of 90 per class to 149. Subsequently, by 1980 there were 18,200 students matriculating in medical school compared to 8,250 in 1956 (Cooper 2003).

Proliferation of Private Insurance Coverage

In 1954, Congress codified what had been an existing practice: permitting employers to deduct from their tax liability the cost of employees' health insurance premiums. Even though ESI had expanded dramatically during World War II, the tax treatment of the premiums paid by employers was uncertain. For the most part, employers relied on a series of private rulings from the Internal Revenue Service permitting them to deduct the cost of premiums for employees' health coverage from their federal income tax. With the passage of the Revenue Act of 1954, however, federal law embedded favorable tax treatment for employers providing health insurance for employees. To this day, that deduction remains in place as an incentive for ESI. Likewise, the predominant way individuals have secured healthcare coverage has been through their employers. Despite this incentive, however, the ever-increasing cost of coverage has caused some employers to re-examine the value of this benefit. Over time, the percentage of Americans receiving health insurance coverage through their employer has diminished from 64.4 percent in 1994 to 58.3 percent in 2012 (Fronstin 2013). The growth in ESI, however, from the end of World War II to the early 1990s was noteworthy, providing the essential underpinning of the US system of financing healthcare (Blumenthal 2006). Exhibit 1.1 provides a snapshot of the history of growth in ESI.

Implementation of Medicare and Medicaid

Universal healthcare coverage has been a policy goal for many people since early in the twentieth century. President Theodore Roosevelt first issued a call for social insurance when he observed that many people could not afford the costs of medical services (Starr 1983).

Exhibit 1.1 Enrollment in Private Insurance in the United States, 1940–1960

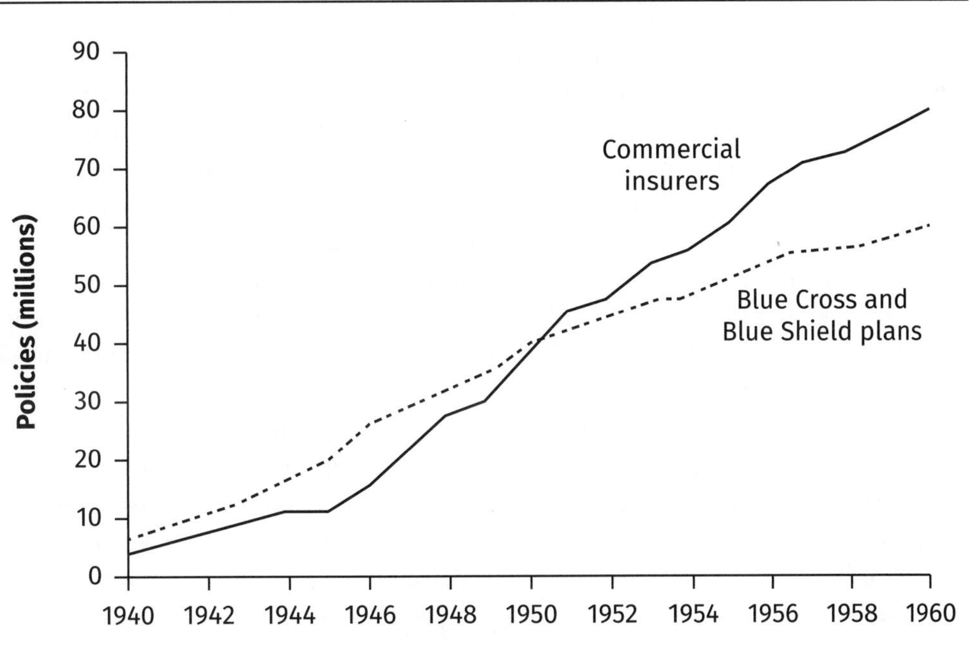

Source: Reprinted from Blumenthal (2006).

Likewise, as discussed earlier, President Franklin Roosevelt ruminated about creating national health insurance in 1934 and 1935. In 1946, President Truman also proposed creating national health insurance—again to no avail (Blumenthal and Morone 2010).

Each of these efforts cited the need for coverage or support because the costs of healthcare services were simply too great to bear for too many people. Invariably, assistance for the poor, elderly, and disabled was at the forefront in making the case for national health insurance. Moreover, while the proposals took several different forms, virtually all failed in the final analysis because healthcare policy was too complicated to explain or because the costs of the proposals were too great (Blumenthal and Morone 2010). Frequently, there were political considerations, such as when the Republican-controlled Congress of the Truman era passed Hill-Burton, in part to blunt the Truman administration's argument about the need for national healthcare coverage.

The recognition that costs were becoming too much to bear for some frequently was rooted in concern for the elderly. Specifically, in 1960, providing assistance with the cost of medical services for the part of the population that was both elderly and poor was the motivating factor behind legislation called "Medical Assistance for the Aged Act," also known as Kerr-Mills for its two sponsors, Senator Robert Kerr (D-OK) and Representative Wilbur Mills (D-AR). This legislation included two important policy decisions. First, the bill created medical assistance for a newly classified group of people, the indigent elderly. The second critical concept, borrowing from Hill-Burton, was the implementation of a matching grant mechanism based on the relative wealth of the state. These concepts became the foundation for what would later become Medicaid (Moore and Smith 2005).

In 1964, the political landscape changed. In the wake of the November 1963 assassination of President John Kennedy, his successor Lyndon Johnson rode to victory on an enormous wave of popular support. The Democrats, in addition to controlling the presidency, controlled both houses of Congress by large margins. If ever there were an alignment of political constellations to move the healthcare coverage needle another step closer to universal coverage, this was the time. It was in this political climate that President Lyndon Johnson and close congressional ally Wilbur Mills (D-AR), chairman of the House Ways and Means Committee, drove through the passage of Medicare and Medicaid. Like all things political, it was necessary to compromise on a number of provisions.

Social insurance
A system of compulsory payments made by everyone to the government to provide assistance to a designated subset of the population for a specific service or set of services. Medicare Part A is a good example: Every employee and employer contributes to the Medicare Trust Fund through a taxing mechanism. Those funds are used to provide hospitalization benefits to everyone older than age 65.

There were, in fact, three separate proposals grounded in different philosophies. One was a **social insurance** proposal mandating coverage for senior citizens. Social insurance takes its name from the concept that it protects individuals from hazards associated with conditions such as old age or unemployment. Coverage is for a particular class of people, paid for by employers and employees as mandated by the government. In other words, everyone pays for a benefit intended for a designated group of people. In this proposal, coverage would include hospitalization charges and physician costs only for inpatient care. In attempting to gain support for the bill, however, the sponsors limited coverage to those older than age 65.

A second proposal emanated from the concept of public assistance, meaning the government would provide coverage only to those who enrolled. The proposal called for coverage only of outpatient physician services. Tax revenues from all taxpayers would subsidize enrollees' premium payments to fund the program.

The third proposal came from the American Medical Association and was called Eldercare. This proposal would have expanded the then-existing Federal-State Medical Assistance for the Aged Program—the Kerr-Mills legislation referenced earlier—that provided a measure of support for the poorest members of the older-than-65 population.

While each of the three proposals competed with the other two, Mills combined them all under one bill to the extent possible. **Medicare** Part A was born from the first proposal, the social insurance concept. The second proposal—the public assistance option—became the foundation for Medicare Part B. And the third proposal became what we now know as **Medicaid**, a program funded by both the federal and state governments to provide health services for the indigent. None of this, of course, had much to do with anticipated future needs and expenditures. It had everything to do with political compromise (Myers 2000).

In the end, the Social Security Act of 1935 provided the legal vehicle for the 1965 passage of Medicare and Medicaid. Title XVIII of the Act is Medicare, while Medicaid has its legal nexus in Title XIX. Medicare and Medicaid were major expansions of the role the federal government plays in people's lives. As noted earlier, the Social Security Act set the policy precedent of the federal government providing a direct benefit to US citizens. Medicare and Medicaid represented expansions on that concept and provided two additional steps on the road to health coverage for all Americans.

Today, Medicare consumes 15 percent of the federal budget, while Medicaid commands 9 percent (Cubanski and Neuman 2018). Combined, they represent 37 percent of **national health expenditures (NHE)**, which is everything Americans spend on healthcare (CMS 2016). These programs have become essential ingredients in the American healthcare system, and the long-term sustainability of each has been, and continues to be, a source of political debate. On average, Medicaid represents 25.6 percent of all state budgets, the largest single category of spending (NASBO 2015). Chapters 2 and 11 will address these programs in detail.

Medicare
The federal program that provides health insurance coverage for people older than 65. Medicare Part A covers hospital costs; Part B covers part of the cost of ambulatory care; Part C is a managed care alternative; and Part D provides a benefit for the partial expense of prescription drugs.

Medicaid
A joint federal–state program that provides insurance coverage for those who cannot afford it. The federal government funds 50 to 75 percent of the costs and controls the broad parameters of the program, which is otherwise administered by the states. The formula that allocates the federal funds is inverse to the relative wealth of the state, meaning that poorer states receive more while richer states receive less.

National health expenditures (NHE)
An economic indicator showing the aggregate amount the United States spends on healthcare each year, frequently expressed as a percentage of the gross domestic product.

The Sum of Postwar Efforts

What might you expect to be the result if you (a) have more hospital beds, (b) more doctors with more areas of specialization, (c) improved diagnostic methods, (d) improved treatment methods, and (e) more widely available insurance? The result, of course, is the delivery of more and better (technologically speaking) healthcare to more people in more places than ever before. Not surprisingly, this translated into astronomical healthcare inflation. Both the cost of care in absolute dollar terms as well as the proportion of gross domestic product (GDP) dedicated to healthcare grew at exponential rates during the 1950s and 1960s.

Expenditures per capita expanded from $147 in 1960 to $356 in 1970 to $1,112 in 1980 (Kaiser Family Foundation 2014). Medical inflation generally ranged from about 7 percent in 1960 to more than 14 percent in 1975 (CMS 2017). These astounding increases presented policymakers with a renewed impetus to "do something" about healthcare costs.

Exhibit 1.2 demonstrates the growth of NHE as a percentage of GDP. NHE includes all healthcare services spending from whatever source, so the graph includes Medicare, Medicaid, commercial insurance, private pay, over-the-counter purchases, and more. Every dollar of healthcare expenditure is included, so you can see the dramatic increase from 1960 onward.

This rampant inflation grabbed the attention of policymakers in the early 1970s, and it has remained a source of concern (and a political issue) ever since. While costs had previously been a motivator to provide coverage for various groups of citizens, overall costs in the system now became a separate, more general source of concern: How long could the country sustain medical inflation at these rates? Thus was born multiple initiatives to curb costs.

1970s to the Affordable Care Act

Earlier, we mentioned President Truman's effort in 1946 to pass National Health Insurance. He was not the only US president to address this issue, but his proposal was the most expansive before the Affordable Care Act of 2010. During his term (1953–1961), President Dwight Eisenhower never tried to institute universal coverage; however, he maintained compassion

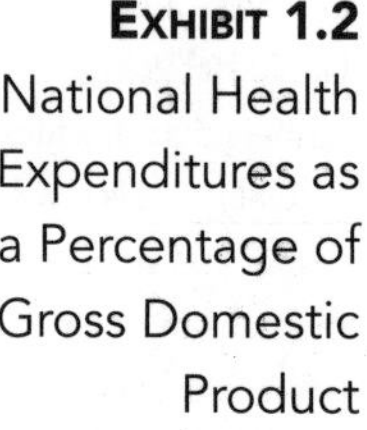

Exhibit 1.2
National Health Expenditures as a Percentage of Gross Domestic Product

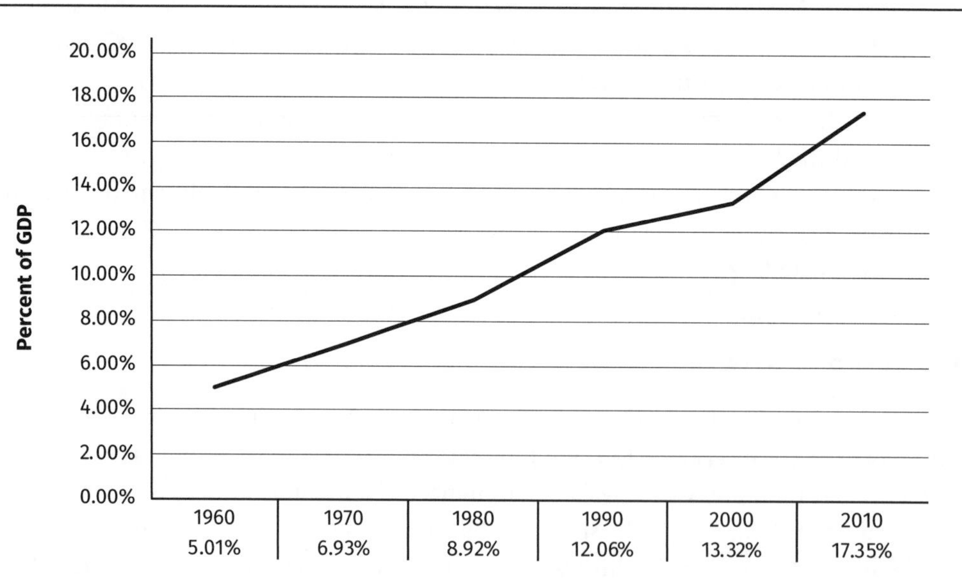

Source: Adapted from CMS (2017).

for those confronting excessive healthcare costs. President John Kennedy (1961–1963) wanted to expand the availability of healthcare services for more people, particularly in the form of Medicare. President Johnson (1963–1969) successfully sought coverage for the aged and the poor in Medicare and Medicaid, as discussed earlier. President Richard Nixon (1969–1974) proposed mandates for employers and individuals to purchase insurance. And President Bill Clinton (1993–2001) proposed universal coverage through "managed competition" of healthcare markets (Blumenthal and Morone 2010).

Responding to Rampant Inflation: 1970s–1990s

Despite policymakers' concerns about the dramatic increases in healthcare costs, they could not seem to control them. Medicare and Medicaid did not address the issue of national healthcare expenditures, but rather focused on ameliorating the impact of the cost of care on specific population groups, the elderly and the poor—and have become major contributors to national healthcare expenditures. Indeed, these two government programs have been among the leading causes of healthcare cost increases (CMS 2017; Kaiser Family Foundation 2014).

As costs exploded throughout the 1970s and beyond, presidents and Congress have struggled, mostly without success, to tame the beast of medical inflation. President Nixon not only proposed insurance mandates, but also suggested the creation and expansion of **health maintenance organizations (HMOs)** as a way of managing costs while providing access to primary care. HMOs were ostensibly a way to limit aggregate spending in the system by restricting access to high-cost specialty care. Insurance companies paid providers a set fee, in advance, to provide care for individuals enrolled in the HMO. These HMOs engaged the primary care physician as a "gatekeeper" for the patient. (HMOs, along with their spinoff **managed care organizations [MCOs]**, will be discussed in detail in chapter 11.) Simply stated, HMO patients could not access specialty care—at least specialty care that would be paid for by their insurance—without the prior referral of their physician. Likewise, some HMOs limited the number of primary care physicians available, so consumers were suddenly limited in their ability to choose their medical care. Consumers began to object to these limits, crescendoing in the late 1990s into a widespread and intense consumer backlash that moved the federal and state governments to pass a wide variety of patient protection acts (Sultz and Young 2014).

Health maintenance organization (HMO)
A healthcare-providing organization that generally has a closed panel (limited number) of physicians (and other providers, including hospitals) that agrees to provide all the medical and hospital care an individual may need, for a fixed, predetermined fee.

Managed care organization (MCO)
A general term applied to a variety of organizations that provide services intended to reduce healthcare costs by managing access to care.

Responding to Rampant Inflation: 1990s–2010

The next major push to realign the healthcare system and how it delivered services came during President Clinton's first term. Before his election, Clinton's political team had taken note of a US Senate special election campaign in Pennsylvania in 1991. Harris Wofford, a Democrat and the state's insurance commissioner, defeated a much better funded, popular

Republican former governor and former US Attorney General, Richard Thornburgh. Wofford's signature line in the campaign: "If criminals have a right to a lawyer, I think working Americans should have the right to a doctor" (Johnson and Broder 1997, 60). It was a stunning upset that captured the attention of the Democratic party leadership as well as the man who would soon become president.

It also captured the attention of the George H. W. Bush administration, which before Wofford's win had been withholding its plan for healthcare reform. Because of Wofford's victory, however, and in an effort to upstage the Democrats as the 1992 presidential campaign took shape, President Bush and his team unveiled a Comprehensive Health Reform Program featuring tax credits and vouchers (Blumenthal and Morone 2010).

Yet after President Bush announced the plan in his 1992 State of the Union address, he never acted on it. Wofford's win moved healthcare access to the forefront of the presidential election of 1992. Governor Clinton campaigned on sweeping reform of the healthcare system, and after winning promised to have a healthcare reform proposal before Congress as one of his first initiatives (Blumenthal and Morone 2010; Johnson and Broder 1997).

Clinton appointed his wife, attorney Hillary Rodham Clinton, to chair the task force charged with developing a comprehensive reform of the American healthcare delivery system. The ultimate product was an intitiative to encourage competition among health insurers, called managed competition. It was a massive upheaval of the insurance markets. Critics derided the proposal as a government takeover of healthcare. After months of debate, the beleaguered plan was withdrawn in the face of overwhelming opposition complicated by other issues on the political agenda (Johnson and Broder 1997).

After eight years in office, the Clinton administration gave way in 2001 to the presidency of George W. Bush without achieving the signature reform on which it had staked so much. The new administration, committed to leaner, less instrusive government, would not venture so far with regard to healthcare reform.

Demographic Changes

In addition to the intense political debate about rising healthcare costs and what to do about them, two significant demographic changes in the American population were creating an increasing demand for long-term care and chronic disease management.

The "baby boom" generation was aging and changing the population pyramid. Born between 1946 and 1964, this extraordinarily large cohort has had an indelible effect on American wants, needs, tastes, and culture. Exhibit 1.3 depicts the age and gender distribution of the US population in 2000, 2025, and 2050. Notice the dramatic growth in the cohorts ages 65 and older over the years. Notice also the dramatic growth in the "85+" age category over time: More people were living longer lives (US Census Bureau 2016). Furthermore, economic mobility meant more families were living farther apart; sons and daughters left home and moved to other regions of the country to pursue their own dreams,

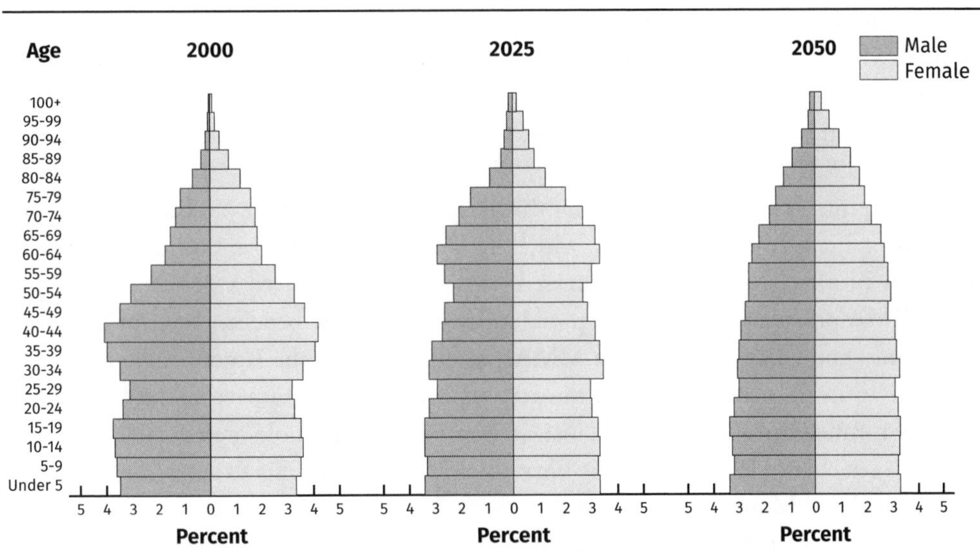

Exhibit 1.3
Age and Gender Distribution of the US Population in 2000, 2025, and 2050

Source: Reprinted from US Census Bureau (2016).

leaving aging relatives to seek help from strangers. "Nursing homes" started to change into "assisted living" and "long-term care" facilities to address the needs of an aging population whose families had dispersed to other parts of the United States.

The growth in the segment of the population of working age also is creating a greater demand for health insurance coverage. At the same time, there has been massive growth in the biotechnology, medical device, and pharmaceutical industries. Money flowing into this "medical industrial complex," combined with increased expenditures on health services by both government and private insurers, exacerbated the overall cost of healthcare coverage and forced employers to begin the process of reconsidering or scaling back the scope of their employee health plans (Rutkow 2010).

Another significant development during this era was the rise of for-profit hospital chains. Traditionally, hospitals had been not-for-profit charitable institutions that provided care for the very ill. As science advanced and improved hospitals' quality of care and outcomes, the facilities began to charge for services. Increasingly, the hospital became a business. A number of entrepreneurs saw an opportunity to provide similar or better service at a lower cost. The for-profit chains were able to generate operational savings through economies of scale when purchasing goods and equipment. Thus, what had been a community service transitioned into a corporate enterprise (Stevens 1999).

The other significant trend that began during this time was hospital ownership of physician practices. Payment systems such as HMOs and preferred provider organizations had begun ratcheting down the number of specialty visits by requiring primary care providers to refer patients to specialists, in order to guarantee that insurers would cover these visits. As this occurred with increasing frequency, hospitals began to acquire primary care practices in the hope of being on the receiving end of these referrals. In addition, hospitals found other ways to align physician practices to maximize referrals to specialists associated with *their* organizations. While this strategy had mixed results, it did presage a movement that would be central to the next wave of realignment in the healthcare system (Stevens 1999).

In terms of health policy during this time, President George W. Bush's initial priority was the enactment of tax cuts, which he largely achieved. The Bush administation eventually proposed—and Congress passed—the Medicare Modernization Act (MMA) of 2003. MMA provided the Medicare population a wholly new benefit: prescription drugs. Commonly known as "Part D," the MMA was at that point the largest single change to Medicare in its 48-year history. Yet the act was controversial, in part because it did not fully pay for medications for seniors, instead creating a "donut hole" gap in coverage. Still, this was a sea change in extending the breadth of Medicare benefits to a new coverage area (Blumenthal and Morone 2010).

Like most of the health policy initiatives targeted at a particular population, the MMA did little to offset the overall level of medical inflation. While it provided a measure of protection to older Americans against the impact of what was then the fastest growing cost in the healthcare market, prescription drugs, the MMA did not offer comprehensive initiatives with regard to overall costs. By the time President Barack Obama took office in 2009, healthcare costs were a stunning 16 percent of the GDP (CMS 2017).

Affordable Care Act to 2018

Affordable Care Act (ACA) Also known as the Patient Protection and Affordable Care Act, legislation that was promulgated by the Obama administration to bring the United States one step closer to "universal coverage," or insurance that covers everyone in the country.

President Obama signed the **Affordable Care Act (ACA)** into law on March 10, 2010, after a bitterly partisan political fight. Chapter 2 includes a more detailed discussion of the ACA and its key provisions, but suffice it to say here that the law represented another expansion of government into the healthcare system. As such, it ignited a heated and protracted debate.

From its introduction, controversy engulfed the ACA that ultimately became intensely partisan. Republicans decried the government "takeover" of healthcare; government interference in the doctor–patient relationship, and the creation of "death panels" intended to control the rising cost of Medicare. There were no "death panels," and the administration countered with the argument that the legislation would insure more people, improve quality of care, and bend the cost curve (Dawes 2016). Ultimately, legislation designated formally as the Patient Protection and Affordable Care Act passed on a straight party line vote in both houses of Congress. Indeed, in the Senate, the Democratic leadership invoked special rules that prevented Republicans from filibustering, further adding to the partisan acrimony.

Because, unlike Medicare and Medicaid, the ACA lacked bipartisan support, the Republican members of Congress have never fully embraced the law. Between 2010 and 2016, the House of Representatives recorded more than 50 votes to repeal the ACA. Largely these were symbolic measures with no practical effect beyond demonstrating the lack of political cohesion underlying the act.

Meanwhile, as the policy debate raged about the prospect of universal healthcare—or anything remotely resembling universal healthcare—the healthcare system itself continued to change in the way it delivered services. Some of these changes were a by-product of reform efforts, while others were natural extensions of clinical measures already in place.

Clinical Integration and Team-Based Care

The development of **electronic health records (EHRs)** facilitated the sharing of patient data across multiple providers. As the traditional "medical chart" morphed from paper to electronic format, it became a database that could be viewed from remote locations by different kinds of providers. Thus, the record of a patient hospitalized for a heart attack could be accessed by his or her primary care provider to review any clinical indicators. The ability to share information in this fashion and act on it is referred to as **clinical integration.** The concept aims to reduce medical errors by coordinating care among multiple providers, eliminating the risk of patients visiting multiple clinicians who might prescribe contraindicated medications or therapy.

Concomitant with this concept is the idea of *team-based care,* which also began to see an upsurge at the turn of the twenty-first century. In the inpatient setting, for example, such a care team might include a surgeon, the attending physician, a pharmacist, a nurse, a social worker, and a nutritionist. In the ambulatory setting, team-based care might include a physician, nurse, social worker, and navigator all working together to care for a patient. This holistic approach implicitly recognizes the need to address multiple systems in a single patient while treating one particular illness or trauma.

Electronic health record (EHR)
A digital record of the care provided to a patient by a healthcare organization, including the patient's up-to-date, real-time health-related information. When the record can be shared among multiple providers, it is said to have *interoperability.* Also called *electronic medical record.*

Clinical integration
The coordinated delivery of patient care by a team across conditions, providers, settings, and time to achieve high-quality care. Best effectuated by a common (electronic) health record to keep all providers informed.

Payment and Structural Changes

Payment and reimbursement strategies also emerged at the beginning of the twenty-first century, spurred by new legislative and administrative policy. These initiatives include pay-for-performance, also referred to as P4P, and bundled payments. These will be explained in depth in chapter 11; in brief, they ask providers to accept more of the risk in financing patient care by incentivizing them to be more efficient and effective in their services.

In addition to changes in the way care was delivered and how it was paid for, the structure and governance of healthcare systems began to change quickly. Mergers and acquisitions continued at a record pace. Healthcare systems became less centralized in a single local hospital and increasingly transformed into large multihospital systems that also provided care in a growing number of ambulatory centers. Chapter 3 will discuss this evolution in more detail.

High Tech and High Touch

Amid these structural and payment changes was another change: the way care quality was measured. While the actual delivery of care was becoming more individualized and high tech, down to the level of the patient's DNA, providers were being asked to focus on the health of whole populations. Reimbursement schemes, such as the accountable care organizations created with the ACA, called for providers to improve the health of communities, not merely individual patients. Payers started to penalize readmissions, for example, prompting healthcare systems to spend more time and resources to manage the care of each patient, offering closer and closer follow-up—an approach known as "high touch." Delivering medical care designed to prevent inpatient admissions and improve a community's overall health status became increasingly important, and hospitals decided that using beds more efficiently was more valuable than having more of them.

Conclusion

The next phase in the evolution of the US healthcare "system" is just beginning. Congress and the executive branch continue to debate and negotiate the "repeal" of the ACA or amending it to reduce the role of government. Once again, the notion of increasing market competition and reducing government involvement has moved to the top of the political agenda. It will be a significant challenge to repeal popular provisions of the ACA, such as ensuring coverage for those individuals with pre-existing medical conditions, or to eliminate coverage for those Americans who only recently received it. Time will tell whether the intensity of political engagement in the healthcare system is waxing or waning. The forces of "greater competition" argue that reducing government activity in the healthcare system is the path to true savings, while others maintain that greater free market influence will result in higher costs, poorer quality of care, and fewer Americans insured.

We began this chapter observing that throughout American history, proponents of greater government engagement and supporters of free market mechanisms have debated their respective philosophies with varying degrees of success. Once again, Americans confront that philosophical choice. The outcome of the debate will influence how the US healthcare system delivers care, at what cost, and to whom. The public debate will address questions of equity: "How fairly is the care being distributed?" That same debate will also address questions of cost: "How much is enough?" And it will also address effectiveness: "How good is the care Americans receive?" Cost of care, quality of care, and access to care form the **iron triangle**. We will explore the inextricable linkage of these three concepts in the next chapter and examine how public policy defines the US healthcare system.

Iron triangle
The interlocking relationships among the cost of care, its quality, and access to it.

Mini Case Study: Medicare's Advantage of Bipartisan Support

Bipartisan support for legislation is important to its long-term survival. Political scientists use the term "legitimacy" to refer to legislation that political actors from all parts of the spectrum support. In the context of Medicaid, Democrats were clearly in control of the presidency and both houses of Congress. President Johnson and his congressional allies developed the national agenda to include the extension of healthcare to segments of the population that could not afford to pay for medical services. In Congress, however, the Republicans eschewed the concept of government-funded healthcare in favor of private markets. On the Ways and Means Committee, Chairman Wilbur Mills, rather than leading efforts to defeat the Republican proposal to create premium-funded coverage, incorporated it as part of a larger legislative initiative. Thus was born Medicaid, as well as Part B of Medicare, a premium-based insurance covering ambulatory services for people older than age 65. It also created Medicare Part A, which is social insurance—that is, inpatient care funded through payroll taxes. By joining the two proposals together, Mills made it easier for Republicans to support Medicare and Medicaid, even if somewhat reluctantly. Consequently, the two systems have enjoyed a 50-year history of bipartisan support and have become a part of the fabric of American healthcare. (This is truer for Medicare than Medicaid, given the proclivity of older citizens to vote.)

Conversely, the ACA passed in 2010 with votes exclusively from Democrats in both houses of Congress. While these majorities, along with President Obama's signature, made the ACA the law of the land, what was then the minority party has never fully accepted the ACA. The Republicans mounted numerous repeal efforts and legal challenges, to no avail. These challenges have undermined the smooth implementation of the ACA. When the GOP next won control of Congress and the presidency, the assault on the ACA continued. In short, the act has never gained the "legitimacy" achieved by Medicare, remaining controversial and the target of vocal critics.

Mini Case Study Questions

1. How did the bipartisan support for Medicare facilitate it becoming a critical part of the US healthcare system?
2. Provide a prognosis for the future of the ACA. What did you describe and why?
3. What might have happened had Wilbur Mills led the outright rejection of the Republican proposal?

Points to Remember

- The US healthcare system is the product of private market and public policy decisions made during the life of the country.
- Scientific development has been central to the types of healthcare services delivered by components of the healthcare system.
- "Germ theory" revolutionized the delivery of care in the United States.
- The Social Security Act fundamentally changed the social contract between the federal government and US citizens by establishing the precedent of federally sponsored services provided directly to individuals in the population.
- The federal government's role in healthcare has grown during the course of history, but not consistently. Government engagement has waxed and waned over time.
- One example of federal government involvement in healthcare is the Hill-Burton Act, which supplied funding for the construction and expansion of hospitals.
- Medicare, Medicaid, and the Affordable Care Act are all examples of federal government engagement in the US healthcare delivery system.

Challenge Yourself

1. Should the federal government's role in the US healthcare system be greater than it is, or should it be less than it is? Explain why in either case.
2. Why is the "germ theory" of medicine still important today?
3. Other than generating a need for more long-term care facilities and organizations, what impact will the continuing aging of the population have on the healthcare system?

For Your Consideration

1. Research the trends regarding employer-sponsored insurance from 1950 through 2000. What did you find? Explain how that trend might affect public policy as it relates to healthcare.
2. Research population trends. Look ahead 30 years, to when you will be in the prime of your career. What will the population graph look like then? Compare the number of people older than 65 to those between 18 and 64. What will this new population distribution mean for your career as a health services administrator?

References

Blumenthal, D. 2006. "Employer-Sponsored Health Insurance in the United States—Origins and Implications." *New England Journal of Medicine* 354 (6): 82–88.

Blumenthal, D., and J. A. Morone. 2010. *The Heart of Power: Health and Politics in the Oval Office.* Los Angeles: University of California Press.

Buchmueller, T. C., and A. C. Monheit. 2009. "Employer-Sponsored Health Insurance and the Promise of Health Insurance Reform." National Bureau of Economic Research Working Paper 14839. Published April. www.nber.org/papers/w14839.pdf.

Centers for Medicare & Medicaid Services (CMS). 2017. *National Health Expenditures.* Accessed January 23. www.cms.gov/Research-Statistics-Data-and-Systems/Statistics-Trends-and-Reports/NationalHealthExpendData/NationalHealthAccountsHistorical.html.

———. 2016. *NHE Fact Sheet.* Accessed March 9, 2017. www.cms.gov/research-statistics-data-and-systems/statistics-trends-and-reports/nationalhealthexpenddata/nhe-fact-sheet.html.

Cooper, R. 2003. "Medical Schools and Their Applicants: An Analysis." *Health Affairs* 22 (4): 71–84.

Cubanski, J., and T. Neuman. 2018. "The Facts on Medicare Spending and Financing." Kaiser Family Foundation issue brief. Published June 22. http://kff.org/medicare/issue-brief/the-facts-on-medicare-spending-and-financing.

Dawes, D. 2016. *150 Years of Obamacare.* Baltimore, MD: Johns Hopkins University Press.

Flexner, A. 1910. *Medical Education in the United States and Canada.* New York City: Carnegie Foundation for the Advancement of Teaching.

Fronstin, P. 2013. *Survey of Health Insurance and Characteristics of the Uninsured.* Accessed January 23, 2017. www.ebri.org/pdf/briefspdf/EBRI_IB_09-13.No390.Sources1.pdf.

Halberstam, D. 1993. *The Fifties.* New York: Random House.

Health Resources and Services Administration (HRSA). 2016. "Get Health Care." Accessed January 23, 2017. www.hrsa.gov/gethealthcare/affordable/hillburton.

Johnson, H., and D. Broder. 1997. *The System: The American Way of Politics at the Breaking Point.* New York: Back Bay Book.

Johnson, S. 2006. *The Ghost Map.* New York: Riverhead Books.

Kaiser Family Foundation. 2014. "National Health Care Expenditures Per Capita, 1960–2023." Published October 23. http://kff.org/health-costs/slide/national-health-expenditures-per-capita-1960-2023.

Lichtenstein, M. 2012. "Health Insurance from Invention to Innovation: A History of the Blue Cross and Blue Shield Companies." Published November 11. www.bcbs.com/node/982#.U3-J2vldU7U.

Millard, C. 2012. *Destiny of the Republic: A Tale of Madness, Medicine and the Murder of a President.* New York: Knopf Doubleday.

Moore, J. D., and D. G. Smith. 2005. "Legislating Medicaid: Considering Medicaid and Its Origins." *Health Care Financing Review* 27 (3): 45–52.

Myers, R. J. 2000. "Why Medicare Part A and Part B as Well as Medicaid?" *Health Care Financing Review* 22 (1): 53–54.

National Association of State Budget Officers (NASBO). 2015. *State Expenditure Report.* Washington, DC: NASBO.

National Institutes of Health (NIH). 2018. "Appropriations History by Institute/Center (1938 to Present)." Accessed June 9. https://officeofbudget.od.nih.gov/approp_hist.html.

Perlstadt, H. 1995. "The Development of Hill-Burton Legislation: Interests, Issues and Compromises." *Journal of Health and Social Policy* 6 (3): 77–96.

Rosenberg, C. E. 1995. *The Care of Strangers: The Rise of America's Hospital System.* Baltimore, MD: Johns Hopkins University Press.

Rutkow, I. 2010. *Seeking the Cure.* New York: Scribner.

Starr, P. 1983. *The Social Transformation of Medicine.* New York: Basic Books.

Stevens, R. 1999. *In Sickness and in Wealth.* Baltimore, MD: Johns Hopkins University Press.

Stille, C. J. 1866. *History of the United States Sanitary Commission.* Philadelphia, PA: Lippincott.

Sultz, H., and K. Young. 2014. *Health Care USA,* 8th ed. Burlington, MA: Jones & Bartlett.

US Census Bureau. 2016. "2000 National Population Projections: Population Pyramids." Revised October 26. www.census.gov/library/visualizations/2000/demo/2000-pop-pyramids.html.

CHAPTER 2

HEALTH POLICY: COST, QUALITY, AND ACCESS

Important Terms

- Administrative rule
- Centers for Medicare & Medicaid Services (CMS)
- Federal poverty level (FPL)
- Gross domestic product (GDP)
- Per capita expenditure
- Special interest group

Learning Objectives

At the end of this chapter, you will be able to do the following:

- ➤ Understand the interrelationship of cost, quality, and access
- ➤ Understand basic elements of the healthcare policymaking process
- ➤ Explain why health policy is important to managers
- ➤ Understand current costs and historical cost trends in the healthcare system
- ➤ Understand the iterative nature of the public policy process

Case Study: Strategy Review

"If there was one clear lesson from the failure of the Clinton plan, this was it. Powerful interests built on the status quo are apt to be threatened by change. And people who are satisfied and familiar with the current arrangements are bound to resist the new and unfamiliar. We saw how Clinton's managed competition plan would have made profound changes in the industry and would have changed the way virtually every individual would purchase insurance or receive medical care. In contrast, Obama's plan minimized the amount of change. It built on the employer-based system and the private market for health insurance, supplemented by existing public programs such as Medicare and Medicaid. Many recommended substantial changes in the delivery system to make the system more efficient and cost effective. Obama acknowledged those ideas, but wisely chose less far-reaching reforms by funding trials and demonstrations. . . .

"Special interests had been the bane of health policy proposals for nearly a century. We saw how the AMA [American Medical Association] opposed universal insurance as early as [the] Teddy Roosevelt [administration] and gave tacit support for smoking in an attempt to derail Medicare. Insurance companies campaigned against every comprehensive reform proposal, as did most business groups. Other health interests, such as pharmaceutical companies, device manufacturers, and hospitals, helped defeat a number of reform initiatives. Conservative political groups opposed nearly any proposal that increased the government role in health care, whereas liberals and labor unions opposed universal [coverage] proposals that were not single-payer.

"Perhaps the key element in the Obama strategy was to bring all the interest groups to the table and to make compromises and deals that would gain their support. . . .

"In a perfect world, a comprehensive health reform proposal would focus on controlling costs as well as expanding access. The Obama plan has been severely criticized for focusing almost exclusively on access and providing only small initiatives to 'bend the cost curve.' The criticism is undoubtedly valid, but, of course, we do not live in a perfect world. Every dollar of reduced cost is a dollar of reduction in somebody's income. That somebody's organization will lobby against the plan, often spending considerable resources to fund the opposition. When Bill Clinton's managed competition morphed into managed competition within a global budget, it threatened to limit revenues across the health system and was opposed throughout the industry.

"Ultimately one has to decide whether his or her preferred approach, which might be politically impossible, is better or worse than a less ideal alternative that is more likely doable. . . . One of the organizers of Kennedy's Workhorse Group was a long-time advocate of single-payer until he realized that all of his efforts had 'not succeeded in getting health insurance to a single person.' . . .

"There is no correct answer as to whether Obama's strategy to largely avoid cost control was preferable even though it certainly was less than ideal. . . . Comprehensive health reform and near-universal coverage would have been impossible to enact if substantial cost control were included. Given the political realities, we believe Obama's strategy was necessary. Nevertheless, there is a clear and evident danger. If Obama, or a subsequent administration, cannot follow up with a reasonably effective way to control cost, the system could fail and his apparent success will have been short-lived." (Altman and Schachtman 2011, 332–334)

Introduction

The chapter-opening case study demonstrates the power of special interests in the policymaking process. In this case particularly, various **special interest groups** associated with healthcare are engaged in defeating, and then to some degree shaping, healthcare reform.

Special interest group
A collection of organizations and individuals dedicated to a particular cause or profession acting in the policymaking arena with the intent of advancing their point of view and seeking an advantage with respect to policy outcomes.

During the period of scientific growth in American medicine, as described in chapter 1, public policy ebbed and flowed. At times, policymakers advocated a greater degree of government involvement in the healthcare system, most remarkably with Medicare. At other times, the public policy apparatus supported greater market influence and less governmental intrusion in healthcare. The refusal of the Roosevelt administration to include health insurance as part of the Social Security Act is a notable example of pushing down the level of government involvement.

In this chapter, we will discuss the policy process and how it affects access to care, quality of care, and cost of care. You will see some of the same ebb and flow of government engagement in the policy debate, the government's impact on the health system, and, importantly, how the policy process works.

Federalism: Layers of Government

This chapter will mostly discuss federal policymaking because of its uniformity across the nation and its impact on the healthcare system. One should not discount, however, the role of the states in crafting healthcare policy. The Tenth Amendment to the US Constitution plays an integral role. This clause, often referred to as the "police power clause," reserves to the states those powers not expressly transferred to the federal government in the constitution (*United States v. Sprague* 1931). Specifically, this means the states have the power to protect the public health and safety of their citizens through licensure and regulatory mechanisms controlling healthcare providers and organizations. In addition, states can mandate certain individual behavior, such as compulsory vaccinations for public school students (Federation of State Medical Boards 2017; *Jacobson v. Massachusetts* 1905).

Consequently, both state and federal governments make policy that affects healthcare providers and systems in their delivery of healthcare services. The state has the power to license providers and discipline them for professional misconduct (Federation of State Medical Boards 2017). States also have the power to regulate the size and location of hospitals and other types of healthcare service organizations (National Conference of State Legislatures

2016). Finally, as an adjunct to the regulation of health services, states have the power to regulate health insurance companies as well (Kofman and Pollitz 2006).

Fundamentally, states have a noteworthy role in determining the supply of healthcare providers and organizations through their power of licensure and regulation. These are policy decisions that affect the public's health and safety as well as its access to care.

In addition, as we will see in the following sections, states have a concurrent authority with the federal government as it relates to Medicaid. The federal government sets the broad parameters and funds up to 75 percent of the program, but the states may make determinations regarding provider fee levels and beneficiary eligibility (Medicaid.gov 2017). (Note that the passage of the Affordable Care Act [ACA] has changed this proportion of costs—increasing the federal contribution—in states that expanded their Medicaid programs.)

Taking notice of state prerogatives is essential. All licensure and regulation affecting the health professions, as well as determinations of medical malpractice, are the province of state governments and state law. As important as these are, however, the focus for the remainder of this chapter will be on the federal government's role, primarily because of its largesse and its ability to influence healthcare through the power of the purse. In addition, provisions in the US Constitution other than the Tenth Amendment, such as the Interstate Commerce clause, permit the federal government to control some aspects of healthcare services delivery.

Healthcare's Iron Triangle: Cost, Quality, and Access

Regardless of political views, the healthcare debate ultimately centers on three fundamental concepts related to health policy: cost, quality, and access. As we saw in chapter 1, these inextricably linked elements form the iron triangle of healthcare. The government cannot take a policy action on one side of the triangle without affecting at least one of the other two. If a state were to expand Medicaid to give more people access to care, for example, federal and state costs would increase. The converse would also be true: If states reduced their Medicaid expenditures, fewer people would have access to care. Likewise, when Medicare refuses to pay hospitals for the costs associated with avoidable readmissions, it is both reducing costs and improving the quality of care by incentivizing hospitals to better care for the patient to avoid the readmission. Exhibit 2.1 is a graphic depiction of these relationships.

While individual organizations certainly can, and do, tinker in the iron triangle arena, our focus is on the larger matter of public policy formation and how each of the three sides of the triangle both motivates, and is driven by, public policy outcomes. No one policy is perfect and completely withstands changed circumstances. The passage of time inevitably brings new perspective, new technology, and new policy demands that motivate change in the existing policy. This means that public policy, including health policy, is iterative in nature. Each "new" policy enactment is born from a previous policy decision. Feedback on

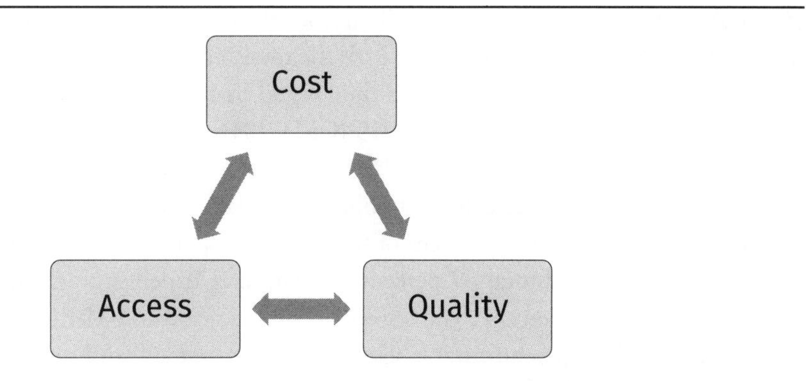

Exhibit 2.1
The Iron Triangle of Healthcare

a policy in place, and the changed circumstances surrounding it, will energize new policy considerations (Longest 2015).

Healthcare Costs: Where the Money Comes From

Before delving into the question of cost, let us review some of the key concepts discussed in the previous chapter, along with a few new definitions that are part of the cost discussion:

Medicare: a federal program to provide insurance coverage for the elderly

Medicaid: a joint federal–state program providing insurance coverage for the poor

Children's Health Insurance Program (CHIP): a joint federal–state program providing insurance coverage for certain categories of children not otherwise eligible for Medicaid

Commercial insurance: insurance frequently offered by employers to provide coverage for their employees. Consumers can also purchase this insurance on the individual market.

Personal expenditure: all out-of-pocket consumer expenditures for health-related goods and services

Other government-sponsored health programs: healthcare for members of the US military, the Indian Health Service, Worker's Compensation, the US Public Health Service, and a host of smaller entities and programs

The most common term used to refer to these costs, as we saw in chapter 1, is *national health expenditures,* or NHE. This is the aggregate of all expenditures from all sources: Medicare, Medicaid, CHIP, commercial insurance, personal expenditures, the Veterans

Centers for Medicare & Medicaid Services (CMS)
The federal government agency that administers the Medicare program and the federal portion of the Medicaid and CHIP programs. CMS is part of the US Department of Health and Human Services. Note that even though the "centers" portion of the name is plural, the CMS acronym is singular.

Gross domestic product (GDP)
The monetary value of all finished goods and services produced in a country by individuals and companies for a specified period of time, usually one year. In 2016, the GDP for the United States was $18.57 trillion. By comparison, the GDP for the second-largest economy in the world, China, was $11.2 trillion.

Per capita expenditure
The total amount spent on healthcare—that is, the national health expenditures (NHE)—divided by the population.

Health Administration, active duty military healthcare, the US Public Health Service, the Indian Health Service, and others. In 2015, the total NHE equaled $3.2 trillion—a growth of 5.8 percent from 2014. This means the United States spent approximately $9,990 per person for all forms of healthcare in 2015 (CMS 2016a). Exhibit 2.2 depicts the source of all 2015 spending.

As you can see in the exhibit, public and private insurance provide the largest share of healthcare spending, at 74 percent of the total. Comparing the two, you will notice that Medicare and Medicaid total 37 percent of healthcare expenditures, while private health insurance provides 33 percent. Said another way, Medicare and Medicaid represent half of the 74 percent of the expenditures labeled "Health Insurance" and more than a third of all healthcare expenditures. What this means is that these programs are important not only to the beneficiaries they serve, but also to the overall system, simply because they are so large. When the **Centers for Medicare & Medicaid Services (CMS)** promulgates an administrative rule governing payment (or nonpayment) for a particular procedure, or when Congress changes Medicare or Medicaid, it has a significant financial impact on the system. Often, commercial insurers follow suit. Note also that the total "Public Insurance" portion of the health insurance slice is 41 percent, including CHIP, the Department of Veterans Affairs, and military spending. The public programs overall, including public health and related activities, constitute 45 percent—nearly half—of all healthcare expenditures. Also, note that "Out of Pocket" is the third-largest category of health expenditures, after the private insurance share of 33 percent, at 11 percent.

Since 2000, healthcare spending in the United States has increased almost 2.5 times, growing from $1.378 trillion to $3.206 trillion in 2015, and it has increased as a percentage of our **gross domestic product (GDP)** (CMS 2016a). Many experts question whether this cost trend is sustainable (OECD 2015). What portion of our GDP *should* be consumed by healthcare? What rate of growth in healthcare spending is sustainable? These are questions that are perennially linked to any debate about healthcare policy. Exhibit 2.3 provides a depiction of the increase in healthcare costs over time as well as the healthcare cost portion of the GDP.

As one might expect, **per capita expenditures** also have risen during this time, on average by about 8 percent per year, as exhibit 2.4 shows.

It is interesting to note, however, that while healthcare costs have continued to escalate overall and per capita expenditures for healthcare costs also have risen, the percentage of costs paid by the individual consumer has decreased. Exhibit 2.5 depicts a shift away from out-of-pocket costs to a greater reliance on public programs, particularly Medicare and Medicaid. Private insurance likewise grew during this time.

There are several explanations for the shift toward greater use of public programs. Some of those are simple demographics; some relate to policy decisions. First, Medicare expenditures are expanding because the population is aging. Remember the population pyramids from chapter 1: The proportion of the population of Medicare-eligible Americans is growing. Approximately 10,000 baby boomers retire every day (Caraher 2014). Second,

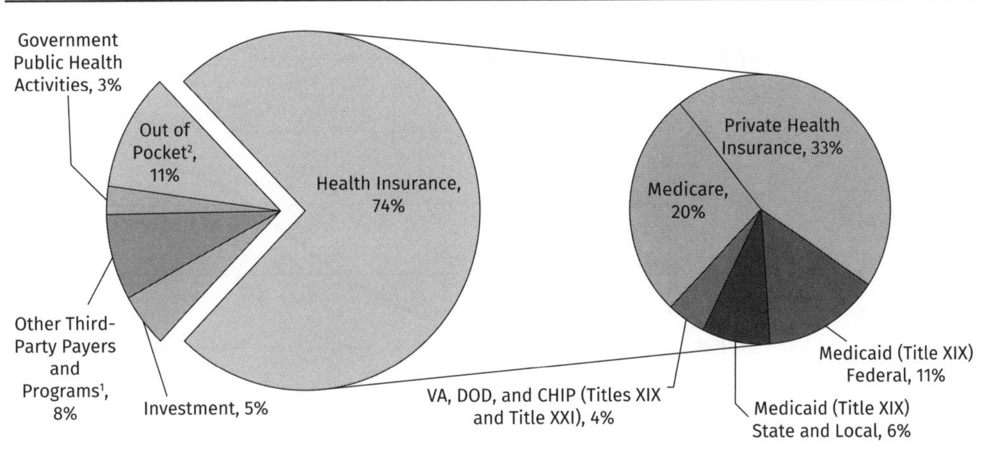

Exhibit 2.2
The Nation's Health Dollar ($3.2 Trillion), Calendar Year 2015: Where It Came From

[1]Includes worksite healthcare, other private revenues, Indian Health Service, workers' compensation, general assistance, maternal and child health, vocational rehabilitation, Substance Abuse and Mental Health Services Administration, school health, and other federal and state local programs.

[2]Includes co-payments, deductibles, and any amounts not covered by health insurance.

Note: Sum of pieces may not equal 100% due to rounding.

Source: Reprinted from CMS (2016a).

Note: VA = Department of Veterans Affairs; DOD = Department of Defense; CHIP = Children's Health Insurance Program.

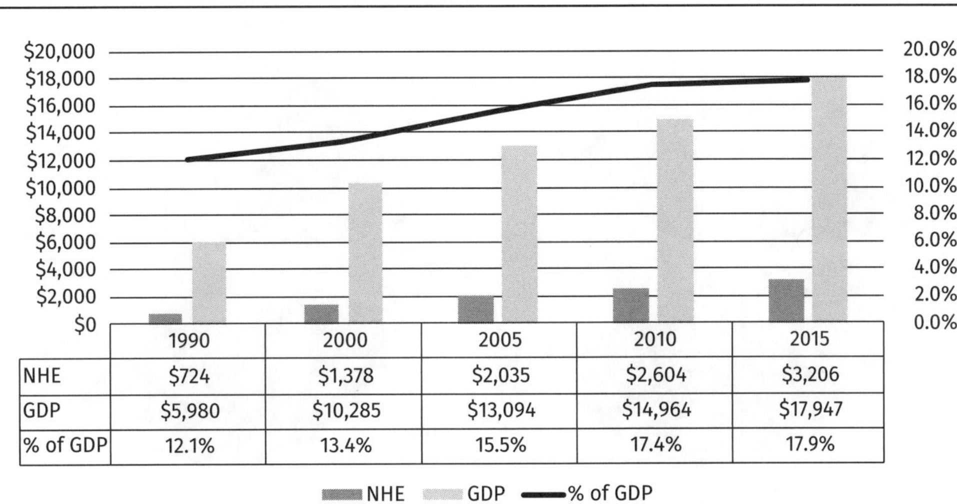

	1990	2000	2005	2010	2015
NHE	$724	$1,378	$2,035	$2,604	$3,206
GDP	$5,980	$10,285	$13,094	$14,964	$17,947
% of GDP	12.1%	13.4%	15.5%	17.4%	17.9%

Exhibit 2.3
National Health Expenditures and Gross Domestic Product, 1990–2015 (Selected Years), in Millions

Source: Adapted from CMS (2016a).

Note: GDP = gross domestic product; NHE = national health expenditures.

Exhibit 2.4
US Per Capita Healthcare Expenditures, 1995–2015 (Selected Years)

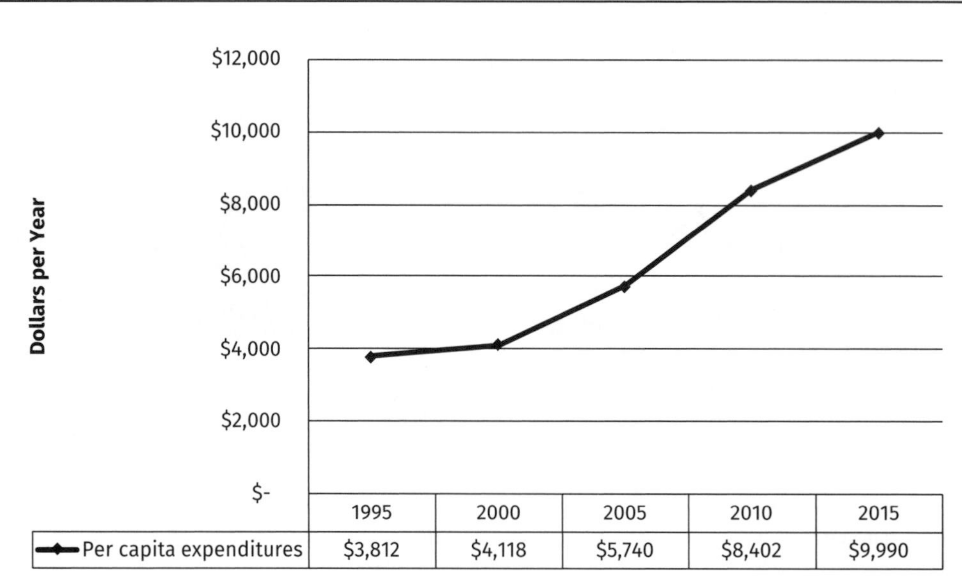

	1995	2000	2005	2010	2015
Per capita expenditures	$3,812	$4,118	$5,740	$8,402	$9,990

Source: Adapted from CMS (2016a).

Exhibit 2.5
Comparison of National Health Expenditures Distribution by Source, 1995 and 2015

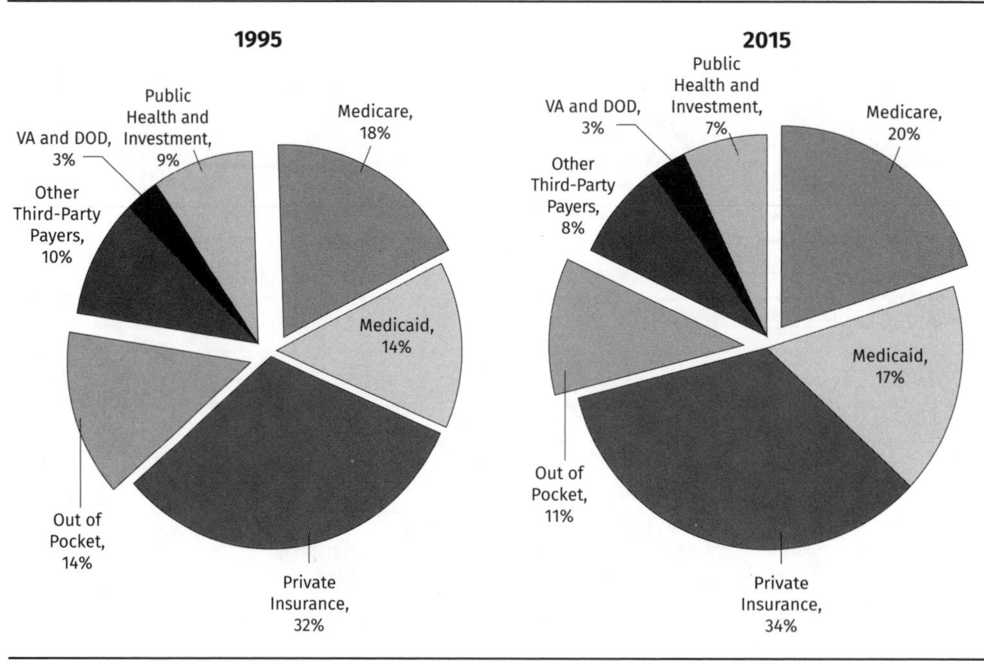

Source: Adapted from CMS (2016a).
Note: DOD = Department of Defense; VA = Department of Veterans Affairs.

as people age they confront more and increasingly severe morbidities and, accordingly, incur higher costs for healthcare (Neuman, Cubanski, and Damico 2015). Increased life expectancy also is a factor in increasing Medicare costs: The longer people live, the longer the period of time for which they require care, leading to higher overall costs (Neuman, Cubanski et al. 2015). Thus, Medicare expenditures are growing because of a greater prevalence of chronic ailments amid the growing and increasingly older population the program serves. To a lesser extent, but also true, is the fact that Medicare now pays for services that previously did not exist or were not covered, such as bariatric surgery for obesity (CMS 2006).

The growth in Medicaid, on the other hand, represents a growth in the number of people the program serves. The ACA initially required all states to expand their Medicaid programs. While the Supreme Court struck down that provision as unconstitutional, as of this writing 32 states have voluntarily expanded their Medicaid programs to include more beneficiaries (Kaiser Family Foundation 2017b). Increased Medicaid expenditures, therefore, are only a natural consequence of these expanded programs.

The decision by Medicare to cover new services, and the decision by many states to expand their Medicaid programs, are policy decisions that change both access to care and its cost. Naturally, when a state expands its Medicaid program, both federal and state costs increase. This is a state-level policy decision, but because of the mixed nature of Medicaid funding, federal costs are also affected. In this particular case, as discussed in the box below, the ACA offered financial inducements to states to expand their Medicaid programs (Antos, Capretta, and Ippolito 2017).

THE AFFORDABLE CARE ACT AND MEDICAID

The chapter's introductory vignette told us how the ACA as proposed by President Obama aimed to build on private insurance structures and expand public programs such as Medicaid. On the private health insurance side, the act required companies employing more than 50 people to provide health insurance for their employees; in addition, it required every individual to purchase health insurance if they were not otherwise covered by a plan. Importantly, the act provided subsidies to purchase health insurance to everyone whose income was between 100 percent and 400 percent of the **federal poverty level (FPL).**

For 2017, the FPL for a family of four was $24,600 (Morgan 2017). So, for 2017, if a family of four had an income between $24,600 and $98,400, that family might be eligible for a subsidy to purchase health insurance. But what about those families who had an income of less than $24,600?

Generally, individuals become eligible for Medicaid when their income is roughly 43 percent of the FPL *or lower* (Kaiser Familly Foundation 2016). For a family of four in 2017, this means

(continued)

Federal poverty level (FPL)
An economic measure used by the federal government to determine the eligibility for certain federal programs intended to assist people living in poverty. The FPL varies with family size and is lower for smaller families and higher for larger families.

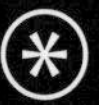

THE AFFORDABLE CARE ACT AND MEDICAID *(CONTINUED)*

they become eligible for Medicaid if they have an income of $10,578 or less. Yet families of four with income between $10,578 and $24,599 are neither eligible for Medicaid nor the subsidies to purchase insurance on the individual market. This was the group of people intended to be covered with the mandated expansion of Medicaid.

But the federal mandate requiring states to expand their Medicaid programs was challenged in federal court. The question ultimately came to the US Supreme Court, which found this provision to be constitutionally coercive, though it permitted the other parts of the ACA—including other provisions affecting Medicaid—to stand (Russell 2012).

This means that the question of a state expanding its Medicaid program became voluntary. Part of the ACA that the Supreme Court found to be constitutional included provisions for the federal government to assume a greater share of the cost for those states that chose to expand their Medicaid programs. If a state agreed to expand coverage, the federal government was to assume 100 percent of that cost for the first three years of the expansion, to be reduced gradually over time to 90 percent of the cost.

In other words, had the ACA provision mandating the states' expansion of Medicaid been allowed to stand, everyone in this income group of 43 percent to 100 percent of the FPL would have been able to secure health insurance through Medicaid. When the Supreme Court struck down the mandate and left the question of Medicaid expansion to the individual states, that coverage only became available based on a person's address. As of 2018, 32 states had expanded their Medicaid programs so this group of people can access care through the Medicaid program (Kaiser Familly Foundation 2017b).

As we move to the issue of how healthcare dollars are spent, consider the paradoxes of access and healthcare expenditures over time. The federal government enacted Medicare and Medicaid in 1965 because the president and Congress consciously decided to provide insurance coverage for two population groups that could not afford the cost of insurance to cover healthcare expenses and were effectively denied access to care. By creating Medicare and Medicaid, the government made a policy decision to expand access for the elderly and the poor by largely assuming the cost of their healthcare. This resulted in new costs for the federal government (and new revenue for providers) and dramatically increased the overall NHE as the government accomplished its policy goal of expanding access to care in creating these programs (Blumenthal and Morone 2008).

Likewise in 2010, the ACA made it possible for approximately 20 million previously uninsured people to have insurance (Cohen, Zammatti, and Martinez 2017). Many gained coverage because of the expansion of Medicaid, while many others were able to purchase insurance through "exchanges" established by the ACA. (Insurance "exchanges" were created by the ACA to provide certain individuals an opportunity to purchase health insurance. There are three kinds of exchanges: state-operated, federally operated, and jointly operated between the federal and state governments. The type of exchange is determined in large measure by the state. For those states choosing not to implement an exchange, the federal government stepped in and operated one there. In other cases, states opted to create their own exchanges or collaborate with the federal government to create one. Individuals eligible to purchase insurance through the exchanges must have an income between 100 percent and 400 percent of the FPL. People falling into this category receive a tax credit to help them afford the cost of the policy.) The federal government made state-level Medicaid expansions possible by assuming a greater share of the cost—the "inducement" referred to earlier (Snyder and Rudowitz 2015). Regardless how the newly insured obtained coverage, the act provided health insurance for people who previously could not afford it. Therefore, we can see the direct relationship between two sides of the iron triangle: The high costs for insurance and healthcare effectively denied many people access to care. The government changed policy to ensure insurance coverage for more people, improving access to care while assuming the burden of the cost, thereby adding to the NHE (Martinez, Ward, and Adams 2015).

Of course, the ACA was—and continues to be—yet another chapter in the history of our ebb and flow with regard to governmental involvement in healthcare. Those who hold the view that healthcare is a "right" for all Americans carried the day—partially—in 1965, with enactment of Medicare and Medicaid, and in 2010, with the ACA. Consequently, the government's role in healthcare has greatly expanded, as reflected in the historical growth of healthcare costs. Those who hold the view that healthcare is a commodity and should be purchased by individuals because their health is an individual matter and not one of larger concern to society have been partly successful: Healthcare remains predominantly a private-sector matter for most Americans, and the complete displacement of the private markets by governmental action has been restrained.

As of this writing, the national debate is focused once again on healthcare costs. This time, however, the emphasis is less about expanding access to care because of costs to the individual than about limiting government expenditures for costs of care. There are clear trade-offs between cost and access. Medicare, Medicaid, and the ACA made the trade-off to expand insurance coverage, and hence improve access to care, while focusing less on what it would cost the public to insulate individuals from high costs. The crux of the current debate is about reducing costs on the public side of the equation, which would result in some people who currently have insurance coverage—and access to care—losing that coverage and having greatly diminished access.

Costs: Where the Money Goes

Because spending $3.2 trillion on health services represents nearly 20 percent of our GDP, or nearly $10,000 per person in 2017, it is important to know where all those dollars were spent. As the vignette at the beginning of the chapter noted, every dollar of cost in the healthcare system is someone else's dollar of revenue. Exhibit 2.6 provides a good graphic depiction of the distribution of healthcare costs in 2015.

Exhibit 2.6 indicates that hospitals represent the largest share of expenses, followed by physicians and clinical services, with prescription drugs representing the third-largest share. Groups representing hospitals, physicians, drug manufacturers, and others such as insurance companies, device manufacturers, and nursing homes are the "special interests" mentioned in the case study at the beginning of this chapter that oppose and often defeat healthcare reform, or modify some of its structure. The professionals in these groups are among those for whom healthcare costs are revenue, and we can expect them to try to fashion the delivery of healthcare services in a manner that best suits their economic needs.

Look at exhibit 2.6 and ask, "Was it always this way?" In other words, if healthcare industry groups were successful in either defeating healthcare reform or shaping it so it is more amenable to their respective interests, would the spending pattern for services provided by these three largest groups change? Exhibit 2.7 provides a partial answer.

You can see in exhibit 2.7 that the physician portion of the healthcare dollar has been remarkably consistent over the years, while spending on prescription drugs has increased, displacing in part some of the spending on hospital care. Hospital expenditures have declined from 38.4 percent of NHE in 1975 to 32.3 percent in 2015, a drop of approximately 16 percent. Some of this shift is a product of improved technology: There are better pharmaceuticals

Exhibit 2.6
The Nation's Health Dollar ($3.2 Trillion), Calendar Year 2015: Where It Went

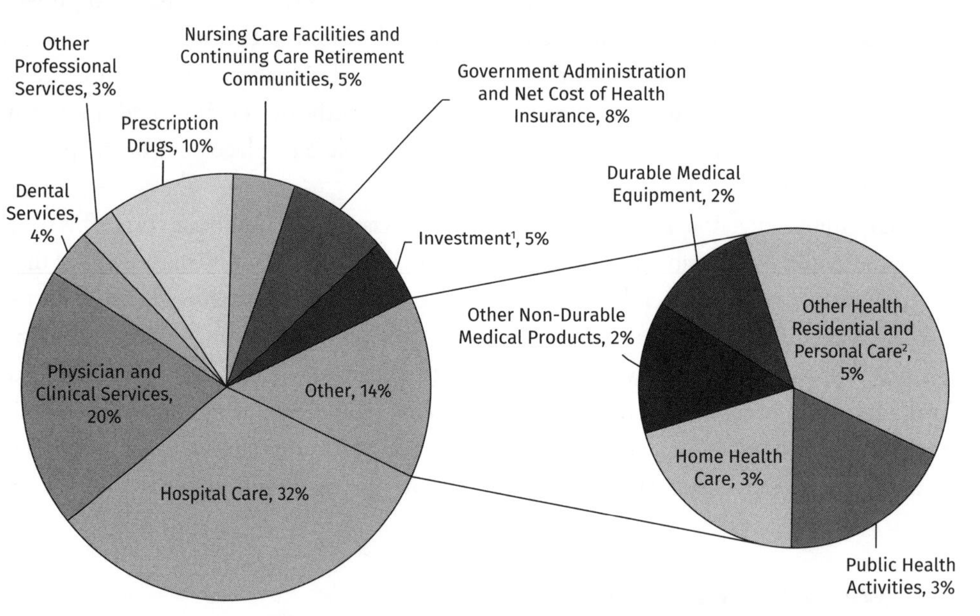

[1] Includes worksite healthcare, other private revenues, Indian Health Service, workers' compensation, general assistance, maternal and child health, vocational rehabilitation, Substance Abuse and Mental Health Services Administration, school health, and other federal and state local programs.
[2] Includes co-payments, deductibles, and any amounts not covered by health insurance.
Source: Reprinted from CMS (2016b).
Note: Sum of pieces may not equal 100% due to rounding.

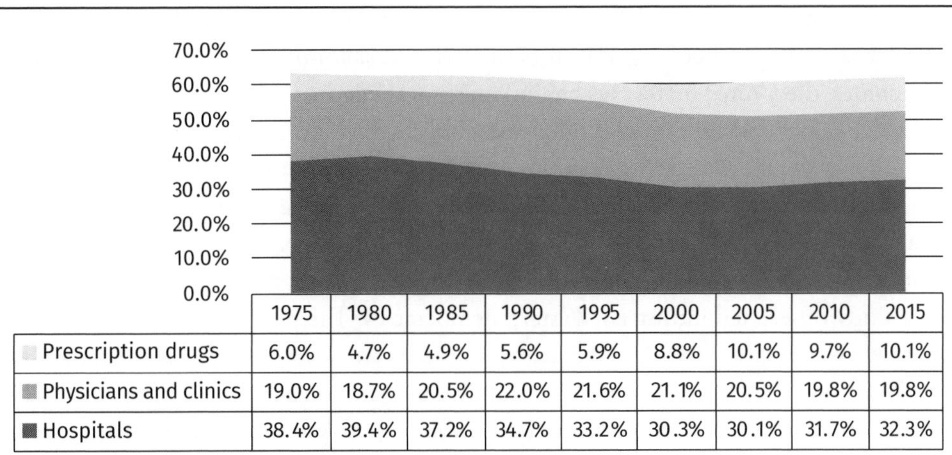

	1975	1980	1985	1990	1995	2000	2005	2010	2015
Prescription drugs	6.0%	4.7%	4.9%	5.6%	5.9%	8.8%	10.1%	9.7%	10.1%
Physicians and clinics	19.0%	18.7%	20.5%	22.0%	21.6%	21.1%	20.5%	19.8%	19.8%
Hospitals	38.4%	39.4%	37.2%	34.7%	33.2%	30.3%	30.1%	31.7%	32.3%

Exhibit 2.7
Percentage of National Health Expenditures by Selected Provider Type, 1975–2015

Source: Adapted from Peterson-Kaiser Health System Tracker (2018).

that can prevent hospitalization (Flaherty et al. 2000). Likewise, many invasive surgeries have moved out of the hospital inpatient setting to outpatient surgical centers (American Hospital Association 2016). This is part of a significant change in the healthcare system that we will revisit in chapter 3.

Hospitals, physicians and clinics, and prescription drugs account for approximately 62 percent of NHE. Indeed, these three groups have consistently accounted for roughly that same percentage of NHE, between 60 and 63 percent, for more than 40 years. What of the other 37 to 40 percent? That amount has been distributed among home health care, public health activity, durable medical equipment, investment in research, dental services, and governmental administration, as shown in exhibit 2.6.

Costs represent only one side of healthcare's iron triangle, but they are always at the heart of any healthcare debate. Does the government spend too much to provide care to those who cannot afford it? Does it spend too little? Should the private market play a greater role in paying for care? If so, how would that work? How do those who cannot afford the price of healthcare pay for it? These are vexing questions, which have been, and will continue to be, the central issues in our national debate. Regardless of the answers, the other two sides of the triangle will always be affected by that same national discussion.

Again, do we really have the best healthcare system on earth? How do we find the answer to that question? We begin that discussion by addressing the next side of the triangle, quality.

Healthcare Quality: The Elusive Element

What do we mean by "quality" in the context of public policy? How do we know we are providing high-quality care *as a country*? The only way to prove or disprove the claim that the United States has the best healthcare system in the world is to compare ourselves to others.

Some data suggest that US health system performance lags behind other countries (Schneider et al. 2017). Looking at factors such as access, administrative efficiency, equity, and outcomes, the United States lags behind many of the industrialized countries in a 2017 study by Schneider and colleagues funded and published by the Commonwealth Fund. See exhibit 2.8 for how the United States ranks overall compared to other industrialized nations.

Indeed, the United States finished last or next to last in all the performance-ranking categories except one, care process. ("Care process" includes measurements in the areas of prevention, patient safety, coordination of care, and patient engagement.) And consider that this is a study of selected industrial Western democracies. The picture does not necessarily improve when comparing the United States to a broader cross section of less affluent nations.

Data from the Organisation for Economic Co-operation and Development (OECD) further illustrate where the United States ranks when we look at two other important measures of health status: infant mortality rate and deaths from cancer. Infant mortality serves as a proxy for quality of prenatal care and for the management of a mother's risk factors (CDC 2016). Exhibit 2.9 shows that the United States is in the bottom third when it comes to infant mortality rate (OECD 2018b). Thirty countries do better than the United States' rate of 5.8 per 1,000, while only 11 countries fare worse on this measure.

Deaths from cancer can also serve as a proxy for both access to and quality of care, as people who are fortunate enough to detect the disease early have a better chance of survival than those who are unable to do so. Exhibit 2.10 tells us that ten OECD countries have a lower rate of death from cancer than the United States (OECD 2018a), which loses 185 out of every 100,000 individuals to the disease. Twenty-five countries have a higher rate.

The meaning of these data is, of course, subject to debate. As mentioned earlier, better access to prenatal care is associated with improved infant mortality (CDC 2016). Likewise, better access to primary care might improve cancer mortality rates. While those arguments may address these two particular indicators from the OECD, the overall performance rating as measured by access to care, administrative efficiency, equity, and health outcomes for the US remains relatively poor. For the United States to improve its performance on those

EXHIBIT 2.8
Healthcare System Performance Rankings

Health Care System Performance Rankings.*

Variable	Australia	Canada	France	Germany	Netherlands	New Zealand	Norway	Sweden	Switzerland	United Kingdom	United States
Overall ranking	2	9	10	8	3	4	4	6	6	1	11
Care process	2	6	9	8	4	3	10	11	7	1	5
Access	4	10	9	2	1	7	5	6	8	3	11
Administrative efficiency	1	6	11	6	9	2	4	5	8	3	10
Equity	7	9	10	6	2	8	5	3	4	1	11
Health care outcomes	1	9	5	8	6	7	3	2	4	10	11

* Rating methods described in Schneider et al.

Source: Reprinted from Schneider et al. (2017).

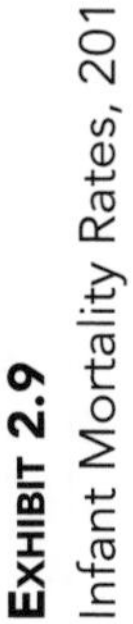

Exhibit 2.9
Infant Mortality Rates, 2014

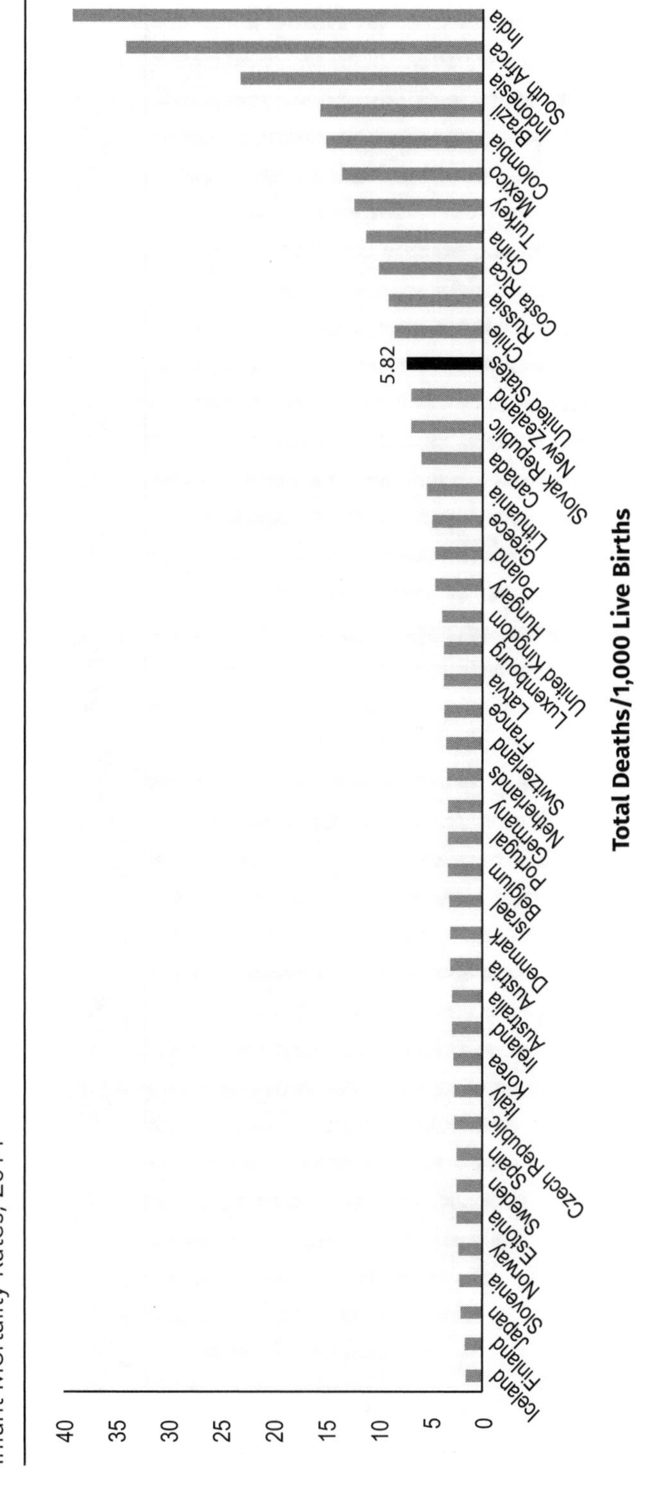

Source: Reprinted from OECD (2018b).

Exhibit 2.10
Cancer Deaths per 100,000 People, 2016 or Most Recent

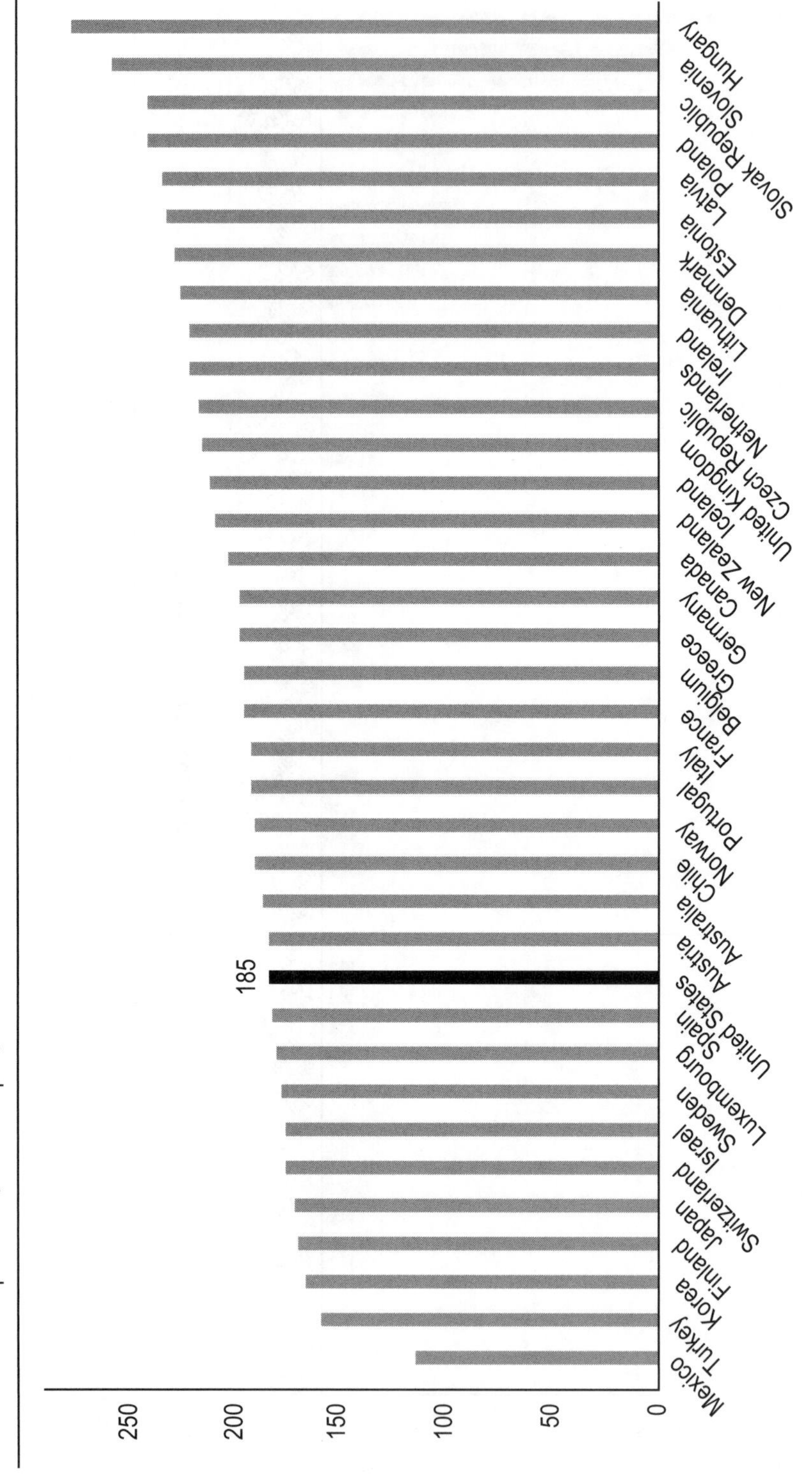

Source: Reprinted from OECD (2018a).

broader, systemic measures would require significant policy changes, especially if we expect to be on equal footing with many of the other industrialized countries.

To that end, we need a deeper examination into what we mean by "quality of care." If the world judges the performance of our healthcare system to be "last," then what do policymakers need to address, and potentially change, to improve? What factors should we consider?

While we will discuss quality in more detail in chapter 14, here let us consider quality of care as a part of the larger policy equation of cost–quality–access. How do we address the rankings developed by the Commonwealth Fund and the OECD? What lessons can we learn and apply from those nations that have "better" healthcare systems?

A close examination of the Commonwealth Fund information, particularly, reveals that the United States lags behind significantly on the standards of "equity" and "access." Should the United States address these issues through the public sector? If so, would such intervention lead to better outcomes and, ultimately, a "better" healthcare system? While it is beyond the scope of this book to examine this statistical relationship, one can see anecdotally from exhibits 2.9 and 2.10 that those countries with better access and a more equitable approach to care have better outcomes. Of the six countries ranking above the OECD average for health outcomes, only France is below average in both access and equity. Of those same six countries, three (Netherlands, Norway, and Sweden) rank above average in both access and equity, while two (Austria and Switzerland) rank above average in equity alone. This would suggest that improved access to care in the United States would lead to better health outcomes. Likewise, because of the relatively heterogeneous nature of the US population, improved access would lead to improved equity, because many people disenfranchised by the current healthcare system are members of minority populations (Elhauge 2010).

As we will see in chapter 14, quality of care at a policy level is vastly different from quality of care at the individual level, yet the two overlap when policy mechanisms promote more effective, and hence better quality, care. From a policy perspective, the answer to improved quality of care may well lie in improved access to healthcare services for all individuals (Schneider and Squires 2017). To date, this has taken the form of Medicare, Medicaid, and the ACA. The policy of denying payment for avoidable readmissions also will improve quality of care. Healthcare organizations have improved processes of care and outcomes since Medicare began denying payment for avoidable readmissions (HHS 2014b).

Expanding the availability of insurance coverage, however, still fails to ensure improved access to care. Insurance is merely one barrier that prevents many Americans from receiving healthcare; it does not guarantee access. In fact, five barriers can affect access to care—barriers that are more profound for some Americans than for others.

Healthcare Access: The Five A's

It is in the realm of improving (or not) access to healthcare services that the government has its most dramatic impact on both cost and quality. We saw earlier in the chapter how in 1965 the federal government made an affirmative decision to provide insurance—and thus eliminate at least some of the cost barrier for the elderly and poor—when it enacted and implemented Medicare and Medicaid. The decision to implement these far-reaching reforms was made fundamentally to pay for the costs of care for those who could not afford basic care for themselves. The force of logic or the embrace of an ideology seldom drives such decisions in an abstract construct. As President Lyndon Johnson said during the great Medicare debate, "You can't treat Grandma this way," referring to the proverbial elderly woman who could not afford to see a doctor (Moyers 2017). Therefore, when the federal government initiated Medicare and Medicaid, it took a major step to improve one of the five aspects of access to healthcare.

The "five A's of Access"—availability, accessibility, affordability, adequacy, and acceptability—determine meaningful access to healthcare. Resolving four of these factors is inadequate; all five must be present for a person to receive high-quality care.

Availability

Availability means the provider needs to be reasonably available to the patient when needed. This does not suggest the doctor should be on call for every whim, but rather that someone in the healthcare system should be available in concordance with the patient's symptoms. Thus, if one calls the physician's office and describes acute, sporadic chest pains that also radiate to the left arm, one might expect the suggestion to get to an emergency room to be seen as quickly as possible. Likewise, if you call to schedule an appointment and are symptom-free, a reasonable delay to get an appointment does not mean the doctor is not "available."

Accessibility

This merely means the provider is physically accessible to the patient. "Accessibility" describes the geographic location of the healthcare service, which should be in reasonable proximity to the patient's location. It also means the office or hospital is physically accessible to a patient who uses assistive devices.

Affordability

It does no good to have the doctor with a wide-open schedule in the office building next door to yours if you cannot afford the fee to see her. Affordability means simply that the patient has the wherewithal to pay for care. This is why insurance is so important: because it is positively associated with making access to care possible (Glied, Ma, and Borja 2017).

Adequacy

Adequacy asks the question, "Is the physician or healthcare service you need adequate for the task and technically competent to render the care you need?" If you need a neurosurgeon to repair a lesion in your upper spine, even the most earnest and dedicated family practice physician will not be able to help you.

Acceptability

Simply put, acceptability means the provider meets the patient on common ground interpersonally. This can describe all manner of things affecting communication between the doctor and patient. Is the provider respectful of the patient's cultural heritage, for example? Does the doctor speak the same language as the patient? This also relates to the interpersonal characteristics of the doctor and the patient: If the patient wants to be actively involved in the decisions affecting her care and the doctor is paternalistic and directive in his manner, then this physician may not be acceptable to her.

To summarize, these are the barriers affecting patients' access to care:

- *Affordability:* The patient cannot afford it (for lack of insurance).
- *Availability:* A limited number of physicians accept their insurance or "self-pay."
- *Accessibility:* The patient does not have adequate transportation.
- *Acceptability:* The patient and provider do not speak the same language.
- *Adequacy*: Their physician cannot provide the specialty care they need.

These constitute real factors that make it impossible for some people to seek care. When that happens, relatively uncomplicated medical conditions can be exacerbated, resulting in more serious illness and ultimately death (Abraham 1993).

Iterative Nature of Public Policy: The Affordable Care Act

Whatever prompted policymakers to act on healthcare in the first place may, or may not, be what causes them to revisit the initial policy in the future. We saw an example of this iterative nature of public policy in chapter 1, in the discussion of how the existing Kerr-Mills Act became the foundation for Medicaid and Medicare. (In the current climate, policymakers see Medicaid as a negative—a major factor in the burgeoning cost of healthcare—so they focus on reducing costs, even if that might reduce access to care.) A more recent example of the iterative nature of public policy is the implementation of the ACA in 2010 (see exhibit 2.11).

Consider the major components of health insurance: private insurance, Medicare, and Medicaid. Remember, these represent nearly three-quarters of all NHE. Now consider that in 2010, even with all those components in place, there were still 49.9 million people without healthcare coverage in this country (Kaiser Health News 2012).

Exhibit 2.11
The Dynamics of the Policy Process

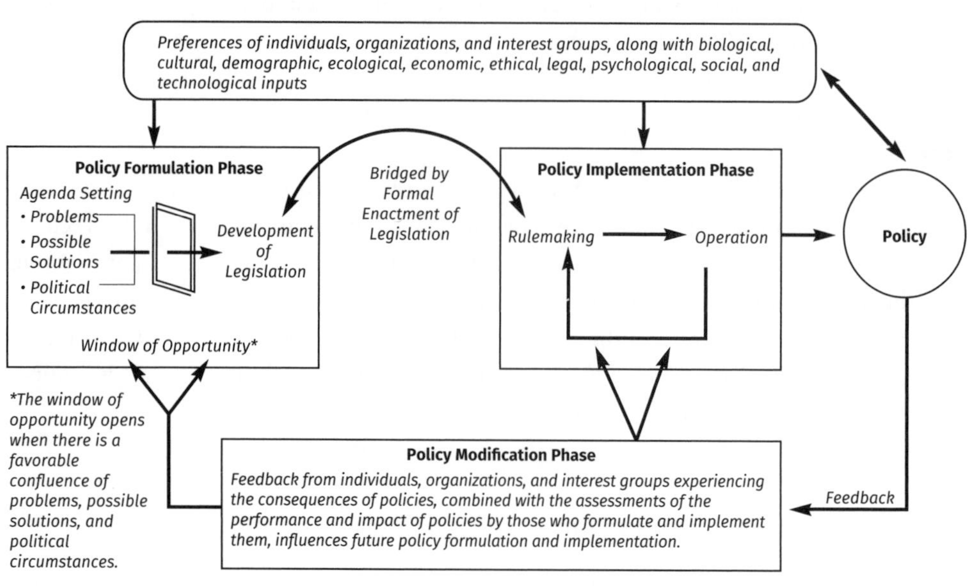

Source: Reprinted from Longest (2015).

In 2008, Barack Obama campaigned, in part, on the promise of healthcare reform, and he converted that promise into a policy initiative when he took office in January 2009. After a year of bitter and partisan debate, he signed the ACA, known formally as the Patient Protection and Affordable Care Act, into law on March 23, 2010 (Altman and Schachtman 2011).

Focus on the "Policy Formulation Phase" in exhibit 2.11. This is where healthcare reform became prominent on the public agenda:

- The problem: 49.9 million uninsured.
- Possible solutions: ranged from a single-payer system, meaning the government would act as insurer to all Americans, to letting individuals buy in to Medicare before age 65, to expanding the private insurance market, or some combination.
- The political circumstances: Democrats controlled the White House and both houses of Congress for the first time since 1993.

This set the stage for a universal healthcare proposal. The question was how to expand healthcare coverage to the nation's 49.9 million uninsured. Rather than draft a complete piece of legislation as President Clinton had done before him, President Obama set forth a number of broad principles that he would support as he challenged Congress to actually write the bill (Altman and Schachtman 2011). This would be the "Development of Legislation" element of the "Policy Formation Phase" of the process. The president proposed a concept and put forth ideas about how it should work. It was up to Congress to develop the legislation.

President Obama's basic principles for healthcare reform legislation included the following (Kaiser Health News 2010):

1. Healthcare should be affordable; no family should need to spend more than 10 percent of their annual income on healthcare.
2. Access to care should be universal; everyone should be able to access necessary healthcare.
3. Health insurance should be portable: A person should be able to keep their health insurance when they change jobs.
4. Individuals should have a choice about where they get their healthcare and healthcare insurance.
5. There should be a new focus on prevention and wellness in the healthcare services delivery system.
6. Healthcare should be safe and of high quality.
7. Any plan should be sustainable over time.

Before we move to the basic elements of the legislation, take a moment to think about why this was happening then. In 2009, Medicare and Medicaid were 44 years old. They had proven track records. Note the box at the bottom of exhibit 2.11: "Policy Modification Phase." After almost half a century, there was plenty of feedback on Medicare and Medicaid because many Americans had experienced the consequences of those two programs. And, as noted in the top box in exhibit 2.11, liberals favored all manner of expansion of healthcare for poor people.

Even with all the help the government could offer through Medicare and Medicaid, after 44 years there were still nearly 50 million people who could not afford even the most basic access to healthcare. Thus, as the political circumstances were so perfectly aligned with the same party in control of all levers of government, an apparent demand for action by Americans, and the yearnings of a multitude of people needing care, the ACA was slowly, laboriously, and at times bewilderingly drafted (Lee 2016). In the case of the ACA, some elements of both the development of legislation in the "Formulation Phase" box and the "Formal Enactment" stage occurred simultaneously. Indeed, exhibit 2.11 is a model of the ideal; the actual policymaking process is more fluid and not quite so tidy.

The "Bridged by Formal Enactment of Legislation" phase in this case consisted of protracted, acrimonious debate. Opponents warned that patients would lose their right to choose their own physician; that the government would ration care through (fictitious) "death panels"; and that requiring individuals to purchase health insurance violated their constitutional rights (Holan 2009). Proponents assured Americans that nothing of the kind was going to take place (Holan 2009).

The Obama presidential campaign of 2008 may be representative of both the top and bottom portions of exhibit 2.11. On the one hand, that campaign was giving voice to "preferences of individuals, organizations," and others, while on the other hand it represented "feedback from individuals . . . experiencing the consequences" of the existing healthcare system. Thus, the political campaign, in part, informed the subsequent policy debate represented by the "Policy Formulation Phase" that began with Obama's inauguration and lasted until late March 2010. Only on March 23, when the ACA was signed into law, did the first phase end.

Administrative Policymaking

When discussing health policy, or any public policy for that matter, there is a general inclination to focus on the legislative process. That is understandable in this particular case because of the intensity and contentiousness of the debate. There is, however, another equally important segment in the policymaking process: implementation by the administration, also known as *administrative policymaking*.

Executive branch action is required to bring any legislative enactment to life and make it a fully developed policy. While our history is laced with discussions about separation of powers between the legislative and executive branches of government, these branches also have a shared responsibility to the citizens of the United States who elected them. Thus, when Congress legislates, the executive branch implements. The agency assigned responsibility for implementing the law (as designated in the law itself) promulgates rules and regulations designed to make legislative mandates effective. This process is called ***administrative rule making***.

Administrative rule
Language written by an agency that explains a piece of legislation in active terms to carry out the law's mandate. It may also be something that describes the agency's process or procedures. This seldom-featured part of the policy-making process is as important as the legislative process that enacted the law.

In the case of the ACA, as noted earlier, Democrats controlled both the White House and Congress. As President Obama collaborated with the congressional Democrats, the provisions of the act were acceptable to him. However, because he also was in charge of the executive branch, congressional Democrats could rely on the Obama administration to interpret and implement the law in ways that would give it maximum effect.

As you might expect, this business of adopting rules and regulations has a process all its own governed by the Administrative Procedure Act of 1946. This law requires an agency to publish proposed rules or regulations in the *Federal Register* and allow time for comment. Special interest groups participate in this process by providing testimony and evidence supporting their perspective. This takes place formally at the public hearing the agency is required to have on any proposed rule. Following publication, comment, and hearing, the agency may revise its draft rule for republication as a final product (Administrative Procedure Act 1946).

In the case of the ACA, numerous rules and regulations were necessary to implement the legislation because of its vast scope. While the case study at the beginning of the chapter credited the Obama administration with not making the proposal overly broad to jeopardize the possibilities for legislative success, it was nonetheless complex legislation that

- provided for either state or federal insurance exchanges in each state;
- called for the expansion of Medicaid, with new payment obligations for the federal government;
- mandated that every individual not covered by an employer-sponsored insurance policy purchase an individual health insurance policy;
- mandated that every employer of more than 50 people provide a health insurance benefit for its employees;
- imposed new minimum benefits that insurance companies would have to provide;
- eliminated an insurance company's ability to deny coverage to an individual with a preexisting health condition;
- allowed children to stay on their parents' health insurance policy until age 26;
- required that Medicare cover wellness visits to physicians;
- established a comparative effectiveness institute to help promote best clinical practices; and more.

Each of the act's provisions required administrative implementation. The US Department of Health and Human Services (HHS) was charged with that responsibility and needed to promulgate rules and regulations for what otherwise would have been a statement of policy (HHS 2014a). This step is the only way to effectuate the intended policy articulated in a piece of legislation.

The administration accomplished that, and the ACA is, as of this writing, the law of the land. That means that, among other features of the act, we have a national policy that

- requires insurance companies to issue policies to patients who have preexisting health conditions that mean higher costs for the insurers;
- provides for expanding Medicaid coverage to people living in those states that decided to expand the program;
- mandates the establishment of statewide exchanges to encourage the individual insurance market; and

- subsidizes the purchase of health insurance for individuals whose income is between 100 percent and 400 percent of the FPL.

However, not all is sanguine. Many critics have complained that insurance companies are leaving the individual markets in many parts of the country, resulting in a small number, sometimes only one and in a few instances no companies at all, offering insurance through the ACA-created exchanges in some counties. As a result, premiums for some individuals have skyrocketed (Cox et al. 2016). Indeed, there has been widespread concern and public condemnation of the ACA on these grounds. This is the early part of the "Policy Implementation Phase" taking place in response to the ACA. Preferences of ACA opponents are still being heard. Thus, this is the beginning of the path to, in the eyes of some, new healthcare cost-control legislation and changes in the reform envisioned in the ACA.

The 2016 general election brought to power a new Congress and a new president with vastly different views about how the government should—or should not—be involved with the expansion of healthcare coverage. The debate now emphasizes measures to control costs even at the expense of impairing access to care for some (Antos and Capretta 2017).

The Policy Formation Network

As you can tell from reading about the ACA, there is often a high level of interaction among interest groups, administrative agencies, and the legislative branch. Taken all together, these members creating all these interactions become a "policy formation network." In our case, we have a particular interest in the health policy formation network. The exchange of information among members of this network is a vital component of the legislative and administrative rule-making processes. In the modern age of politics, the exchange of money has joined the process in the form of political contributions. Examination of the flow of money is beyond the scope of this book. Instead, let us examine how each of the members of the health policy formation network behaves in the process.

Special Interest Groups: What Are They and What Is Their Role?

Special interest groups play a significant role in the legislative process. As we saw at the beginning of the chapter, in the initial formation of its health policy, the Obama administration called many groups together to help craft a universal health insurance proposal.

Many consider the term *special interest group* to be pejorative and decry the groups' influence on the legislative process. No doubt there is some truth to this perspective, particularly as it relates to the campaign contributions just mentioned. That aside, however, consider that nearly everyone in the healthcare community is a member of one or more such groups:

Physician	➔	American Medical Association
Administrator	➔	American Hospital Association
Pharmaceutical company	➔	Pharmaceutical Research and Manufacturers of America
Nurse	➔	American Nurses Association
Physician practice administrator	➔	Medical Group Management Association
Ambulatory surgery center	➔	American Surgery Center Association
Health insurance executive	➔	America's Health Insurance Plans
Senior citizen	➔	AARP
Long-term care facility	➔	American Health Care Association
Durable medical equipment representative	➔	Medical Equipment Suppliers Association

We are just scratching the surface to name ten special interest groups. You most likely will become a member of at least one as a healthcare administrator, so already you are at the table. Are you wondering about the group for the general public? Keep in mind that while nearly every participant in the healthcare process is a "member" of one group or another, there are only a small handful of groups that represent "the patient" exclusively. The list shown here is a small, representative sample of *some* of the interest groups active in health policy.

As unseemly as some may find these groups, the constitution generally protects them and their activities. The First Amendment of the US Constitution guarantees free speech, freedom of association, and the absolute right to petition the government for redress of grievances. These three concepts taken together guarantee a place in our society—and, more important, our political process—for special interest groups.

Interest groups are frequently the source of expert information. One would expect the American Medical Association to know more about "doctoring" than most other groups, save perhaps a handful of specialty practice groups. This expertise is a source of power. If a legislator or member of the executive agency wants to learn how a specific disease might be treated, who better to help explain it than those actually associated with the treatment of the disease? In short, the members of the special interest groups can bring a wealth of information to any health policy discussion.

Legislators

Legislators (and their staffs) are consumers of information. Frequently, they need to understand the implications of their intended votes, and this knowledge then forms the rationale for their decision and the talking points used to explain it to their constituents. Because the stakes are so high, the information must be accurate and truthful. To be sure, the interest group information may come with a bias, but the information will be accurate and truthful if that group expects to have a working relationship with that particular legislator. Likewise, the legislator has influence over the special interest group with the way he or she votes on legislation. While the interest group attempts to persuade the legislator to their particular point of view, whether or not the legislator agrees will influence the behavior of the interest group. As we saw in the vignette at the outset of the chapter, the groups garnering revenue from the current system have little inclination to change it, unless they can be engaged to change it to a way beneficial to them, or that at least insulates them from economic harm. Thus, the work of special interest groups may easily lead to legislative or policy inertia, as the vignette suggests.

The relationships between legislators and administrative agencies also are important. Agencies rely on Congress for appropriations to continue their work. Likewise, legislators rely on agencies for information, often for help with individual constituent matters and sometimes for enforcing the rule in a particular way. It is a symbiotic relationship, as the agencies also rely on the legislators.

Administrative Agencies

Last, but certainly not least, are the administrative agencies, whose officers write the rules that interpret the legislation. They interpret those rules to regulate any fact or situation, and they govern the behavior of those they regulate through their interpretations. Thus, special interest groups want to influence regulators' views, and legislators may seek to influence how the agency interprets the legislation it is implementing. This discretion is even written into many significant laws, including the ACA, which empowered the Secretary of HHS to grant states waivers from key provisions of the law so they could experiment with innovative structures for improving access to care (42 U.S.C. Sec. 18052). Because administrative agencies depend on legislators for funding and authority, the legislator is likely to get a friendly ear from the agency. It is through this ongoing exchange of information and influence that policy is initiated, implemented, criticized, and changed again, reinforcing the iterative nature of both the outcome—no policy is ever "final"—and the process. See exhibit 2.12 for a depiction of the policy-formation network.

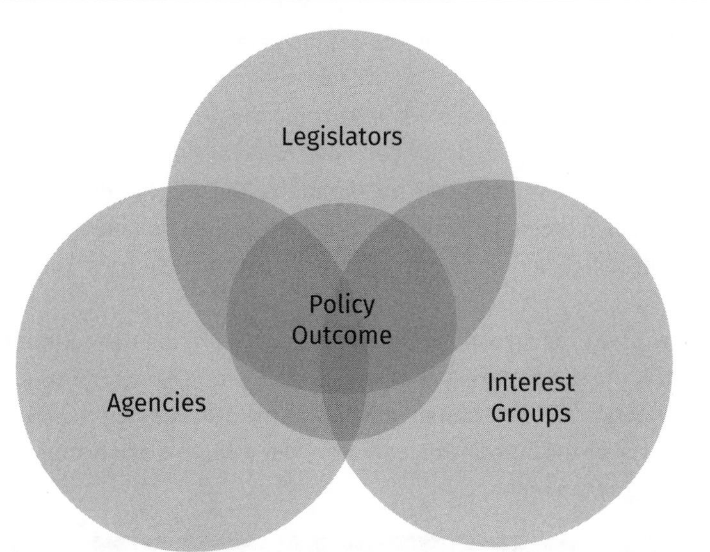

Exhibit 2.12 The Policy–Network Interaction

Conclusion

There is little doubt that efforts to amend, repeal, or replace "Obamacare" will be forthcoming. There is no single perfect policy that can withstand the test of time and the accompanying changes in circumstances.

It has happened before. There was the Kerr-Mills legislation, enacted to provide care for the poorest individuals among the elderly. Then in 1965 came sweeping changes that implemented Medicare for senior citizens and Medicaid for the impoverished. This was followed in 2006 with the Medicare Prescription Drug, Improvement and Modernization Act that created a first-ever benefit for prescription drugs within Medicare (Kaiser Family Foundation 2016, 2017a). Next came President Clinton's unsuccessful effort to advance universal healthcare (Blumenthal and Morone 2010), which was followed by President Obama's advocacy for universal coverage, leading to the ACA in 2010.

There are ebbs and flows in the sea of change with respect to government involvement in our healthcare system. Over time, despite occasional retrenchments toward less governmental intervention, the arc of history suggests an ever-increasing governmental role to make healthcare coverage more equitable and, thus, the delivery of healthcare services more universal. In the wake of the ACA, the movement in favor of reducing the government's role has gained strength. The next round of policymaking in this arena could well see a reduction in the scope of government intervention and a renewed focus on free market forces to drive a greater portion of the health insurance and health services markets.

Because of this ebb and flow, and because the policy process is never complete, it is important that healthcare administrators understand the process so they can knowledgeably observe and participate in it. The policy decisions made at the federal and state levels have far-reaching implications for healthcare organizations. Those policy decisions are part of the milieu in which the healthcare administrator functions professionally. Failure to understand the importance of policy decisions, and how they continually evolve, can have disastrous consequences.

In chapter 1, we examined the historical development of the US healthcare system. Here, we have seen how the policymaking apparatus works, why it is important to the healthcare system, and how it contributes to system changes. In the next chapter, we will review what the system looks like today: the outcome of multiple policy decisions and historical developments since the beginning of the republic.

Mini Case Study: Mandates and a Quid Pro Quo

Even though the Obama administration and Congress built the ACA on the existing system of employer-sponsored insurance, it had significant ramifications for much of the healthcare system. Under the mandates of the ACA, (1) insurance companies were required to provide coverage for people with preexisting conditions, (2) payments to hospitals for accepting a higher number of economically disadvantaged patients were phased out, (3) doctors were required to adapt to new payment models, (4) reimbursements for hospitals and health plans were reduced, and (5) benchmarks were used to penalize hospitals for not performing up to certain standards.

One part of the healthcare industry that favored the ACA and voluntarily contributed funds to help defray its cost was the pharmaceutical industry. Prices for prescription drugs continue to rise. Requirements for Medicare to use its negotiating power to reduce drug prices were scrapped from the legislation before it was drafted. The law did not include provisions to allow the re-importation of drugs from Canada, where prices for prescription medicines are much lower. For all practical purposes, the pharmaceutical industry continues to conduct business just as it did before the enactment of the ACA.

Mini Case Study Questions

1. Why did other segments of the healthcare industry seemingly make greater sacrifice than prescription drug manufacturers?
2. Would it have been possible to alter the way drug companies do business as part of the ACA and still succeed in enacting the law? Why or why not?

Points to Remember

- Special interest groups have long played a role in shaping US health policy.
- Health policy, like all public policy, has no "end point." Policy is changed because of new information or circumstances applied to existing policy.
- Because of our federalist system, healthcare providers need to be aware of both federal and state laws that may influence their behavior.
- In terms of outcomes, the United States lags behind many of its peers, as other developed countries have longer life expectancies and lower infant mortality rates.
- National health expenditures always increase and never decrease. The rate of growth may vary, but the NHE always goes up.

Challenge Yourself

1. Why was it important for the Affordable Care Act ("Obamacare") to build on the existing system of employer-sponsored insurance? Would it have been easier to scrap the existing system and start over?
2. What role did special interest groups play in helping to fashion the final version of the ACA?
3. Why must we always change public policy? Why does it seem like policymakers are continually debating the same set of issues or causes? Are they really the same?

For Your Consideration

1. Research which states have expanded Medicaid since the passage of the Affordable Care Act. How many are there? Have any states reversed course and repealed (or attempted to repeal) the expansion? What were their reasons?
2. Find several news articles about healthcare and health policy. What are the key issues? How do the issues you have identified relate to the ACA?

References

Abraham, L. 1993. *Mama Might Be Better Off Dead.* Chicago: University of Chicago Press.

Administrative Procedure Act. P.L. 79-404, 60 Stat. 237 (1946).

Affordable Care Act. 42 U.S.C. Sec. 18031 (2010).

Altman, S., and D. Schachtman. 2011. *Power, Politics and Universal Health Care.* Amherst, NY: Prometheus Books.

American Hospital Association. 2016. *Trends Affecting Hospitals and Health Systems: Chartbook 2016*. Accessed August 9, 2017. www.aha.org/research/reports/tw/chartbook/ch3.shtml.

Antos, J., and J. Capretta. 2017. "The CBO's Updated Estimate of the AHCA." *Health Affairs Blog*. Published June 6. http://healthaffairs.org/blog/2017/06/06/the-cbos-updated-estimate-of-the-ahca/.

Antos, J., J. Capretta, and B. Ippolito. 2017. "The Basis for Compromise on Medicaid Reform and Expansion." *Health Affairs Blog*. Published June 15. http://healthaffairs.org/blog/2017/06/15/the-basis-for-compromise-on-medicaid-reform-and-expansion/.

Blumenthal, D., and J. Morone. 2008. "The Lessons of Success—Revisiting the Medicare Story." *New England Journal of Medicine* 359 (22): 2384–89.

———. 2010. *The Heart of Power: Health and Politics in the Oval Office*, 2nd ed. Los Angeles: University of California Press.

Caraher, L. 2014. *Millennials & Management*. New York: Routledge.

Centers for Disease Control and Prevention (CDC). 2016. "Reproductive Health: Infant Mortality." Updated January 2018. www.cdc.gov/reproductivehealth/maternalinfanthealth/infant mortality.htm.

Centers for Medicare & Medicaid Services (CMS). 2016a. "National Health Expenditure Data: Historical." Updated January 2018. www.cms.gov/Research-Statistics-Data-and-Systems/Statistics-Trends-and-Reports/NationalHealthExpendData/NationalHealthAccountsHistorical.html.

———. 2016b. "National Health Expenditures, 2016 Highlights." Accessed July 5, 2018. www.cms.gov/Research-Statistics-Data-and-Systems/Statistics-Trends-and-Reports/NationalHealthExpendData/Downloads/highlights.pdf.

———. 2006. "National Coverage Determination (NCD) for Bariatric Surgery for Treatment of Morbid Obesity (100.1)." Accessed June 15, 2018. www.cms.gov/medicare-coverage-database/details/ncd-details.aspx?NCDId=57&bc=AgAAgAAAAAAA&ncdver=3.

Cohen, R., E. Zammatti, and M. Martinez. 2017. "Health Insurance Coverage: Early Release of Estimates from the National Health Interview Survey, 2016." National Center for Health Statistics, National Health Interview Survey Early Release Program. Released May 2017. www.cdc.gov/nchs/data/nhis/earlyrelease/insur201705.pdf.

Cox, C., M. Long, A. Semanskee, R. Kamal, G. Claxton, and L. Levitt. 2016. "2017 Premium Changes and Insurer Participation in the Affordable Care Act's Insurance Marketplaces." Updated November 1. Henry

J. Kaiser Family Foundation. www.kff.org/health-reform/issue-brief/2017-premium-changes-and-insurer-participation-in-the-affordable-care-acts-health-insurance-marketplaces.

Elhauge, E. 2010. *The Fragmentation of US Healthcare: Causes and Solutions*. New York: Oxford University Press.

Federation of State Medical Boards. 2017. "The Role of the State Medical Board." Accessed August 8. www.fsmb.org/Media/Default/PDF/Advocacy/role_of_state_medical_boards.pdf.

Flaherty, J., H. Perry, G. Lynchard, and J. Morley. 2000. "Polypharmacy and Hospitalization Among Older Home Care Patients." *Journal of Gerontology* 55 (10): 554–59.

Glied, S. A., S. Ma, and A. Borja. 2017. "Effect of the Affordable Care Act on Health Care Access." The Commonwealth Fund. Published May 8. www.commonwealthfund.org/publications/issue-briefs/2017/may/effect-aca-health-care-access.

Holan, A. 2009. "PolitiFact's Lie of the Year: 'Death Panels.'" PolitiFact. Published December 18. www.politifact.com/truth-o-meter/article/2009/dec/18/politifact-lie-year-death-panels/.

Jacobson v. Massachusetts, 197 U.S. 11 (1905).

Kaiser Family Foundation. 2017a. "The Medicare Part D Prescription Drug Benefit." Published October 2. www.kff.org/medicare/fact-sheet/the-medicare-prescription-drug-benefit-fact-sheet/.

———. 2017b. "Status of State Action on the Medicaid Expansion Decision." Accessed August 17. www.kff.org/health-reform/state-indicator/state-activity-around-expanding-medicaid-under-the-affordable-care-act/.

———. 2016. "Who Is Impacted by the Coverage Gap in States That Have Not Adopted the Medicaid Expansion?" Updated November. www.kff.org/slideshow/who-is-impacted-by-the-coverage-gap-in-states-that-have-not-adopted-the-medicaid-expansion/.

Kaiser Health News. 2012. "Number of Uninsured Americans Drops by 1.3 Million." *KHN Morning Briefing*. Published September 13. http://khn.org/morning-breakout/census-numbers-2/.

———. 2010. "Full Text: Obama's Health Care Proposal." Published February 22. http://khn.org/news/obama-health-care-proposal/.

Kofman, M., and K. Pollitz. 2006. "Health Insurance Regulation by States and the Federal Government: A Review of Current Approaches and Proposals for Change." Georgetown University

Health Policy Institute. Published April. www-tc.pbs.org/now/politics/Healthinsurance reportfinalkofmanpollitz.pdf.

Lee, M. 2016. "Who Drafted the Bill That Became the Affordable Care Act: Obama or Congress?" Quora. Published November 22. www.quora.com/Who-drafted-the-bill-that-became-the-Affordable-Care-Act-Obama-or-the-Congress.

Longest, B. 2015. *Health Policymaking in the United States*, 6th ed. Chicago: Health Administration Press.

Martinez, M., B. Ward, and P. Adams. 2015. *Health Care Access and Utilization Among Adults Aged 18–64, by Race and Hispanic Origin: United States, 2013 and 2014*. NCHS Data Brief. Published July. www.cdc.gov/nchs/data/databriefs/db208.pdf.

Medicaid.gov. 2017. *Medicaid & CHIP: Strengthening Coverage, Improving Health*. Published January. www.medicaid.gov/medicaid/program-information/downloads/accomplishments-report.pdf.

Morgan, R. B. 2017. "2017 Federal Poverty Guidelines." National Conference of State Legislatures. Published May 30. www.ncsl.org/research/health/2014-federal-poverty-level-standards.aspx.

Moyers, B. 2017. "LBJ Launches Medicare: 'You Can't Treat Grandma This Way.'" Salon. Published August 5. www.salon.com/2017/08/05/lbj-launches-medicare-you-cannot-treat-grandma-this-way_partner.

National Conference of State Legislatures. 2016. "CON—Certificate of Need State Laws." Published August 25. www.ncsl.org/research/health/con-certificate-of-need-state-laws.aspx.

Neuman, P., J. Cubanski, and A. Damico. 2015. "Datawatch: Medicare Per Capita Spending by Age and Service." *Health Affairs* 34 (2): 335–39.

Neuman, T., J. Cubanski, J. Huang, and A. Damico. 2015. "The Rising Cost of Living Longer: Analysis of Medicare Spending by Age for Beneficiaries in Traditional Medicare." Kaiser Family Foundation. Published January 14. www.kff.org/medicare/report/the-rising-cost-of-living-longer-analysis-of-medicare-spending-by-age-for-beneficiaries-in-traditional-medicare/.

Organisation for Economic Co-operation and Development (OECD). 2018a. "Deaths from Cancer." Accessed June 18. https://data.oecd.org/healthstat/deaths-from-cancer.htm.

———. 2018b. "Infant Mortality Rates." Accessed June 18. https://data.oecd.org/healthstat/infant-mortality-rates.htm.

———. 2015. "Healthcare Costs Unsustainable in Advanced Economies Without Reform." Published September 24. www.oecd.org/health/healthcarecostsunsustainableinadvanced economieswithoutreform.htm.

Peterson-Kaiser Health System Tracker. 2018. "Webcast: Why Are Healthcare Prices So High, and What Can Be Done About Them?" Forum held May 9. www.healthsystemtracker.org/?sfid=4356&_sft_category=access-affordability,health-well-being,spending,quality-of-care.

Russell, K. 2012. "Court Holds That States Have Choice Whether to Join Medicaid Expansion." SCOTUS Blog. Posted June 28. www.scotusblog.com/2012/06/court-holds-that-states-have-choice-whether-to-join-medicaid-expansion.

Schneider, E., D. O. Sarnak, D. Squires, A. Shah, and M. M. Doty. 2017. *Mirror, Mirror 2017: International Comparison Reflects Flaws and Opportunities for Better U.S. Health Care*. The Commonwealth Fund. Published July. www.commonwealthfund.org/interactives/2017/july/mirror-mirror.

Schneider, E., and D. Squires. 2017. "From Last to First—Could the U.S. Health Care System Become the Best in the World?" *New England Journal of Medicine* 377 (10): 901–904.

Snyder, L., and R. Rudowitz. 2015. "Medicaid Financing: How Does It Work and What Are the Implications?" Kaiser Commission on Medicaid and the Unisured. Published May. http://files.kff.org/attachment/issue-brief-medicaid-financing-how-does-it-work-and-what-are-the-implications.

United States v. Sprague, 282 U.S. 716 (1931).

US Constitution. First Amendment. Available at www.law.cornell.edu/constitution/first_amendment.

———. Tenth Amendment. Available at www.law.cornell.edu/constitution/tenth_amendment.

US Department of Health and Human Services (HHS). 2014a. "HHS Regulations Toolkit." Reviewed July 1. www.hhs.gov/regulations/regulations-toolkit/index.html.

———. 2014b. *New HHS Data Shows Major Strides Made in Patient Safety, Leading to Improved Care and Savings*. Published May 7. https://innovation.cms.gov/Files/reports/patient-safety-results.pdf.

Waiver for State Innovation. 42 U.S.C. Sec. 18052 (2010).

CHAPTER 3

THE HEALTHCARE SYSTEM TODAY

Important Terms

- Academic health center (AHC)
- Accountable care organization (ACO)
- Activities of daily living (ADL)
- Acute care
- Ambulatory surgery center (ASC)
- Assisted living facility
- Bundled payment
- Centers for Medicare & Medicaid Services (CMS)
- Clinical integration
- Community hospital
- Explanation of benefits (EOB)
- Fee-for-service
- Graduate medical education
- Health Resources and Services Administration (HRSA)
- Home health agency
- Hospice
- Hospital outpatient department
- Instrumental activities of daily living (IADL)
- Licensed practical nurse (LPN)
- Long-term care facility (LTC)
- Nurse practitioner (NP)
- Pay-for-performance
- Pharmacy benefit manager (PBM)
- Physician assistant (PA)
- Public hospital
- Registered nurse (RN)
- Rehabilitation hospital
- Residential care community
- Retail clinic
- Shared savings program
- Teaching hospital

Learning Objectives

After reading this chapter, you will be able to do the following:

➤ Give a general overview of the US healthcare system

➤ Describe the differences between acute care and ambulatory care

- Describe the different types of hospitals and their missions
- Describe the difference between a hospital and an ambulatory surgery center and the movement of care from inpatient to outpatient
- Understand the differences between long-term care, assisted living, and rehabilitation hospitals
- Understand how "extenders" work and describe the differences between them
- Discuss in general terms how healthcare is financed
- Describe the difference between Medicare and Medicaid
- Describe evolving payment systems

Case Study: The Evolving Healthcare System—What It Looks Like Today

Barbara, an active 81-year-old resident of a suburban area in a mid-Atlantic state, recently wrote an e-mail to a friend:

"Have been so busy trying to get things straightened out from the move my family doctor made. He closed his practice after 30 years and merged with another internal medicine group. Problem being he didn't have his records on the computer and didn't do too much electronically. He and his wife have a practice together but she has her patients and he has his patients. My problems started with the prescriptions. He hand-wrote everything and I had paper scripts that I sent in for my 90-day supplies. Now it is all done by fax [and] the group put the responsibility on the patient to take care of figuring out what to do. I have gotten so many wrong answers from their office help and am about ready to scream. . . . Hopefully, by the end of the weekend I will have all of the prescriptions at the right place and if they have problems they can call the practice and fix it up. But as far as technology goes, they can scrap it. Never had such problems in my life. I like the 'country doctor' method."

Introduction

Barbara's frustration is surely understandable given such a big change in how she accesses her medical care and prescriptions. Her situation—the migration from "country doctor" to larger, integrated providers—is, however, becoming increasingly common as the healthcare delivery system continues to evolve. Moreover, Barbara likely will experience even greater change when she next makes an appointment or needs to schedule a diagnostic test.

In the previous two chapters, we reviewed the growth of science in medicine and the policy processes that drive development of the healthcare system. Understanding the scientific background of the current healthcare delivery system and the policy mechanisms that help shape it set the stage for a thorough examination of the healthcare delivery system as it is today. In this chapter, we will explore how the healthcare delivery system continues to evolve and how the delivery of clinical care in the United States is changing. In examining that evolution, we will explore the changes that continue to affect the delivery of "how" and "where" in healthcare and, importantly, the quality of care.

Current Trends

Several trends are changing the look of our healthcare system. These result from a combination of forces, including market forces, policy decisions, and the movement away from sporadic individual care toward population health. In short, we have fewer hospitals and more clinics; fewer primary care physicians, but more specialists. Hospitals are merging with other organizations to become "systems," or systems are acquiring hospitals. In many cases, there may not be an actual "acquisition," but rather an agreement for management of the hospital by the larger system. Furthermore, it has become increasingly untenable for smaller hospitals to survive. That is because attempts to ameliorate cost increases while improving quality and expanding access to care have caused the environment to move toward integrated records and emerging payment models that incentivize multiple layers of integration and increased collaboration across traditional clinical boundaries.

As hospitals merge, acquire one another, or otherwise join forces, they create "systems" in which they deliver health services. By the end of 2016, there were 626 such systems in the United States. These systems include multiple kinds of hospitals as well as physicians and other types of services and professionals to provide them. Exhibit 3.1 shows the coalescing trend from 1994 to 2014, while exhibit 3.2 highlights important facts about these multi-organizational care-delivery systems from 2016.

Exhibit 3.1 Number of Hospitals Belonging to Health Systems, 2004–2014

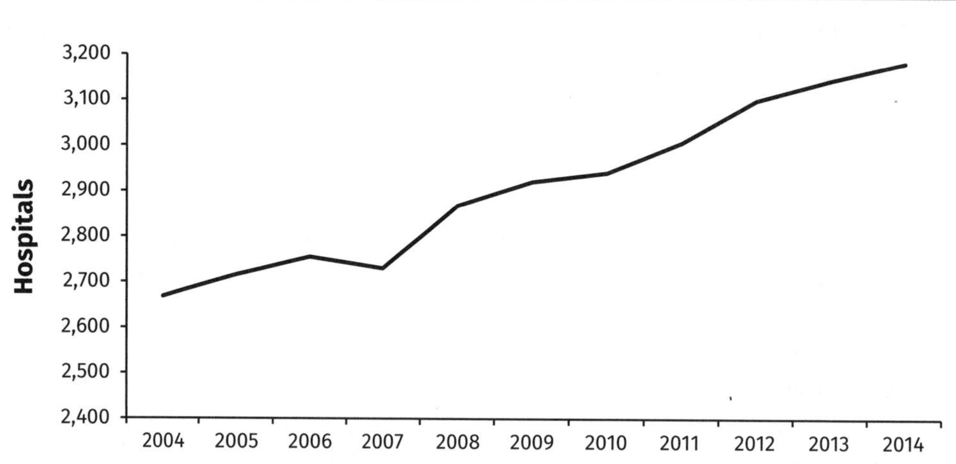

Source: Reprinted from American Hospital Association (2017c).

Exhibit 3.2
US Hospitals and Physicians Belonging to Health Systems

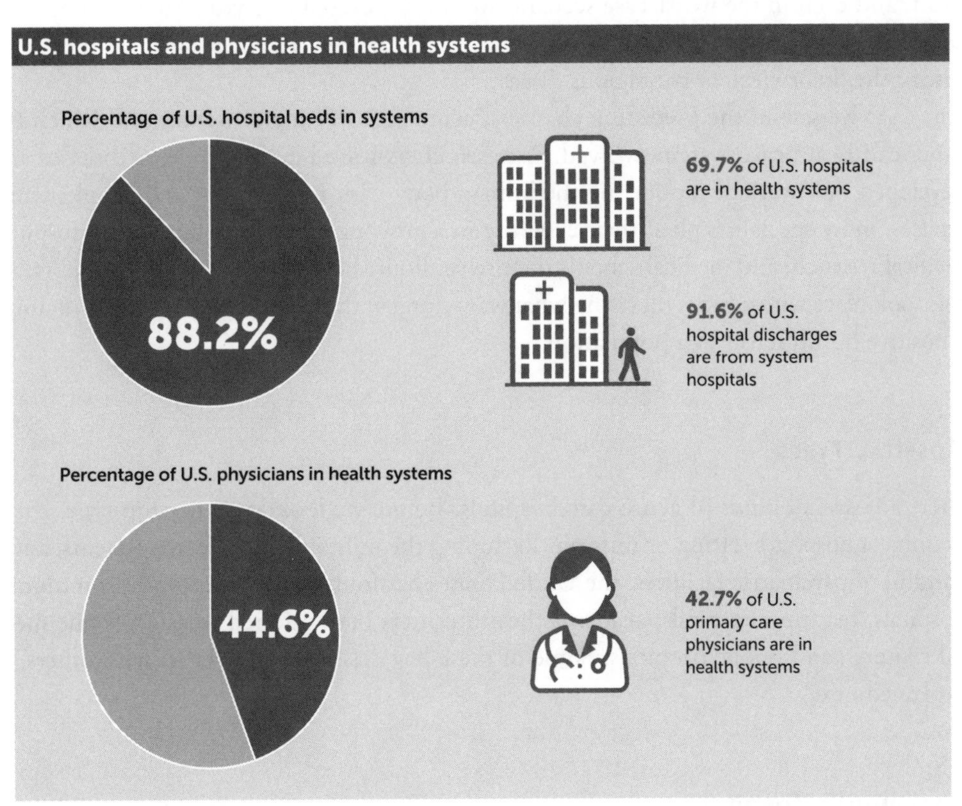

Source: Reprinted from Agency for Healthcare Research and Quality (2017).

What does this mean for the patient? It means that despite her frustration, Barbara is most likely going to receive care facilitated by a medical record shared between her local hospital and her physician, and one that is accessible to any specialist associated with that system in the event she requires care beyond the scope of her primary care physician. And, if her physician and hospital are part of a larger network of different provider organizations, Barbara will have access to a wide range of health services should she need them, without having to carry medical records or images such as MRIs or X-rays with her.

Still, what makes up a system? The answer to that question can vary widely, so let us begin by examining the component parts of US healthcare overall.

Acute Care

Acute care
Short-term care for patients who have a relatively severe illness.

Acute-care hospitals are the backbone of the US healthcare system. What is **acute care**? It is the care provided to treat severe trauma or illness for which the patient needs a procedure or medical care as an inpatient. Furthermore, the duration of this kind of care is relatively short, and even in the worst-case scenario would not exceed one year. Some examples of acute care include heart surgery, joint replacements, and severe illness such as an extreme case of the flu or virulent contagious disease.

As we saw in the preceding chapters, acute care was the center around which the American healthcare system evolved. As researchers found cures for more diseases and developed new ways of supporting the human body with replacement and supplemental devices, more specialists plied their expertise in a growing number of hospitals. Hospitals, medical research, and medical schools themselves flourished with government support. All this took place with a focus on fixing what was wrong with the individual, not maintaining a positive health status in a population.

Hospital Types

There are several kinds of acute-care hospitals. Before we look at ownership type, let us examine a hospital's setting or mission. Excluding the military and veterans systems, and a handful of psychiatric facilities, the United States has four kinds of hospitals: community hospitals, teaching hospitals, academic health centers (also referred to as academic medical centers), and public hospitals. Some of these key designations overlap with others, as explained next.

Community hospital
Hospitals, ranging from large teaching hospitals to small inpatient facilities, that provide medical services to their communities.

Community Hospitals

Community hospitals are the most common hospital type in the United States. They can be large teaching hospitals (which, as we will discuss next, are not the same as academic health centers) like Hartford Hospital in Connecticut, or they can be small hospitals located in relatively small communities like Titusville General Hospital in Titusville, Pennsylvania. Regardless, these hospitals provide needed medical services to their community. Thus, obstetrics, orthopedics, general surgery, and nonsurgical medical cases form the large majority of their services. In many cases, cancer care also is a part of the community hospital portfolio. The primary mission for these facilities is providing care for the residents of the community in which they are located.

Teaching hospital
A hospital that provides care for the citizens of its local community and residency training programs for medical school graduates preparing to enter a specialty.

Graduate medical education
Formal education in residency programs available to physicians who have graduated from medical school.

Teaching Hospitals

Approximately 1,000 of the nation's community hospitals are also considered **teaching hospitals** (American Hospital Association 2017a). In addition to their mission of providing care for citizens in their local communities, they also support **graduate medical education**. This means they host residency programs for medical school graduates preparing to enter a specialty. There might be one program for just one specialty, or there might be several residencies for various specialties. This is a critically important mission, as it is where surgeons train to be surgeons, cardiologists train in cardiology, and the like. Advanced training for all medical specialties, including primary care fields such as internal medicine and family practice, takes place in residency programs located either at teaching hospitals or at academic health centers. In addition, a teaching hospital also may sponsor limited research projects to advance the science of care. A nonteaching community hospital focuses exclusively on providing care and has virtually no teaching or research activities.

Academic Health Centers

Approximately 120 of the country's 1,000 teaching hospitals are **academic health centers (AHCs)** (American Hospital Association 2017a). These are the citadels of the American healthcare system: They exist to train physicians. However, in addition to the teaching role, AHCs engage in research that adds to the store of knowledge about the human body. Studies conducted at AHCs are responsible for new pharmaceutical compounds that help treat disease; new implantable devices and prosthetics that help keep the body whole; and new methods for treating all the morbidities that can afflict a human being.

Academic health center (AHC)
A teaching hospital that provides healthcare services to the community, trains physicians, and engages in medical research.

Historically, new medical procedures and techniques have been developed at AHCs. Part of the AHCs' mission is to disseminate improvements in care to more providers. As other providers learn the new method, the procedure migrates outward, first to teaching hospitals, then community hospitals, and then, in some cases, **ambulatory surgery centers (ASCs)** (Anderson, Steinberg, and Heyssel 1994). A good example of this process is knee replacement surgery. A variety of techniques and materials were studied in many AHCs, both in the United States and in Europe, with each building on the work of others. As scholars published journal articles and presented at professional conferences on their approaches, surgeons at other AHCs began to contribute to the process. As the process of trial and error proceeded, certain materials, designs, and techniques became more prevalent. Surgeons were trained in the new techniques at AHCs. As those students graduated and entered into practice in other locations, and as other surgeons learned the techniques from colleagues, the idea of knee replacement migrated to community hospitals. Today, knee replacement is a common procedure at community hospitals, and, indeed, in many instances it is considered a "day surgery" that does not require a 24-hour hospital stay (Song et al. 2013). Advanced pain medications and new medicines for increasingly exotic diseases also are products of America's AHCs.

Ambulatory surgery center (ASC)
A facility capable of performing surgery on an outpatient basis, with a patient's arrival and departure on the same day.

Public hospital
Publicly owned medical facility found mostly in major metropolitan areas, though sometimes in rural counties as well; frequently treats uninsured patients or those insured through Medicaid.

Public (or "Safety Net") Hospitals

Publicly owned hospitals exist mostly in major metropolitan areas. The cost of owning and operating a hospital is overwhelming and, thus, **public hospitals** are not sustainable in rural areas with a smaller tax base. Examples are John H. Stroger Jr. Hospital of Cook County, Illinois, and Los Angeles County/USC Hospital in California. Both of these hospitals serve as "safety nets" for their respective communities, meaning that the bulk of their patients are either insured through Medicaid or Medicare or are uninsured. Some states also own hospitals, usually associated with medical schools, that are also safety net facilities. Examples include the Medical University of South Carolina (MUSC) Hospital and the University of Kansas Medical Center (UKMC).

Overlapping Missions

Notice, in the previous section, how hospital missions can overlap: Stroger of Cook County and Los Angeles County/USC are both public hospitals and teaching hospitals, but not AHCs, while MUSC and UKMC are both AHCs and public hospitals.

Even though all hospitals are some form of "community hospital," many limit themselves to certain functions. Said another way, consider that all nonfederal hospitals are "community hospitals." Of that group, some are AHCs, some are teaching hospitals, and some are hospitals that focus on providing care to the community they serve and have teaching missions. Graphically, this would look something like exhibit 3.3.

Number of Hospitals by Ownership and Trends

Adding another dimension to the picture is hospital ownership structure, of which there are several categories:

Exhibit 3.3 Conceptual Depiction of Hospital Relationships by Type

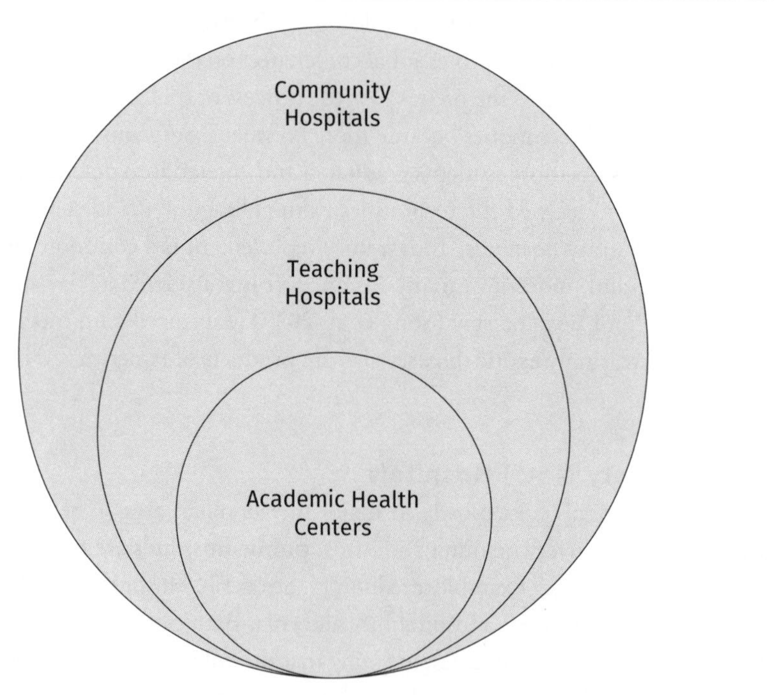

- Nongovernmental not-for-profit
- Investor-owned (for-profit)
- State and local government–owned

Exhibit 3.4 illustrates the number of hospitals by ownership category.

In addition, approximately 700 hospitals are *not* community hospitals and fall into three additional categories, as shown in exhibit 3.5.

As science continued to find new ways to fight disease, and as cost pressures continued to increase over time, the trend of building new hospitals began to abate. The outpatient setting increasingly became the venue of choice for delivering a wide variety of medical procedures.

Exhibit 3.4 Number of Community Hospitals by Ownership Type

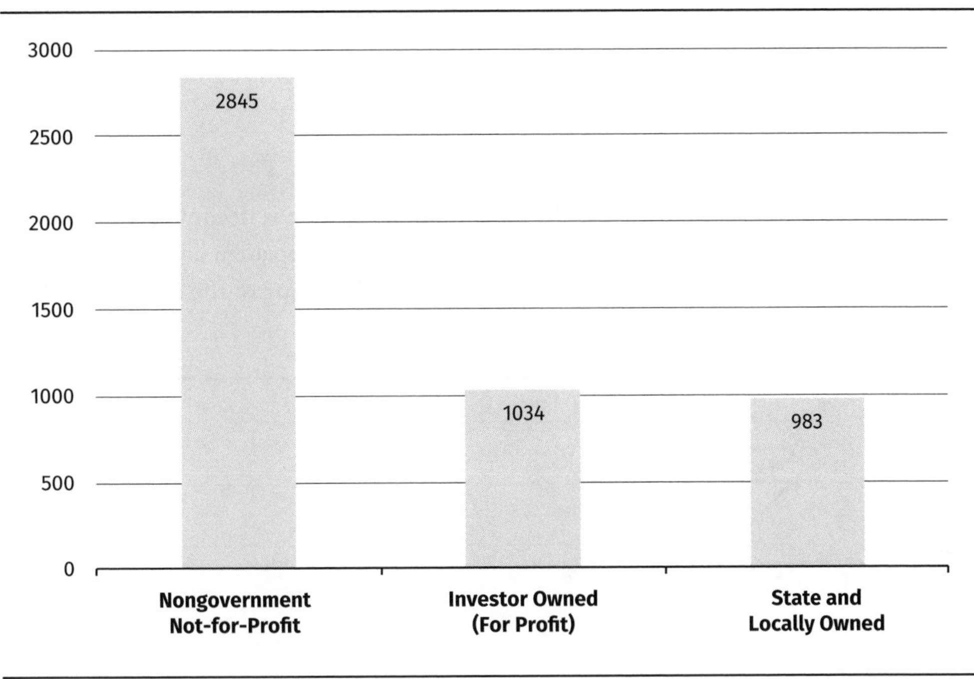

Source: Adapted from American Hospital Association (2017b).

Exhibit 3.5 Numbers of Additional Noncommunity Hospitals

Federal government hospitals	212
Nonfederal psychiatric hospitals	401
Nonfederal long-term care hospitals	79

Source: American Hospital Association (2017b).

In general, the number of hospitals in the United States has been declining since the mid-1990s. Exhibit 3.6 shows this trend in detail. Some hospitals have merged with others and may still be operating, but under a single license. Others have merged and been transformed into freestanding emergency suites or immediate care centers. Still others have closed. The cost pressures in healthcare make it particularly difficult for smaller, rural hospitals to survive.

Hospitals (and physicians, as we shall see later) have increasingly joined, or in some way come to be within the ambit of, a "system," while others have closed entirely. Certainly, shrinking reimbursements and other changes in the payment system are substantial reasons for this continued restructuring. Additional reasons are shorter hospital stays and, critically, fewer of them.

Hospitals and health systems are finding that more of their revenue is coming from outpatient activity, while inpatient activity (and revenue) decline. The migration of care from inside the hospital to the clinics and ASCs is quickening in pace, as demonstrated by exhibit 3.7.

Ambulatory Care

As you can see from exhibits 3.6 and 3.7, inpatient, acute care is declining. Increasingly, various procedures have moved from the inpatient setting to outpatient clinics and surgery centers. Surgical procedures such as cataract removal, arthroscopy of the knee, and a host

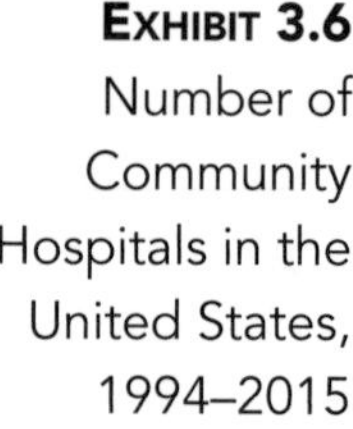

Exhibit 3.6
Number of Community Hospitals in the United States, 1994–2015

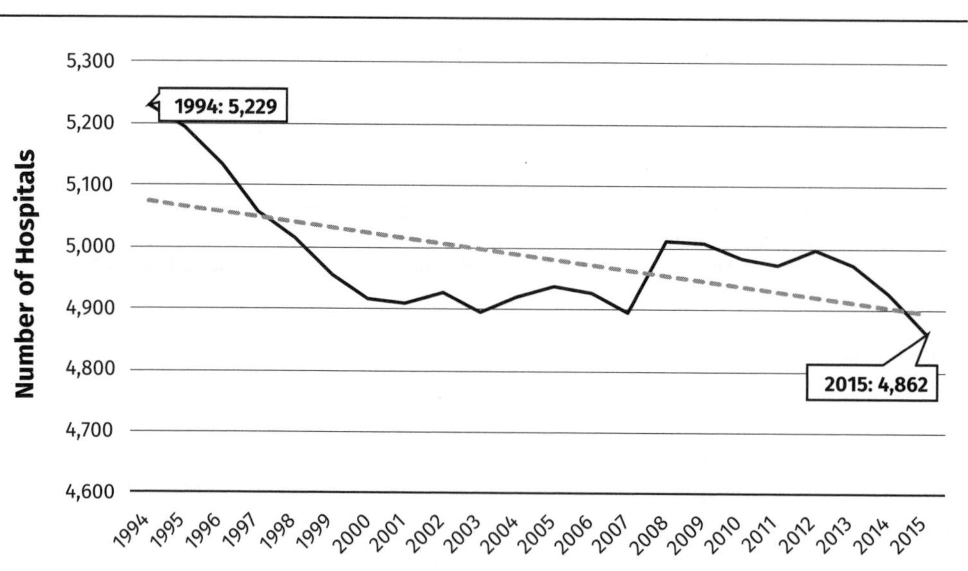

Source: Adapted from American Hospital Association (2017b).

Exhibit 3.7 Distribution of Hospital Outpatient and Inpatient Revenues, 1994–2014

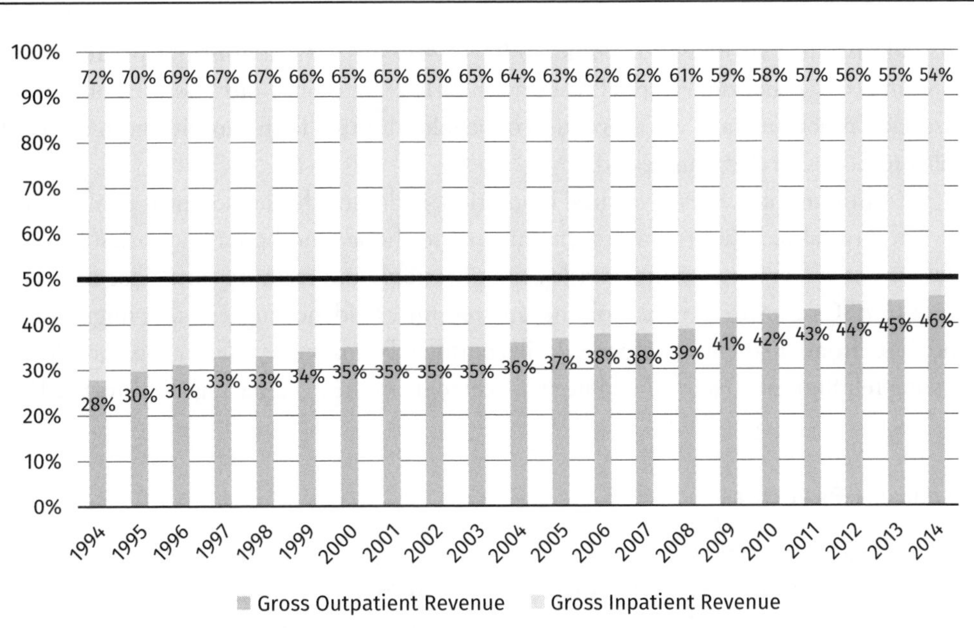

Source: Adapted from American Hospital Association (2017c).

of others no longer require inpatient care. These procedures may be performed in smaller, more cost-efficient surgery centers and do not require an overnight hospital stay. This long-term trend shows no sign of diminishing. In addition, remote monitoring and the use of telemedicine techniques continue to change the delivery of healthcare in the United States (Wiler and Harish 2017).

Ambulatory Surgery Centers

As the number of inpatient procedures has declined, and outpatient procedures have increased, the number of places providing outpatient care also has ramped up dramatically over the last two decades, climbing from 3,028 ASCs in 2000 to 5,446 in 2014 (MedPAC 2016). As of 2016, there were 5,480 Medicare-certified ASCs, with each one housing an average of 15,262 square feet of space and four operating rooms (Rechtoris 2017). ASCs are frequently freestanding facilities that limit patient stays to less than 24 hours, so the procedures performed there are informally known as "day surgeries." To be clear, an ASC is not the same as a **hospital outpatient department**, which may offer many of the same services, but is located within a hospital (or on hospital grounds) and cares for medically more complex patients (MedPAC 2016). The Centers for Disease Control and Prevention reported that, in 2010, 48.3 million outpatient surgical and nonsurgical procedures were performed during 28.6 million visits to ASCs and hospitals combined (Hall et al. 2017). By

Hospital outpatient department
A part of a hospital designated for the treatment of outpatients: people with health problems who visit the hospital for diagnosis or treatment, but who do not need to be admitted for overnight care.

comparison, the number of inpatient hospital surgeries fell from 9,833,938 in 1994, with 118.0 admissions per thousand people, to 9,015,467 on 103.7 admissions per thousand people in 2016 (American Hospital Association 2017c). In other words, hospital utilization for surgical procedures and the proportion of people admitted to the hospital both declined while procedures at ASCs increased.

Continuing advances in medical innovation, including the development of minimally invasive surgical techniques, improvements in anesthesia, and better analgesics for pain relief—all of which reduce surgical risks, complications, and recovery time—together contribute to ASCs' growth in visits, volume, and revenue. Evidence suggests that migration of procedures from inpatient to outpatient will continue. For example, Medicare is considering allowing reimbursements for total knee replacements in the ASC setting (Rechtoris 2017).

Physician Practices

Most ambulatory care takes place in offices staffed by physicians or other healthcare providers. Historically, physicians practiced in small groups or as "solo practitioners." In the 1980s and early 1990s heyday of **fee-for-service** reimbursement, this arrangement was more economically viable. In recent years, however, hospitals have been acquiring physician practices, and in 2015, hospitals or health systems employed approximately 38 percent of all practicing physicians (Physicians Advocacy Institute 2016).

This trend has significant implications. For Barbara in the case study at the beginning of the chapter, it means her physician has better access to information that helps him care for her. Conversely, as we can see from the case, patients and doctors need to adjust to new ways of doing things. Barbara is not happy with the new ways associated with this change of ownership and use of new technology. Still, it is clear that, in an effort to improve care quality and efficiency, patients and physicians will have to adapt to a greater use of technology in the future.

Post-Acute Care

Post-acute care (PAC) includes rehabilitation or palliative services that beneficiaries receive after, or in some cases instead of, a stay in an acute-care hospital. Depending on the intensity of care the patient requires, treatment may include a stay in a facility, ongoing outpatient therapy, or care provided at home. The Medicare Payment Advisory Commission analyzes trends in care and spending in PAC settings and makes payment policy recommendations to Congress and the Medicare program (MedPAC 2018).

There are three kinds of residential PAC facilities: nursing homes or **long-term care (LTC) facilities**, **rehabilitation hospitals**, and **residential care communities**, which can be either an **assisted living facility** or a hybrid combining independent living, assisted living, and LTC. These residential communities are increasingly important in an era when

Fee-for-service
A method of paying physicians for services in which each service carries a fee.

Long-term care (LTC) facility
A facility that provides rehabilitative, restorative, or ongoing skilled nursing care to patients or residents requiring assistance with activities of daily living.

Rehabilitation hospital
A hospital devoted to the rehabilitation of patients with various neurological, musculoskeletal, orthopedic, and other medical conditions following stabilization of their acute medical issue with a goal of restoring all or most of their pre-acute care functioning.

Residential care community
A facility that provides room, board, housekeeping, supervision, and personal care assistance with basic activities such as personal hygiene, dressing, eating, and walking for people generally older than age 60.

the population is aging and baby boomers are retiring at the rate of 10,000 people per day (Social Security Administration 2013).

Assisted living facility
A living arrangement for older adults who can live independently but require some non-nursing support with some activities of daily living in order to do so.

Long-Term Care Facilities

LTC facilities, also sometimes called nursing homes, serve people who are frequently in very advanced years and declining health. An LTC facility provides a wide range of assistive services for people who are unable to perform several of the six **activities of daily living (ADLs)**: eating, bathing, dressing, toileting (getting on and off the toilet), transferring (e.g., being able to get out of a bed or chair), and continence (controlling one's bladder and bowel). Residents in LTC facilities frequently require help with several of these functions. On the recommendation of a physician or family member, the individual will be assessed by a social worker to determine the level of need. Based on that judgment, the facility may then admit the patient, who will receive care according to a protocol addressing his or her needs.

Activities of daily living (ADLs)
Functions that are generally done for oneself, such as eating, bathing, dressing, grooming, and taking care of bodily functions.

Rehabilitation Hospitals

Rehabilitation hospitals, as the name suggests, provide rehabilitation services to patients who may not be able to recover at home. Admission to a hospital usually includes an evaluation by a case manager or caseworker that includes an appraisal of the patient's physical needs and support network. Specifically, if a patient undergoes joint replacement or heart surgery, the case manager will want to know if a family member will be available at home to help provide care afterward; if not, the patient may need services on an inpatient basis at a facility where they can receive therapy on a regular basis. Rehabilitation hospitals do not provide surgical procedures, nor are they appropriate settings for someone with a severe medical illness. These highly specialized organizations only provide care for patients discharged from an acute-care setting and supply important physical and occupational therapy to help the patient regain full functioning.

Instrumental activities of daily living (IADLs)
Essential activities of daily living, as well as more specialized activities such as shopping, preparing meals, handling money, doing housework and laundry, and driving or using public transportation.

Residential Care Communities

Social workers and case managers use the **instrumental activities of daily living (IADLs)** to assess the appropriateness of a patient entering some form of residential care community. IADLs include shopping, cooking, managing medications, looking up phone numbers and using the phone, doing housework and laundry, driving or using public transportation, and managing finances. People who are fully able to perform ADLs, but may require some help with some of the activities listed here, are usually good candidates for moving into an assisted living arrangement.

Some organizations, known as continuing care retirement communities (CCRCs), combine independent living with assisted living and LTC in different facilities across a single campus. Patients may live in an apartment or house until they require help with IADLs, at which point they will move from their independent living arrangement into the CCRC's assisted living facility. They receive an assessment and subsequent support according to the protocol that best addresses their needs. Finally, as their health deteriorates with advanced age, they might move into the LTC space and receive a broader range of services to support their living. Thus the name, *continuing care* retirement community.

Home health agency
An organization that provides medical and other health services in the patient's home.

Hospice
A program that assists with the physical, emotional, spiritual, psychological, social, and financial needs of a dying patient and the patient's family. This service may be provided in the patient's home or in a facility.

Other Options

Not all LTC is provided to residents of a facility. Many patients receive care at home or in day centers designed to serve the elderly. Providers of these services fill the gaps in the care continuum, either through these alternative locations or by providing a less intensive kind of care or support. Adult day care centers, **home health agencies**, and **hospice** providers each play an important role in the panoply of services aimed at supporting the elderly, individuals with disabilities, and people who are terminally ill.

There are approximately 15,600 LTCs, 12,400 home health agencies, 4,000 hospice providers, and 30,200 residential care communities in the United States (Harris-Kojetin et al. 2016). As the population continues to age, there will be an increasing demand for these kinds of services and the professionals who provide them. In addition, because it is common for older people to have multiple illnesses, this population will put an increasing stress on all forms of the healthcare system: acute inpatient care, ambulatory care, and elder care, which is specialized care for older people most commonly provided in LTCs and similar organizations discussed earlier.

Behavioral Health Care

Specialized behavioral health services have become a priority for providers across the United States. Behavorial health issues—which include substance abuse, mental disorders, Alzheimer's disease, and other dementias—have become the country's most expensive category of disease, costing nearly $221 billion in 2014 and prompting many healthcare providers to try to mitigate some of these costs (Johnson and Meyer 2018). Expenditures for this category are expected to exceed $280 billion in 2020, up from $171.9 billion in 2009 (SAMHSA 2014).

A patient's primary care provider is the ideal first contact for obtaining care for behavioral health concerns. Nearly 70 percent of behavioral health patients also have a cooexisting medical condition, or comorbidity (Johnson and Meyer 2018), and the association between mental and physical well-being makes managing their overall health a complex challenge. Delivering care in the most appropriate setting is essential. While behavioral health care historically has been administered on an inpatient basis, care may be more effective when employing outpatient or ambulatory options (Thorpe, Jain, and Joski 2017). There is a growing body of evidence and support for integrating some treatment of behavioral health into primary care (Asarnow et al. 2015; Zeiss and Karlin 2008). Some commentators suggest that integrating behavioral health and traditional medical care could save the industry $26 billion to $48 billion annually (Arndt 2017).

Despite the projected cost increases from 2009 to 2020, overall projected costs for combined mental health and substance abuse are expected to lag behind other healthcare spending through 2020 and beyond. This is not to say behavioral health care costs will not increase; they will increase more slowly and become a smaller portion of the national health expenditures over time. The fact that many drugs used to treat mental illness are losing patent protection and being replaced with less costly generic drugs is a primary contributor to this projection (SAMHSA 2014). Likewise, the closure of state-owned psychiatric hospitals, a long-term trend, is also contributing to slower spending growth in behavioral health (SAMHSA 2014).

The **Centers for Medicare & Medicaid Services (CMS)** Innovation Center has begun to look toward launching a behavioral health payment model to meet the needs of Medicare, Medicaid, and Children's Health Insurance Program (CHIP) beneficiaries (Dickson 2017). Medicare, Medicaid, and dual beneficiaries—that is, patients eligible for more than one insurance program—account for nearly one-third of all adults treated for behavioral health symptoms in the United States (Thorpe, Jain, and Joski 2017).

Centers for Medicare & Medicaid Services (CMS)
The federal government agency that administers the Medicare program and the federal portion of the Medicaid and CHIP programs. CMS is part of the US Department of Health and Human Services. Note that even though the "centers" portion of the name is plural, the CMS acronym is singular.

Behavioral health is fraught with challenges. Diagnoses are often not as clear-cut as with physical issues, which often makes reimbursement problematic. Because of questionable reimbursement, there are shortages of both providers and appropriate inpatient placements. Behavioral health frequently is seen as the stepchild of the healthcare system, and there is little evidence that status will change in the near future.

The Healthcare Workforce

Perhaps more important than the location of care is the issue of who delivers it. This raises the question of how many healthcare providers the United States will need in the future. What kind? How will the number of physicians and other providers affect equity in access to care and its quality?

Physicians

Between 2000 and 2016, the number of physicians in the United States grew from 603,100 to 649,850 (US Bureau of Labor Statistics 2017)—a rate of 7.76 percent. Meanwhile, the rate of population growth for those same years was 14.8 percent, from 281.42 million to 323.13 million (US Census Bureau 2018), which suggests a serious shortage of physicians in the future.

The mix of those in the profession, however, is changing. The number of general practitioners, general internists, and surgeons actually declined, while other subspecialties such as anesthesiology, radiology, dermatology, psychiatry, and oncology grew (US Bureau of Labor Statistics 2017). The trend of growth in the number of subspecialists, combined with an aging and growing population, gives rise to the question about having an adequate supply of primary care physicians to meet the anticipated demand. There is considerable concern about a long-term physician shortage (Dall et al. 2017).

Registered nurse (RN)
A healthcare professional who, having graduated from formal training, has been licensed by the state to ensure a specific level of competence in rendering nursing care.

Nurses: RNs and LPNs

The total number of nurses climbed from approximately 2.19 million in 2000 to 2.85 million in 2016. Based on existing supply, nursing education trends, and the expected demand for nursing services, the Health Resources and Services Administration (HRSA) projects a surplus of **registered nurses (RNs)** by 2030 (HRSA 2017; US Bureau of Labor Statistics 2017). However, despite this nationwide projected surplus, HRSA also projects RN shortages in specific states, with a more widespread shortage of **licensed practical nurses (LPNs)** in at least 30 states (HRSA 2017). LPNs are licensed by the state in which they practice and can provide routine care for a patient under the supervision of an RN. An RN has a higher level of education and can provide a wider array of services for the patient.

Licensed practical nurse (LPN)
A person licensed by the state to carry out specified nursing duties under the direction of a registered nurse.

Physician assistant (PA)
A healthcare professional with advanced training who is licensed to practice medicine under the supervision of a physician.

Physician Assistants and Nurse Practitioners

Physician assistants (PAs) and **nurse practitioners (NPs)** have become increasingly important in recent decades. Commonly referred to as "extenders" or "midlevels," PAs and NPs provide an important array of caregiving services, including ordering lab tests and imaging to provide the patient and physician a preliminary diagnosis (Slee, Slee, and Schmidt 2008). They frequently fulfill duties formerly performed by physicians, thereby extending the physician's practice, hence the moniker "extender." Together, PAs and NPs provide care that falls between what an RN is licensed to do and what a physician does.

Nurse practitioner (NP)
A registered nurse who has completed additional educational requirements (a master's degree or higher) and has qualifications that permit conducting an extended evaluation of the patient with a focus on primary care and patient education.

To be clear, the PA and NP occupy different roles. A PA is usually required to practice under the "direct supervision" of a physician. This means different things in different states, with some states requiring closer control than others. Under this supervision, the PA can examine a patient, diagnose disease, presecribe medication (with some limitations, depending on the state), and do things incidental to the care of the patient. A PA can "practice medicine on teams with physicians, surgeons, and other healthcare workers. They examine, diagnose, and treat patients" (US Bureau of Labor Statistics 2018b).

A "nurse practitioner" is a particular designation within a larger group referred to as advanced practice registered nurses (APRNs). An APRN can, depending on training, be a nurse anesthetist, a nurse midwife, or an NP. An NP can "coordinate patient care and may provide primary and specialty healthcare. The scope of practice varies from state to state" (US Bureau of Labor Statistics 2018a), but a key concept is "may provide primary . . . healthcare." In many states, an NP can examine a patient, diagnose illnesses, and prescribe medications independently of a physician, while the remainder still require some level of physician supervision.

You might encounter NPs at **retail clinics** in your drugstore, supermarket, or college student health center because of their relatively independent status. Because neither PAs nor NPs can bill at the same rate as physicians, they may become a relatively low-cost way to expand the availablity of primary care and constrain costs at the same time.

Retail clinic
A "walk-in" clinic usually located in a drugstore or other retail store, most often staffed by a nurse practitioner who can provide a variety of primary care services and diagnoses.

Barbara, from the chapter-opening vignette, may encounter a PA or NP at some point, even outside a retail clinic or similar establishment. PAs, in particular, are being used increasingly to screen primary care medical issues in physicians' offices. In addition, it is common to see a PA in a specialist's office before seeing the physician. The PA can focus on the relevant symptoms and help the physician finalize the diagnosis more quickly. Barbara may find this frustrating because she is accustomed to seeing her physician or the specialist to whom her physician referred her.

Emerging Models of Care and Payment

Earlier in the chapter we pointed out three important trends in healthcare. First, the number of hospitals is declining, either through closure or through merger and consolidation of licenses. Second, concomitant with consolidation, we noticed that the number of hospitals considered part of a "system" has increased in recent decades. Finally, we saw that hospitals' inpatient revenue is declining while outpatient revenue is increasing. These trends are evidence of new, emerging models of care.

We are witnessing the confluence of several important developments. Thanks to better pain management medications and the miniaturization of technology—which enables surgeons to perform complex procedures through tiny incisions, reducing the risk of blood loss and other complications—many surgical procedures have migrated from hospital operating rooms to ambulatory settings. At the same time, payers, notably the federal government in the form of Medicare, have initiated new payment models intended to encourage better quality of care while reducing the volume of care. This "pay-for-performance" movement, combined with newer, better technology, has yielded the trend known as **clinical integration**.

Clinical integration
The coordinated delivery of patient care by a team across conditions, providers, settings, and time to achieve high-quality care. Best effectuated by a common (electronic) health record to keep all providers informed.

Clinical integration refers to the coordination among providers to provide comprehensive care for the patient across settings, conditions, and time, relying on an electronic health record that helps eliminate duplicated tests and services (Wilson 2016). (If a specialist can see the results from a test already conducted by a previous provider, there is no need for the patient to undergo—and the payer to pay for—that same test a second time.) Beyond the mere exchange of information, however, the idea behind clinical integration is

Accountable care organization (ACO)
A form of health services delivery organization that includes multiple kinds of providers who work together to improve care delivery to the individual patient as well as to improve the health status of a particular population, such as a group of employees or Medicare enrollees. The providers work as a team because of a reimbursement mechanism that incentivizes improvement in patient outcomes.

Shared savings program
A payment strategy that incentivizes healthcare providers to reduce spending for a defined patient population by offering them a percentage of any net savings realized because of their efforts.

Explanation of benefits (EOB)
A statement sent by a health insurance company to covered individuals explaining what medical treatments and services were paid for on their behalf.

to incentivize providers to render care that is safe, efficient, patient-centered, timely, effective, and equitable. In short, clinical integration aims to improve the overall patient experience by improving the quality of care, reducing its cost, and ensuring better access to care (Institute for Healthcare Improvement 2018).

Clinical integration was truly put into practice with the introduction of **accountable care organizations (ACO)**, which were authorized under the Affordable Care Act (ACA). ACOs encourage the seamless exchange of information among providers by making all of them jointly responsible for the care of a Medicare patient. For example, the patient's primary care physician, cardiologist, and ophthalmologist will all have access to the patient's records so they can coordinate their care—such as by making sure a heart medication does not cause the side effect of blurred vision—and better manage the individual's overall health.

The providers are financially motivated to cooperate because of the Medicare **shared savings program**, which also was created by the ACA. Shared savings means that, if the ACO can improve the health status of a population while also saving money for the payer—in this case, Medicare—the providers share in the financial benefit. Frequently, this process involves the use of a bundled payment mechanism.

Before we delve into bundling, consider the traditional method of billing for a knee replacement. This complex surgery involves multiple types of care and services, resulting in multiple costs to the patient and an overwhelming number of bills and related documentation from the insurance company and each of the many providers. For example, providers historically have billed separately for the following services:

- Anesthesia
- Coordination of care
- Durable medical equipment
- Hospitalization
- Injections
- Pharmacy
- Physical therapy
- Postoperative outpatient care
- Surgery

This process means the patient and insurance company receive numerous bills along with a similar number of **explanation of benefits (EOB)** forms. The EOB is a document that specifies provider charges, insurance payments, and the patient's financial responsibility.

With **bundled payments**, in contrast, and a bundled billing mechanism, there is only one bill covering all the services associated with the knee replacement process. This kind of billing serves two purposes: (1) It saves money by eliminating administrative costs associated with multiple bills and EOBs, and (2) it encourages better coordination among the providers. Better coordinated care, meaning more of a team approach and sharing of information, results in reduced chance of medical error and, therefore, better quality of care for the patient. Moreover, the whole experience is much less confusing to the patient.

Bundled payment
Payment to providers based on expected costs for clinically defined episodes of care.

This approach is called clinical integration, and it requires not only a shared electronic medical record but also some overarching governing mechanism to engage all these varied providers in a shared endeavor. The relationship among the providers can be common ownership, or it can exist by a contractual relationship among various entities. While it is possible for clinical integration to exist outside the formal designation of an ACO, the combination of providers in this context frequently is referred to as an ACO. Some ACOs, depending on how they are organized, bear the entire financial risk of producing better health outcomes than were achieved previously. The trade-off for assuming that risk is that if the care provided actually saves money compared to what would have been spent using the old model, the provider organization shares in the savings. The savings cannot be calculated on a case-by-case basis but rather are calculated in the aggregate for a defined population.

There are approximately 560 ACOs in the United States, all of which participate in the Medicare Shared Savings Program. While they may apply clinical integration techniques for all patients, the Shared Savings Program from Medicare provides a substantial financial impetus to become designated as an ACO. The determination of whether an organization will share in the losses depends on the contractual options it chooses when enrolling in the ACO program with CMS (2016, 2018).

Financing of Healthcare

We will more fully address the financing of healthcare in chapter 11; however, discussing certain elements here is necessary in examining the structure of our healthcare system. How healthcare is financed, and how payment mechanisms are structured, influences how and where care is delivered (Rosenthal et al. 2004).

Suffice it to say that, in this era of reform, we are moving away from traditional fee-for-service, in which the insurance company pays the provider an agreed-upon fee for the specific service provided. The major concern with this form of payment mechanism is that is encourages patients and providers to overutilize the system. This means that we—those of us who pay insurance premiums and who pay taxes to support Medicare and Medicaid—are paying for unnecessary medical services performed on patients who do not need them. This has led to a tremendous growth cycle in expenditures, as we saw in chapter 2.

Pay-for-performance A financial reward system for healthcare providers in which a portion of their monetary compensation is related to improvement in patient outcomes and other indicators of improved performance.

In an effort to curb the ever-rising costs of healthcare services, insurers, providers, and governments have been devising new payment structures that will provide an incentive to provide *quality* care as opposed to simply *more volume* of care. To that end, CMS and commercial insurance companies are experimenting with bundled payment mechanisms and other **pay-for-performance** mechanisms that reward better quality of care instead of higher volumes. In the example of the knee replacement mentioned earlier, we saw how bundled payment would work to replace fee-for-service.

Pharmaceutical Industry

As we saw in chapter 2, the fastest-growing component of healthcare expenditures is pharmaceuticals. Prescription drug spending in the United States skyrocketed from $121 billion in 2000 to $324.6 billion in 2015 (National Center for Health Statistics 2017).

The aggregate cost increase is attributable to several factors. First, utilization of prescription drugs continues to increase. Second, new and expensive drugs, mainly for cancer treatment, have arrived on the market. Third, the length of patents on brand-name drugs makes it difficult to bring a generic equivalent to market. Finally, some companies continue to engage in monopoly pricing (Schumock and Vermeulen 2017).

Pharmacy benefit manager (PBM) A company used by managed care providers and insurers to improve the efficiency of providing patients the drugs covered by their plan.

Efforts to constrain these costs have been plentiful and led to the advent of the **pharmacy benefit manager (PBM)**. A PBM is a third party used by insurers and managed care companies to increase the efficiency of providing drugs to the insured consumer. PBMs profit by gaining manufacturer rebates and encouraging the use of generic drugs whenever possible (Slee, Slee, and Schmidt 2008).

To provide a small sample of the dimensions of this industry, the top ten pharmaceutical manufacturers (ranked by sales) had total sales of $338,478,000 in 2016 while they spent $63,451,700 on research and development of new drugs (Christel 2017). One of the trends as seen in chapter 2 is the displacement over time of hospital costs with pharmaceutical costs. As the healthcare system increases its focus on population health, chronic disease maintenance, and prevention, we can expect this trend to continue.

Conclusion

The US healthcare system is large and complex. It is also constantly evolving. As we saw in Chapter 1, the system began as a cottage industry founded on myth and driven by snake-oil salesmen and charlatans. Today's healthcare is grounded in science and increasingly reliant on technology.

The system continues to be challenged by issues of cost, quality, and access. New organizational structures and payment mechanisms aim to improve quality while constraining continued cost increases. Concomitantly, care continues to move from inpatient settings to ambulatory facilities. Advanced pharmaceuticals have replaced rising hospital costs.

As the population ages, there will be increasing demand for a variety of LTC services. The post-acute care industry is poised for growth, ready with a variety of organizations to serve the needs of baby boomers as they retire in record numbers.

New types of providers will extend primary and specialty care while electronic medical records facilitate the sharing of information among various providers. As you will see in the next chapter, the relatively new focus on "team"-oriented care and an emphasis on patient-centeredness while integrating provider roles more closely is the future model of care that is beginning now. The confluence of new technology, better drugs, new kinds of providers, and new ways of working together give hope for a system to address the ongoing challenges of cost, quality, and access.

Mini Case Study: One Sad Example

Katherine O'Donnell, a 29-year-old nurse, presented for a minor elective sinus surgery at the North Haven Surgery Center in Connecticut. She was in good health when she arrived.

Shortly after being administered general anesthesia, just before 11 a.m., O'Donnell's blood pressure started to fall. By 11 minutes after the hour, her blood pressure was unobtainable. In addition, the pulse oximeter was not reading. The surgery continued even while CPR was administered.

The ambulance company's records reflect it received a call at 11:40 a.m., indicating a 29-minute delay in summoning emergency help. O'Donnell was transported to Yale–New Haven Hospital (YNNH) and arrived at 12:22 p.m. Efforts to revive her were unsuccessful, and she was pronounced dead approximately an hour later.

Medical records conflict regarding how long the surgical team continued operating on O'Donnell after her blood pressure and oxygen levels began to drop.

Government reports indicate she received epinephrine, a heart stimulant, at 11:10 a.m., soon after surgery began. A code blue emergency was not initiated until 26 minutes later, at 11:36 a.m. At that time, O'Donnell's pulse rate was recorded at just 42 beats per minute.

An expert's review of medical records, included in the subsequent lawsuit, cites conflicting accounts of what happened in the interim. One case note says that all anesthetic medications were discontinued at 11:15 a.m., that surgery was stopped, and that CPR was started. Another emergency-related document says surgery was halted at 11:22, but then resumed at 11:30.

There were several other important conflicts in documentation related to the amount of epinephrine administered and the time at which O'Donnell was transferred to YNNH.

This case raises questions about how well equipped freestanding surgical centers are to handle emergencies, and what sanctions they face for alleged lapses in care. The subsequent lawsuit alleged that the center and the anesthesia provider failed to respond properly by stopping the surgery immediately and calling a code blue emergency when O'Donnell's blood pressure and oxygen levels plummeted (Chedekel 2016).

Mini Case Study Questions

1. Surgical procedures performed in ambulatory surgery centers are considerably less expensive than surgeries performed in hospitals. Given this, if you were a policymaker, would you make it easier to start ASCs? Harder? Why?
2. If you were a healthcare regulator, what precautions would you require of freestanding ASCs?

Points to Remember

- The total number of hospitals is continuing to decline, but the number of hospitals belonging to healthcare systems is increasing. Some hospitals are simply closing.
- New payment methodologies are helping to address excessive spending in the healthcare system while aligning provider interests to improve the quality of care.
- Hospitals are garnering an increasing share of their revenue from ambulatory care, while inpatient revenue continues to decline.
- Ambulatory surgery centers continue to grow in number and in the kinds of procedures they undertake.
- Long-term care will be in larger demand in the future as members of the baby boom generation continue to retire in large numbers.

Challenge Yourself

1. How can the healthcare system adequately provide primary care for Americans if there are not enough physicians?
2. Is the current trend of hospitals becoming part of larger health systems a positive development? Why or why not?
3. Is the development of walk-in clinics in drugstores (and other locations) helpful to the clinical integration of care for the patient? Why or why not?

For Your Consideration

1. Research the acquisitions of pharmacy benefit managers by insurance companies. What does this mean for the future of healthcare?
2. Select three prescription medications you see advertised on television. Research ways to obtain those same medications through Canadian websites. What do you observe about the price differences?

References

Agency for Healthcare Research and Quality. 2017. "Compendium of U.S. Health Systems, 2016." Reviewed December. www.ahrq.gov/chsp/compendium/index.html.

American Hospital Association. 2017a. *Academic Medical Centers and Teaching Hospitals.* Accessed January 8, 2018. www.aha.org/content/17/teaching-value17.pdf.

———. 2017b. *Fast Facts on US Hospitals.* Accessed October 28. www.aha.org/research/rc/stat-studies/101207fastfacts.pdf.

———. 2017c. *TrendWatch Chartbook 2016.* Accessed September 28. www.aha.org/search?q=trendwatch&search_type=aha&site=redesign_aha_org%7CHPOE.

Anderson, G., E. Steinberg, and R. Heyssel. 1994. "The Pivotal Role of the Academic Health Center." *Health Affairs* 13 (3): 146–58.

Arndt, R. 2017. "Accessing Behavioral Health Through Primary Care." *Modern Healthcare.* Published November 25. www.modernhealthcare.com/article/20171125/TRANSFORMATION03/171119895.

Asarnow, J. R., M. Rozenman, J. Wiblin, and L. Zeltzer. 2015. "Integrated Medical-Behavioral Care Compared with Usual Primary Care for Child and Adolescent Behavioral Health: A Meta-analysis." *JAMA Pediatrics* 169 (10): 929–37.

Centers for Medicare & Medicaid Services (CMS). 2018. "Performance Year 2018 Medicare Shared Savings Program Accountable Care Organizations—Map." Accessed July 17. https://data.cms.gov/Special-Programs-Initiatives-Medicare-Shared-Savin/Performance-Year-2018-Medicare-Shared-Savings-Prog/7zis-nzdf.

———. 2016. *Accountable Care Organizations: What Providers Need to Know.* Accessed January 31, 2018. www.cms.gov/Medicare/Medicare-Fee-for-Service-Payment/sharedsavingsprogram/Downloads/ACO-Providers-Factsheet-ICN907406TextOnly.pdf.

Chedekel, L. 2016. "Lawsuit Filed After Death at Surgery Center." *Hartford Courant.* Published March 7. www.courant.com/health/hc-surgical-center-lawsuit-20160307-story.html.

Christel, M. 2017. "Pharm Exec's Top 50 Companies 2017." PharmExec.com. Published June 28. www.pharmexec.com/pharm-execs-top-50-companies-2017.

Dall, T., R. Chakrabarti, W. Iacobucci, A. Hansari, and T. West. 2017. *2017 Update: The Complexities of Physician Supply and Demand: Projections from 2015 to 2030.* Association of American Medical Colleges. Published February 28. aamc-black.global.ssl.fastly.net/production/media/filer_public/a5/c3/a5c3d565-14ec-48fb-974b-99fafaeecb00/aamc_projections_update_2017.pdf.

Dickson, V. 2017. "CMS Looks to Launch Behavioral Health Pay Model." *Modern Healthcare.* Published July 20. www.modernhealthcare.com/article/20170720/NEWS/170729990.

Hall, M., A. Schwartzman, J. Zhang, and X. Liu. 2017. "Ambulatory Surgery Data from Hospitals and Ambulatory Surgery Centers: United States, 2010." *National Health Statistics Reports* 102 (February): 1–15.

Harris-Kojetin, L., M. Sengupta, E. Park-Lee, R. Valverde, C. Caffrey, V. Rome, and J. Lendon. 2016. *Long-Term Care Providers and Services Users in the United States: Data from the National Study of Long-Term Care Providers, 2013–2014.* National Center for Health Statistics. Published February. www.cdc.gov/nchs/data/series/sr_03/sr03_038.pdf.

Health Resources and Services Administration (HRSA). 2017. *Supply and Demand: Projections of the Nursing Workforce: 2014–2030.* Published July 21. bhw.hrsa.gov/sites/default/files/bhw/nchwa/projections/NCHWA_HRSA_Nursing_Report.pdf.

Institute for Healthcare Improvement (IHI). 2018. *Triple Aim Initiative.* Washington, DC: IHI.

Johnson, S., and H. Meyer. 2018. "Behavioral Health: Fixing a System in Crisis." *Modern Healthcare.* Accessed June 15. www.modernhealthcare.com/reports/behavioral-health/.

MedPAC. 2018. "Post-Acute Care." Accessed June 15. www.medpac.gov/-research-areas-/post-acute-care.

———. 2016. *Report to Congress: Medicare Payment Policy.* Washington, DC: US Department of Health and Human Services.

National Center for Health Statistics. 2017. *Health, United States, 2016.* Published May. www.cdc.gov/nchs/data/hus/hus16.pdf.

Physicians Advocacy Institute. 2016. "Hospital Ownership of Physician Practices Increases Nearly 90 Percent in Three Years." Press release published September 7. www.physiciansadvocacyinstitute.org/Portals/0/assets/docs/Physician-Acquisition-Study-Release9-6-16.pdf.

Rechtoris, M. 2017. "51 Things to Know About the ASC Industry." *Becker's ASC Review*. Published February 21. www.beckersasc.com/asc-turnarounds-ideas-to-improve-performance/50-things-to-know-about-the-asc-industry-2017.html.

Rosenthal, M., R. Fernandopulle, R. HyunSook, and B. Landon. 2004. "Paying for Quality: Providers' Incentives for Quality Improvement." *Health Affairs* 23 (2): 126–41.

Schumock, G., and L. Vermeulen. 2017. "The Rising Costs of Prescription Drugs: Causes and Solutions." *Pharmacotherapy* 37 (1): 9–11.

Slee, D. A., V. N. Slee, and H. J. Schmidt. 2008. *Slee's Health Care Terms*, 5th ed. Sudbury, MA: Jones & Bartlett.

Social Security Administration. 2013. *Annual Performance Plan for Fiscal Year 2013 and Revised Final Performance Plan for Fiscal Year 2012*. Accessed January 28, 2018. www.ssa.gov/agency/performance/.

Song, E., J. Seon, J. Moon, and J. Yim. 2013. "The Evolution of Modern Total Knee Prostheses." In *Arthroplasty Update*, edited by P. Kinov, 183–95. InTechOpen. Published February 20. www.intechopen.com/books/arthroplasty-update/the-evolution-of-modern-total-knee-prostheses.

Substance Abuse and Mental Health Services Administration (SAMHSA). 2014. *Projections of National Expenditures for Treatment of Mental and Substance Use Disorders, 2010–2020*. Rockville, MD: SAMHSA.

Thorpe, K., S. Jain, and P. Joski. 2017. "Prevalence and Spending Associated with Patients Who Have a Behavioral Health Disorder and Other Conditions." *Health Affairs* 36 (1): 124–32.

US Bureau of Labor Statistics. 2018a. "What Nurse Anesthetists, Nurse Midwives, and Nurse Practitioners Do." Updated April 13. www.bls.gov/ooh/healthcare/nurse-anesthetists-nurse-midwives-and-nurse-practitioners.htm#tab-2.

———. 2018b. "What Physician Assistants Do." Updated April 13. www.bls.gov/ooh/healthcare/physician-assistants.htm#tab-2.

———. 2017. "Occupational Employment Statistics." Updated March 2018. www.bls.gov/oes/tables.htm.

US Census Bureau. 2018. "Quick Facts." Accessed July 17. www.census.gov/quickfacts/fact/table/US/PST045217.

Wiler, J., and N. Harish. 2017. "Do Hospitals Still Make Sense? The Case for Decentralization of Healthcare." *NEJM Catalyst.* Published December 20. catalyst.nejm.org/hospitals-case-decentralization-health-care.

Wilson, J. K. 2016. *Clinical Integration: A Roadmap to the Future?* Medical Group Management Association. Published July 19. www.mgma.com/MGMA/media/files/fellowship%20papers/FACMPE-Paper-Clinical-Integration-FINAL.pdf.

Zeiss, A. M., and B. E. Karlin. 2008. "Integrating Mental Health and Primary Care Services in the Department of Veterans Affairs Health Care System." *Journal of Clinical Psychology in Medical Settings* 15 (1): 73–78.

CHAPTER 4

MEDICAL AND HEALTHCARE ENVIRONMENTS

Important Terms

- Accountable care organization (ACO)
- Community health center
- Coordination of care
- Disease prevention
- Federally qualified health center
- Health promotion
- Interprofessionalism
- Patient-centered medical home
- Patient's role on the healthcare team
- Population health
- Post-acute care facility
- Quadruple Aim
- Rehabilitation
- Social determinants of health
- Triple Aim

Learning Objectives

After reading this chapter, you will be able to do the following:

- ➤ Understand the various sites of healthcare practice and the categories of healthcare services
- ➤ Explain care coordination
- ➤ Explain population health management
- ➤ Define patient-centered medical homes
- ➤ Understand the role of interprofessionalism

- Describe the importance of the health services manager's participation as an equal member of the interprofessional team
- Define patient experience
- Explain the role of the patient as a member of the healthcare team

Case Study: Maryland's LOFR Teams

In 2014, Maryland formed Local Overdose Fatality Review Teams (LOFRTs) with the purpose of reviewing overdose fatalities in the state (Rebbert-Franklin et al. 2016). In 2013, there were 858 reported drug overdose deaths in Maryland, which was more than the number of deaths caused by car accidents (509), homicides (420), and suicides (559) (Rebbert-Franklin et al. 2016). With the governor's support and state legislation that developed guidelines for the team, as well as financial assistance from the US Department of Justice's Harold Rogers Grant, professionals from public health, a local hospital, emergency medical services, county behavioral health services, and law enforcement, along with healthcare experts specializing in substance abuse and treatment, formed 15 LOFRTs to serve as multidisciplinary teams that evaluated about 200 overdose fatalities (Rebbert-Franklin et al. 2016).

Perhaps a key element to the success of this interprofessional effort was the legal stance that enabled the team to require agencies to provide information about each death. That is, criminal, healthcare, and counseling agencies had to provide—by law—information pertaining to the overdose fatality. However, it is important to note that the requirement to provide information was accompanied by the LOFRT members' commitment and adherence to confidentiality of information, including personal health information (Maryland Department of Health 2017).

The LOFRT program did not aim to initiate or extend the investigation of past deaths by state or local authorities. Instead, it focused on establishing trust among team members to foster an open and candid discussion. In addition, it set out to prevent future deaths by (Baier 2015)

- identifying missed opportunities for prevention and gaps in the system;
- building working relationships between local stakeholders on overdose prevention;
- recommending policies, programs, and laws to prevent overdose deaths; and
- creating a local overdose and opioid misuse prevention strategy.

The teams' findings revealed that existing care coordination efforts needed improvement, as many of the deceased had had contact with each department (social services, criminal justice, and healthcare entities). In particular, older drug users were found to have had co-occurring chronic health issues (Baier 2015). The teams concluded that if a person has an overdose history, improved coordination and communication among these public and healthcare agencies might help improve the referral system and change intake questionnaires to more fully assess the patient's risk of overdosing. The LOFRT members were able to come to this realization because of their ability to communicate, ask questions, and gather and analyze data.

The experience demonstrated that the better team members' contributions, the more likely data-driven decisions with input from professionals of varied backgrounds were made. This process of engaged, diverse team members may help decrease the number of future overdose fatalities so patients get to the right professionals for treatment and follow-up before they overdose. Maryland's LOFRTs illustrate the value of **interprofessionalism**, as defined by the Institute of Medicine (2003, 54): "An interdisciplinary team is composed of members from different professions and occupations with varied and specialized knowledge, skills, and methods."

Interprofessionalism
An interdisciplinary healthcare team comprising members from different health professions.

To belong on an interprofessional team, members must abide by six key principles (Hammick et al. 2009, 36):

1. The willingness and capability to work both collaboratively and inclusively
2. An understanding of the nature and extent of their duty of care, both to those who use their services and to their colleagues
3. Maintaining respect, confidence, engagement, willingness to negotiate, and readiness to share in relationships with colleagues and clients
4. The willingness and capability to communicate clearly what you want and believe and to listen to what others want and believe
5. The commitment and capability to develop and deliver mutually acceptable shared plans
6. The willingness and capability to contribute to shaping change and to welcome contributions from a spectrum of other stakeholders in the services you offer

Coordination of care
Deliberate communication and organization of healthcare actions between two or more providers and the patient to ensure better health outcomes.

In this interprofessional learning environment, each team member adds her knowledge, skills, and methods in collaboration with others. Hence, while the team of professionals who comprised the Maryland LOFRTs came from different organizations, they exhibited the key principles of interprofessionalism and were therefore able to make recommendations with the aim of improving **coordination of care** and of care delivered to the person in order to reduce drug overdose fatalities.

Introduction

The case study that opened this chapter illustrates the power of interprofessionalism—the way that experts from different disciplines interact and communicate to address a public health concern. The team members in Maryland exhibited mutual respect and trust in each other and collaborated to share pertinent information. In particular, this case demonstrates how various professionals associated with the public engaged in identifying trends and then helped to shape interventions to reduce drug dependency and influence policies and procedures to prevent future overdose fatalities.

While the previous chapter analyzed healthcare by the numbers, this chapter will describe the industry in terms of the places and teams in which healthcare professionals work. We will discuss the concept of population health management, which is employed to improve patients' experiences and outcomes throughout their healthcare interactions, and we will examine some of the work settings students may want to consider when determining their place in the field of healthcare services management. We also will explain the need for healthcare professionals to take an interprofessional approach to patient care, and, importantly, see how population health management helps achieve patient-centered access, team-based care, care management, care coordination, and quality improvement.

Categories of Health Services

The healthcare system offers services aimed to promote wellness, prevent disease, diagnose and treat illness, and provide rehabilitation care.

Health Promotion and Disease Prevention

Health promotion
Activities designed to influence individual behaviors that affect personal health.

Disease prevention
The result of education and other health-promotion efforts designed to help people become healthier and stay healthy.

The focus of **health promotion** and **disease prevention** is to keep people healthy by encouraging them to adopt a healthier lifestyle and helping them increase their health literacy—that is, boosting their ability to make informed decisions about their healthcare. Some people may boost their wellness by taking responsibility for their health, such as by eating nutritious (plant-based) foods, avoiding tobacco (including e-cigarettes), exercising regularly (60 minutes per day), getting enough sleep (about eight hours per night), and taking action to prevent injuries (e.g., not texting while driving).

One example of a health promotion campaign is the World Health Organization (WHO) Framework Convention on Tobacco Control (FCTC), which launched in 2005 as the world's first public health treaty (WHO 2015). One hundred and eighty countries pledged to increase taxes on tobacco products to discourage their purchase, ensure smoke-free workplaces, put health warning labels on tobacco products, prohibit tobacco advertising and packaging that presents false claims, offer support for tobacco cessation initiatives, and engage in public awareness actions about tobacco and health (WHO 2015). Despite these efforts, WHO has noted that tobacco still kills more than half its users, and each year about seven million people in the world die from smoking or related diseases (WHO 2017b). In the United States, cigarette smoking is *the* leading cause of preventable disease, and tobacco-related illnesses cause about 480,000 deaths annually (CDC 2016). Still, the outcomes of the FCTC show positive change. In the United States, for example, in 2005 when the treaty was launched, 23 percent of high school students and about 21 percent of adults smoked cigarettes. By 2016, the percentage for high school smokers had declined to 8 percent while in 2015, about 15 percent of adults reported smoking (CDC 2016, 2017b).

As the tobacco example illustrates, health promotion efforts can have positive effects on disease prevention, the first category of health services. Professionals who work in health promotion and disease prevention include clinical providers, administrators, and information managers. Smokers rely on a team of experts. A cardiologist will see the patient regularly to find, treat, and prevent heart disease, and a pharmacist may recommend medication to aid in smoking cessation (American College of Cardiology 2017). Other clinicians, such as a registered dietitian, will advise patients on nutrition and eating habits that may help prevent the weight gain associated with quitting smoking. Moreover, registered dietitians will help patients tailor a nutrition plan for better overall health (Academy of Nutrition and Dietetics 2017). Meanwhile, a hospital's public relations and marketing manager may be in charge of planning the smoking cessation meetings as part of the hospital's community outreach programs, and a mental health professional, such as a psychologist, may lead the group of smokers to quit smoking successfully (Munsey 2008). Together, these efforts to reduce the number of smokers rely on an interprofessional team to help bring about better outcomes.

At the same time, however, it is incumbent upon the individual—the smoker in this example—to take ownership of his or her own health and healthcare. Several healthcare systems have even listed what responsibilities a patient should assume. In the late 1990s, President Bill Clinton appointed the Advisory Commission on Consumer Protection and Quality in the Health Care Industry to draft a healthcare consumer's bill of rights (President's Advisory Commission 1997a), which included a statement of patient responsibilities, such as the following (President's Advisory Commission 1997b):

- Take initiative and adopt more healthy habits, such as exercising regularly, eating a healthy diet, and not smoking.
- Become involved in specific healthcare decisions.
- Work collaboratively with healthcare providers to develop and carry out agreed-upon treatment plans.
- Disclose relevant information and clearly communicate wants and needs.
- Use the health plan's internal complaint and appeal processes to address concerns that may arise.
- Avoid knowingly spreading disease.
- Recognize the reality of risks and limits of the science of medical care and the human fallibility of the healthcare professional.

- Be aware of a healthcare provider's obligation to be reasonably efficient and equitable in providing care to other patients and the community.
- Become knowledgeable about health plan coverage and plan options (when available), including all covered benefits, limitations, and exclusions, rules regarding use of network providers, coverage and referral rules, appropriate processes to secure additional information, and the process to appeal coverage decisions.
- Show respect for other patients and healthcare workers.
- Make a good-faith effort to meet financial obligations.
- Abide by administrative and operational procedures of health plans, healthcare providers, and government health benefit programs.
- Report wrongdoing and fraud to appropriate resources or legal authorities.

UCLA Health was one of the hospitals to adopt the commission's advice and list its patients' responsibilities on its website. Located in Los Angeles and Santa Monica, California, UCLA Health was at the time one of the largest health science centers in the United States, with two medical centers housing a combined 846 patient beds, a neuropsychiatric hospital, a children's hospital, and an outpatient medical plaza (UCLA Health 2017a). UCLA Health patient responsibilities include the following (UCLA Health 2017b):

- The most effective plan is the one to which all participants agree and that is carried out exactly. It is your responsibility to tell your healthcare provider whether or not you can and want to follow the treatment plan recommended for you.
- It is your responsibility to ask your healthcare provider for information about your health and healthcare. This includes following the instructions of other health team members, such as nurses and physical therapists who are linked to this plan of care. The organization makes every effort to adapt a plan specific to your needs and limitations.
- Continue your care after you leave UCLA Health. This includes knowing when and where to get further treatment and what you need to do at home to help with your care.
- Accept the consequences of your own decisions and actions if you choose to refuse treatment or not to comply with the care, treatment, and service plan offered by your healthcare provider.

Each of these points underscores the fact that the **patient's role on the healthcare team** is essential for achieving optimal outcomes. Along those lines, eastern North Carolina provider Vidant—a private, not-for-profit system comprising Vidant Medical Center (900 beds), seven community hospitals (total of 530 beds), a medical group, home health and hospice, and three wellness centers (Vidant Health 2017a)—published on its website a list of patient responsibilities similar to the Commission's report and UCLA Health's list, but with the addition of one key point (Vidant Health 2017b): "Recognize that your lifestyle and behaviors affect your health."

Patient's role on the healthcare team
Patients' responsibilities to be proactive regarding becoming healthier, staying healthy, and actively engaging with their healthcare team when appropriate.

Patients are considered to be active members of the healthcare team; thus, speaking up, asking questions, and fully understanding that lifestyle and behaviors affect their own health ensure that patients are among the experts dedicated to their health and well-being. It is important to note, however, that the prevention of illness is not just attributed to lifestyle and behaviors. People who do eat properly, exercise, and are active members of their healthcare team also may become ill or injured. When that occurs, the health system also provides diagnosis, treatment, and rehabilitation services.

Diagnosis, Treatment, and Rehabilitation

Diagnosis and treatment are the most widely used healthcare services, as people tend to seek medical care when they are not feeling well. Diagnoses typically involve physician visits and, if necessary, diagnostic procedures such as laboratory tests or digital imaging. Technological advances that facilitate diagnoses and treatment have brought about better care, but at a price.

Healthcare economists estimate that 40 to 50 percent of annual healthcare costs may be attributed to the use of new and established technologies (Callahan 2008). Consider, for example, the development of computer-assisted artificial limbs and their potential use for military personnel serving in Afghanistan and Iraq. In 2014, 1,558 amputations were performed on soldiers (Brinkerhoff 2014). When wounded veterans receive a computer-assisted artificial limb, the benefit is life-changing, enabling individuals such as retired marine William Gadsby to walk, hike mountain trails, and climb stairs more easily than with a conventional prosthetic (Burke 2012). As Gadsby said, "It's really changed my life. . . . It's the closest thing I've ever seen to being a real person again. Psychologically, this is a big deal as well" (Burke 2012).

However, consider that the Department of Veterans Affairs spent $70,000 on Gadsby's prosthetic leg, illustrating how the benefits of this technology are costly. You probably would agree that this cost is worth it, particularly given that Gadsby is a veteran who lost his limb in service to his country. But, you also need to recognize that increased technological benefit brings with it an increase in costs to the payer.

Rehabilitation
Therapies that help restore someone to normal or close-to-normal life.

In addition to the cost of the limb itself, **rehabilitation** services are needed to restore a person to normal or near-normal life through training and therapy. The care team for a

US Army amputee includes physical and occupational therapists who help patients learn to maximize their physical abilities and navigate their environments (Potter and Scoville 2006). Psychosocial services also are needed, along with vocational training to help patients prepare to return to duty or enter the civilian working world. Altogether, the rehabilitation efforts require a group of professionals such as physicians, nurses, pharmacists, therapists, social workers, psychologists, dietitians, vocational rehabilitation counselors, and healthcare administrators who work as an interprofessional team, with each individual offering their specific expertise to contribute to better care and outcomes.

Social Determinants of Health

In chapter 2, we discussed healthcare's iron triangle of cost, quality, and access. Some people enjoy more quality of care than others. They have insurance or have the financial ability to pay for healthcare. Other people cannot afford the benefits of technology to help them improve their health, or they may have unreliable transportation to travel to healthcare services. Consequently, the conditions in which people live influence their health. These conditions are referred to as **social determinants of health** and help explain why some of us are not as healthy as we could be. We will now explore these social determinants in detail and discuss efforts to address them.

Social determinants of health
The conditions in which people live and work that affect their access to appropriate healthcare and their ability to be an effective and responsible patient.

WHO points out that people's living conditions are shaped by income inequalities, power distribution, and the resources available to them, including money, time, knowledge, and the ability to influence public policy (WHO 2018). For example, access to a necessary service such as clean water is more likely to be found in locations where residents are wealthier, more highly educated, and have resources. Take the case of Flint, Michigan. Beginning in 2014, lead seepage into the drinking water caused a health crisis in a city where 40 percent of residents live in poverty (Kennedy 2016). In California's Central Valley, an analysis of drinking water between 2005 and 2007 found that communities with lower rates of home ownership (an indicator of income) had higher water arsenic levels than areas where residents owned their homes (Balazs et al. 2012).

Earlier, we discussed smoking and tobacco cessation efforts to illustrate the concepts of health promotion and disease prevention. But individuals' choices and habits may not be the only factors affecting whether they pursue unhealthy behaviors. The Centers for Disease Control and Prevention (CDC) reported on a 2012 national survey about drug use and health. The survey respondents indicated their educational attainment, and when we compare adult smokers who did not finish high school with smokers who graduated from college, the difference is significant: Adults with less than a high school education were more than three times more likely to smoke than those with a college diploma (CDC 2017a, 2017c).

These examples suggest that something besides personal choice and individual behavior—social determinants—affects health. Healthy People 2020, a government program launched to improve the nation's health, classifies these social determinants into five domains:

economic stability, education, health and healthcare, neighborhood and built environment, and social and community context (HealthyPeople.gov 2018). The underlying theme of Health People 2020 is that increased access to safe housing, affordable and healthy food, clean drinking water, education, healthcare, and so on bring about better health outcomes.

Initiatives have been established to spur reduction in health disparities. For instance, the CDC distributed Preventive Health and Health Services (PHHS) Block Grants to all 50 states, the District of Columbia, two American Indian tribes, and eight US territories to promote health equity (CDC 2017b). This funding is one response to the issues outlined by Health People 2020. (See exhibit 4.1 for the distribution of the 2017 funds.)

Previous initiatives funded in 2015 by PHHS Block Grants included training by the Virginia Department of Health healthcare providers on the CDC's best practices for drug overdose prevention, school dental screening to help reduce tooth decay in North Carolina, and "Fit and Fall Proof" exercise classes for older adults in Idaho (CDC 2017b).

Efforts to increase health equity take into account the importance of place. That is, where we educate people about good health habits, such as the schools in the North Carolina 2015 PHHS program, or physician clinical settings where diagnoses may occur, or hospitals where treatment may be given: All rely upon the presence of healthcare providers and administrators to provide necessary services. Let us now turn our attention to place and discuss *where* healthcare professionals provide care.

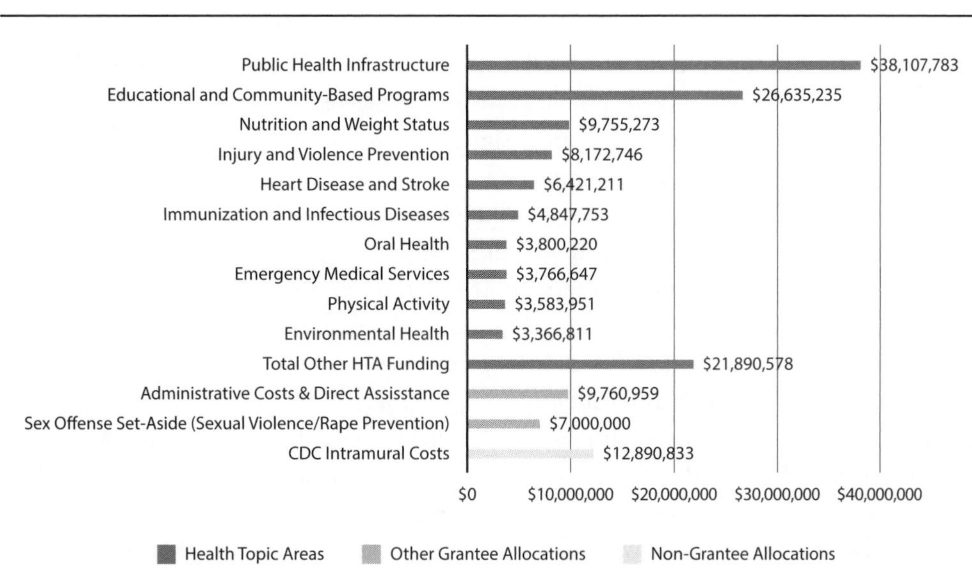

EXHIBIT 4.1 Total PHHS Block Grant Funding Allocation, Fiscal Year 2017 $160,000,000

Source: Reprinted from CDC (2017b).
Note: CDC = Centers for Disease Control and Prevention; HTA = health topic area; PHHS = Preventive Health and Health Services.

Health Service Settings

The places where healthcare professionals work continue to evolve to offer various sites that provide healthcare for patients with differing needs. These sites include community health centers and clinics, hospitals, outpatient surgery centers, post-acute care facilities, residential care communities, and medical group practices. This variety affects the work conducted by health services managers, as relationships between and among providers and administrators change when employment status and place of care change. These changes also prompt the need for effective interprofessional efforts and care coordination so professionals can be successful in their health promotion, disease prevention, diagnosis and treatment, and rehabilitation efforts.

Community Health Centers and Clinics

Community health center (CHC)
One of a network of clinics designed to provide patient care in a designated area.

Federally qualified health center (FQHC)
A clinic designated to serve an underserved area or population, offering a sliding fee scale and comprehensive healthcare services.

Health Resources and Services Administration (HRSA)
The federal agency that deals with issues relating to access, equity, quality, and cost of care. It is part of the Department of Health and Human Services.

Community health centers (CHCs) have the mission to serve those who have less access to healthcare because they have a lower income, are underinsured or uninsured, or otherwise lack the ability to pay. CHCs typically are private, nonprofit organizations that provide healthcare to residents of a defined geographic area that is medically underserved—that is, fewer providers are locally available to administer healthcare services. Both public and private sources fund CHCs. According to the National Association of Community Health Centers (NACHC), CHCs receive funding from state and local sources, such as Medicaid (NACHC 2014). Additional funding comes from private insurance, Medicare, self-pay patients, and federal grants. A center that is known as a **federally qualified health center (FQHC)** receives funds from the **Health Resources and Services Administration (HRSA)** Health Center Program to provide primary care in underserved areas (NACHC 2014). Care is focused on primary and preventive care designed to promote wellness and prevent disease, but diagnosis and treatment are also provided in the clinic setting.

The term *clinic* refers to a variety of settings, such as retail clinics. For example, CVS Caremark Corporation operates MinuteClinics in 33 states and the District of Columbia (CVS 2017). Patients do not need an appointment but simply walk into their clinic in a CVS or Target store to be diagnosed and treated for minor illnesses and conditions (CVS 2017).

Other clinic types include specialty clinics in which a group of healthcare providers offers specialty services such as fertility, eye care, nephrology, or rehabilitation (including occupational, physical, and speech therapy). Specialty clinics may be part of a healthcare system or stand alone, and they may receive self-referral patients or patients referred by another medical provider. General outpatient clinics describe community-based primary care, and they may be affiliated with a health system. And free clinics, as the name implies, are free or low cost to patients. They offer primary, chronic, and acute care services to those who cannot afford to pay to receive the services elsewhere.

Hospitals

WHO (2017a) defines hospitals as

> health care institutions that have an organized medical and other professional staff, and inpatient facilities, and deliver services 24 hours per day, 7 days per week. They offer a varying range of acute, convalescent and terminal care using diagnostic and curative services.

In the United States, hospitals vary by ownership type. For instance, 85 percent of all hospitals are community hospitals, and most of these are nonprofit (58.5 percent), some are for-profit (21.3 percent), and others are owned by state or local governments (20.2 percent) (Kaiser Family Foundation 2015). (Hospital types are discussed in more detail in chapter 3.) Hospital utilization trends indicate that Americans are spending fewer days as inpatients and instead are receiving healthcare more and more on an outpatient basis. Also, the older US population is opting to receive care via home health options and residential communities, such as assisted living, rather than moving into nursing homes. Further, providers such as physicians are shifting away from solo practice to medical group practices and from being self-employed with hospital privileges to being employed by hospitals.

Let us look at utilization in more detail. To begin, the average length of stay by patients in community hospitals has declined from 6.7 days in 1994 to 5.5 days in 2014 (AHA 2016a), while the number of outpatient surgeries has increased. Outpatient surgery centers are what the name implies: They provide specialized surgical procedures on an outpatient basis. When the American Hospital Association (AHA 2016b) analyzed community hospitals, they found the trend in surgeries performed moving from inpatient services to outpatient settings (see exhibit 4.2). These data do not include outpatient procedures performed in freestanding ambulatory surgery centers (ASCs), which also are experiencing growth. In a study of Medicare outpatient surgeries at ASCs, researchers Hollenbeck and colleagues (2014) found the proportion of all outpatient procedures administered at ASCs increased from 28.5 percent in 2001 to 37.4 percent in 2010.

Exhibit 4.2 United States Inpatient vs. Outpatient Utilization in Community Hospitals

Year	Inpatient (*N*) and as Percentage of Total Surgeries Performed (Inpatient Plus Outpatient)	Outpatient (*N*) and as Percentage of Total Surgeries Performed (Inpatient Plus Outpatient)
1995	9,833,938 (43%)	13,154,838 (57%)
2004	10,050,346 (37%)	17,351,490 (63%)
2014	9,015,467 (34%)	17,386,061 (66%)

Source: Data from AHA (2016a, 2016b).

Post-acute care facilities

Post-acute care (PAC) facility
A facility that offers a continuum of care depending on patient or resident need.

Post-acute care (PAC) facilities offer a continuum of care, depending on patient or resident need. PAC providers include skilled nursing facilities, home health agencies, inpatient rehabilitation facilities, and long-term care hospitals. They are designed for patients who have been released from a hospital to a rehabilitation site, nursing home, or hospice facility to ensure recovery from an acute illness or to provide palliative care. The role of PAC is no small matter, as the percentage of Medicare beneficiaries discharged from hospitals to PAC facilities increased from 37.5 percent in 2008 to 42 percent in 2013 (AHA 2015). Also, in 2013, the AHA reported that patients discharged from a hospital to a post-acute setting were more likely to go to a skilled nursing facility (19.5 percent) or receive care from a home health agency (16.8 percent) (AHA 2015).

The need for healthcare, particularly long-term care, also is expected to increase as baby boomers get older. The largest cohort ever in the United States, totaling 76 million births between 1946 and 1964, "boomers" will all be older than age 65 by 2030 (Colby and Ortman 2014; Vincent and Velkoff 2010). At that point, they all become eligible for Medicare. In addition, the Centers for Medicare & Medicaid Services (CMS) notes that overall healthcare expenditures for people older than 65 will increase, as boomers who are Medicaid recipients will continue to age and decline in health (Wilensky 2017). Moreover, as boomers age, they continue to spend more money on healthcare. In 2010, people age 65 and older spent about $18,424 on their healthcare, which is about three times more than the average amount spent by working adults younger than 65 (Lassman et al. 2014).

The large baby boomer cohort also is affecting the demand for long-term care. As we age, we are more likely to experience chronic health conditions that may result in daily activity limitations. Daily activities require a degree of physical and mental acuity, including the ability to prepare meals, eat, bathe, dress, and pay bills. The Congressional Budget Office (2013) reported that about one-third of people between ages 65 and 84 and two-thirds of people 85 or older had at least one limitation in their daily activities. Healthcare providers for this age group work in residential care communities or provide home health services. Nursing homes are still an option for those with medical issues, but the number of nursing home residents declined by about 50 percent from 1977 to 2014, which suggests that the growth in services provided will rely more on coordination of care among providers at healthcare sites such as hospitals and residential care communities and home health care options (National Center for Health Statistics 2017).

Medical Group Practices

Changes have also occurred in physician practices, shifting from the solo physician office model to medical groups. Between 1983 and 2014, the percentage of physicians who practiced alone declined from 41 percent to 15 percent (Squires and Blumenthal 2016). By 2017, more than half of all physicians had joined larger practices, and about one-third of physicians were employed by a hospital-owned practice (Kacik 2017). Medical group practices may be wholly or partially owned by hospitals or remain independent. Currently, about 25 percent of practices are hospital-owned (MacDonald 2016).

Patient-Centered Medical Homes

With this variety of healthcare locations and services, care coordination and interprofessionalism are essential to improve patient care. As the chapter-opening case study on Maryland's LOFRTs indicated, professionals from different occupations who work together are more likely to identify potential improvements, such as changes that can reduce the number of people dying from overdoses. Once again, this situation ties into the iron triangle of access, cost, and quality. Simply put, on a patient care basis, interprofessional efforts help identify and implement ways to provide the right care for the patient at the right time at the right price. In order to provide these "rights," interprofessional efforts have focused on ways to improve primary care delivery so a patient has access to and receives quality care with the costs contained. Two models have been developed to help providers offer a broad range of healthcare services while being mindful of costs to the consumer: the patient-centered medical home and accountable care organizations. Both of these models serve to promote and implement care coordination on behalf of the patient.

First, let us look at the **patient-centered medical home (PCMH)** model, which is based on care being provided by an interdisciplinary team. PCMHs are designed to deliver five core functions of patient-centered primary healthcare (AHRQ 2018):

Patient-centered medical home (PCMH)
A healthcare delivery model in which the primary care provider ensures the patient receives the right treatment at the right time by the right provider in a way they can understand and that helps them be an active participant in their care.

1. Comprehensive care—including prevention, education, diagnosis, and treatment
2. Patient-centered care—that is, healthcare that includes the patient and family (as appropriate) on the healthcare team, and ensures healthcare providers know patients as individuals and are aware of their health history
3. Coordinated care—ensuring all places where you receive care have the information providers need about your health, and emphasizing open communication among caregivers, patients, and families
4. Accessible services—so patients are able to receive the appropriate attention and treatment when needed
5. High-quality and safe care—providing patient-centered care and engaging in behaviors that ensure high quality and patient safety

Early research suggests the PCMH model leads to better patient care and health outcomes. One study found that diabetic patients valued patient-centered care and accessible services, and that these factors motivated them to take an active role in managing their chronic condition (Bilello et al. 2018). Another study found that the presence of an on-site pharmacist who belonged to the interprofessional team encouraged more patients to receive influenza vaccinations (an example of disease-prevention efforts) than PCMH sites without a pharmacist present (Luder et al. 2018). In addition, the National Committee for Quality Assurance (2018) reported that patients belonging to PCMHs have better health outcomes. This may be because they benefit from health-promotion and disease-prevention care and education (e.g., cancer screenings), or because they are seen at a place where providers know them and their history (the patient-centered care model) as opposed to their having to access care via a hospital emergency department.

Accountable care organization (ACO)
A form of health services delivery organization that includes multiple kinds of providers who work together to improve care delivery to the individual patient as well as to improve the health status of a particular population, such as a group of employees or Medicare enrollees. The providers work as a team because of a reimbursement mechanism that incentivizes improvement in patient outcomes.

Accountable Care Organizations

Accountable care organizations (ACOs), introduced in chapter 3, are a set of healthcare providers "who are jointly held accountable for achieving measured quality improvements and reductions in the rate of spending growth" (McClellan et al. 2010, 982). ACOs focus on providing clinically integrated care across the spectrum. Thus, while individual ACOs vary, they may provide primary and specialty care as well as inpatient, outpatient, and home health services. The goal of this coordinated care is to provide appropriate services to patients while ensuring that providers communicate, which helps avoid duplication of services and medical errors (CMS 2017).

The number of ACOs is increasing. The United States had 64 in 2011 (Whitman 2017), but by 2017, there were more than 900 (Kaufman et al. 2017). A review of the literature regarding the impact of ACOs indicates that the presence of an ACO helps decrease emergency department visits and increase preventive care, health promotion, and chronic disease management (Kaufman et al. 2017).

So what is the difference between a PCMH and an ACO? Data suggest that accessibility is key to patient outcomes in both models. But while PCMHs are accountable to themselves and invest in personalized care, ACOs involve a consortium of providers who sign an agreement regarding how each facility will work with the others to provide care and receive payment (Bresnick 2015). What is similar about PCMHs and ACOs is that they are components of a larger picture regarding population health management, which focuses on the healthcare outcomes of a group.

Population health
The health outcomes of a designated population, including the distribution of such outcomes within this population.

Population Health

According to Kindig and Stoddart (2003, 380), the term **population health** refers to

> the health outcomes of a group of individuals, including the distribution of such outcomes within the group . . . . The field of population health includes health outcomes, patterns of health determinants, and policies and interventions that link these two.

In 2008, Donald Berwick, president and CEO of the Institute for Healthcare Improvement (IHI), along with Thomas Nolan and John Whittington, two other senior fellows at IHI, proposed that barriers to integrate care in the United States were not technical but political, and they suggested that improving the US healthcare system required efforts on three aims simultaneously (Berwick, Nolan, and Whittington 2008):

- Improving the experience of care
- Improving the health of populations
- Reducing the per capita cost of healthcare

Accomplishing this "**Triple Aim**" relied on a practice of cost control, patient-centered care, integration and coordination of health services, and a focus on health promotion to keep the population healthy (IHI 2009). This is similar to how PCMHs and ACOs keep patients from going to the emergency department for care that can be provided in a less costly setting, as well as how these models have increased patient access to preventive measures, such as vaccinations, and provided help for managing chronic diseases, such as diabetes.

Triple Aim
The goals of improving the patient experience and health of the population while reducing healthcare costs.

Physicians Bodenheimer and Sinsky (2014) have identified a fourth goal and created healthcare's "**Quadruple Aim**." While acknowledging that IHI's Triple Aim has become accepted as "a compass to optimize health system performance" (p. 573), they caution that physician and staff burnout also warrant attention. As a healthcare manager, the responsibilities are yours to help create a work environment that discourages worker burnout and encourages job satisfaction. Chapter 12 will explore how to establish this environment and why it is worth investing the time and resources to do so. For now, understand that this fourth factor of quality care for providers is important for healthcare managers to address.

Quadruple Aim
The goals of improving the patient experience, the health of a population, *and* the provider's experience while reducing healthcare costs.

Conclusion

We opened this chapter with a discussion of the state of Maryland's LOFRT program. There, the presence of interprofessional teams allowed for informed, open, and candid discussions about the need for care coordination to bring about better patient care, which, in turn, could help reduce overdose fatalities in the state. Coordinated care is necessary in all places where healthcare is delivered, and working together is key for the effective delivery of health promotion and disease prevention services, as well as diagnosis, treatment, and rehabilitation. Understanding how and where healthcare is delivered is important for students of healthcare management. Possessing the knowledge that where people live influences their health (the social determinants of health), and a thoughtful attention to the Triple and Quadruple Aims to improve our healthcare system, will help you as you enter the field of healthcare management. As stated earlier, the Triple Aim has become a compass for better health performance, but a fourth aim—caring for caregivers—also is important to consider. CenteringPregnancy was a model of care for pregnant women developed in the 1990s by the Centering Healthcare Institute that has come to meet this Quadruple Aim of improving the patient care experience, the provider experience, and the health of populations, all while reducing costs. The Centering Healthcare Institute is a nonprofit organization based in Boston dedicated to changing healthcare delivery and outcomes by focusing on providing care via Centering groups. By 2018, Centering Healthcare Institute models had been adopted by more than 500 healthcare organizations (Centering Healthcare Institute 2018).

Mini Case Study: CenteringPregnancy: Meeting the Quadruple Aim in Prenatal Care

Operating in North and South Carolina, CenteringPregnancy offered women prenatal care in a group setting. Groups of 8 to 12 pregnant women had the opportunity to network with other expectant mothers with similar due dates. The program also encouraged the women to take their own vital signs and engaged them in provider-directed discussions about the health of their pregnancies (Strickland, Merrell, and Kirk 2016). The groups met for 10 two-hour sessions, which included time for patients to interact with each other and providers. Patients also met individually with providers for one-on-one care. Afterward, their reviews indicated satisfaction with the experience (Strickland, Merrell, and Kirk 2016, 395):

> We started on time and ended on time and something happened the whole time we were there.
>
> I loved the program because every time you come you can share your story.

CenteringPregnancy met the first goal of the Quadruple Aim: improving the experience of care. It also showed positive results in terms of the second aim of population health, in that women had fewer preterm births and were more likely to breastfeed and use birth control following birth as well as attend postpartum follow-up medical appointments.

To elaborate, among 777 women at seven CenteringPregnancy sites in North Carolina in 2015, the rate of preterm births was 8.9 percent, while the general statewide rate was 9.7 percent. In addition, this reduction in preterm births helped reduce the number of babies requiring neonatal intensive care. Low birth weight was present in 5.6 percent of babies born to CenteringPregnancy participants, compared to the overall North Carolina rate of 8.5 percent, and 87 percent of CenteringPregnancy participants breastfed compared to 73.2 percent of new mothers statewide (Strickland, Merrell, and Kirk 2016). Overall, participation in the CenteringPregnancy model led to better health outcomes.

Exhibit 4.3 Centering-Pregnancy Outcomes in South Carolina

Health Outcome	*N* Saved from Poorer Health Outcome Because of Participation in CenteringPregnancy	Cost Savings per Infant in Health Expenditures	Total Cost Savings
Lower birth weight	57	$29,627	$1,688,739
Premature births	51	$22,667	$1,156,017
NICU care	42	$27,249	$1,144,458

Source: Data from Gareau et al. (2016).
Note: NICU = neonatal intensive care unit.

In South Carolina, a review of 1,262 CenteringPregnancy births from 2009 to 2013 found that pregnant women who had participated in CenteringPregnancy had healthier babies, saving the state millions of dollars (Gareau et al. 2016). Exhibit 4.3 shows the poor health outcomes avoided and health costs saved as a result of the program.

South Carolina's overall investment in CenteringPregnancy was $1.7 million; the return on that investment was $2,289,214 (Gareau et al. 2016), with better health outcomes for the state and reduced Medicaid expenditures. In addition, evidence from the North and South Carolina programs indicates that CenteringPregnancy met the second and third aims: improving the health of populations and reducing per capita costs of healthcare.

Last, let us look at CenteringPregnancy and the fourth aim—improving the provider experience. In 2009, three family physicians were interviewed separately for about 60 minutes regarding their provider experience with CenteringPregnancy in Calgary, Canada. They were asked six questions about their experiences, positive and negative, providing the group prenatal care (McNeil et al. 2013). Overall, the physicians reported that they enjoyed getting to know the patients better, as they had more time with them, and that even though they spent more time with each patient, they found the process of providing care more efficient. For example, one physician commented that she appreciated not having to repeat the same instructions to each patient individually throughout the day; rather, she could explain something once in the group care setting (McNeil et al. 2013). Certainly, the sample size for this study was small. Nonetheless, the physicians' positive responses indicate that CenteringPregnancy may be meeting the fourth aim as successfully as it is meeting the first three.

Mini Case Study Questions

1. How does CenteringPregnancy address the fourth aim as presented by Bodenheimer and Sinsky (2014)?
2. Explain how CenteringPregnancy is a model that enhances the patient experience. (Refer to Strickland, Merrell, and Kirk [2016] regarding the North Carolina study.)
3. Explain how CenteringPregnancy reduces healthcare costs. (Retrieve the publication by Gareau and colleagues [2016] regarding their South Carolina study.)

4. What other healthcare initiatives might take advantage of lessons learned from CenteringPregnancy to improve the patient and provider experience?

Points to Remember

- Various sites offer healthcare practice. The trend is moving from inpatient to outpatient care and a focus on health promotion and prevention.
- While individuals must take responsibility for their own health, social determinants of health affect their ability to do so.
- Social determinants of health are shaped by income inequalities, power distributions, and the resources available.
- Patient-centered medical homes and accountable care organizations emphasize care coordination, and interprofessionalism is important for improving patient care and containing costs.
- Improvement to the US healthcare system involves our meeting the Quadruple Aim of care, health, cost, and finding meaning in work.

Challenge Yourself

1. As you prepare to become a healthcare manager, explain how you envision your role on an interprofessional team. Give an example to illustrate.
2. As a student in a healthcare management program, what do you think are important factors to consider when selecting your internship site? What type of work environment do you prefer (e.g., patient-centered medical home)? Why did you select that environment?
3. Identify a health promotion activity conducted by your local health center, hospital, or clinic. Read the organization's website regarding what it is doing about that health promotion activity. How is it trying to reach out to its audience (e.g., how is the site reaching out to smokers)? What information is it telling the reader?

For Your Consideration

1. Conduct a library search for "CenteringPregnancy" to locate research published in your current year of study or the year before. Summarize the study. Are the researchers finding continued support for CenteringPregnancy to help meet one or more of the Quadruple Aims? Offer examples from the study to illustrate what you found.
2. One of the aims for better health performance is improving the patient experience of care. Consider this aim in relation to the following scenario:

Jesse Murray had been working as a patient advocate at Community Hospital for two years. He served as a liaison between patients and hospital staff, meeting with each patient or with a patient's family members after the patient had been admitted to the hospital. Jesse loved his job. He was able to talk with the people who used the hospital's services and to improve their stays. He frequently dealt with patient concerns regarding diet ("the food arrived cold") and timely medication distribution ("the nurse took too long to give me my pain shot") and spent time with the patients and their families so they knew they had an advocate during the hospital stay. When Jesse heard about a complaint, he would investigate it and then meet with hospital personnel to try to come to a workable solution. More often than not, a reasonable solution could be found, which increased patient satisfaction.

Recently, Jesse had been hearing patients complain of long wait times in the radiology department. Inpatients reported that they would be wheeled down to X-ray and sit there for hours, waiting for their exam. Jesse met with Rayna Radcliffe, the radiology supervisor, and asked if she had noticed an increase in wait times. Rayna said they were understaffed in the unit, so patient wait times had increased. "But," she added, "I don't think this has anything to do with patient satisfaction. It is just a consequence of staffing."

Jesse decided to assess Rayna's assertion by conducting in-house research. He distributed a survey each day for two weeks to patients who had gone to the radiology department (see exhibit 4.4).

Judging from the survey results, what is the problem in this situation? What would you recommend that Jesse do?

Exhibit 4.4 Patient Satisfaction with Radiology and Imaging Department Survey Results

	Very Satisfied	Acceptable	Dissatisfied
Length of time waiting in radiology department before you were seen	20%	30%	50%
Time spent with your provider	60%	30%	10%
Technical skills of your provider—thoroughness, carefulness, thoughtfulness	90%	10%	N/A
Personal manner of your provider—courtesy, respect, sensitivity, friendliness	10%	10%	80%
Your time spent in radiology department overall	10%	20%	70%

References

Academy of Nutrition and Dietetics. 2017. "What an RDN Can Do for You." Published September 22. www.eatright.org/resource/food/resources/learn-more-about-rdns/what-an-rdn-can-do-for-you.

Agency for Healthcare Research and Quality (AHRQ). 2018. "5 Key Functions of the Medical Home." Accessed July 11. https://pcmh.ahrq.gov/page/5-key-functions-medical-home.

American College of Cardiology. 2017. "Your Health Care Team." Accessed December 19. www.cardiosmart.org/Heart-Basics/Your-Health-Care-Team.

American Hospital Association (AHA). 2016a. "Trendwatch Chartbook 2016: Trends in Inpatient Utilization in Community Hospitals, 1994–2014." Accessed June 16, 2018. www.aha.org/research/reports/tw/chartbook/2016/table3-1.pdf.

———. 2016b. "Trendwatch Chartbook 2016: Supplementary Data Tables, Utilization and Volume, Tables 3.3 and 3.4." Accessed December 28, 2017. www.aha.org/research/reports/tw/chartbook/2016/table3-4.pdf.

———. 2015. "TrendWatch Report: The Role of Post-Acute Care in New Care Delivery Models." Published December. www.aha.org/research/reports/tw/15dec-tw-postacute.pdf.

Baier, M. 2015. "Overdose Fatality Review." Accessed December 18, 2017. bha.health.maryland.gov/OVERDOSE_PREVENTION/Pages/OFR-.aspx.

Balazs, C., R. Morello-Frosch, A. Hubbard, and I. Ray. 2012. "Environmental Justice Implications of Arsenic Contamination in California's San Joaquin Valley: A Cross-Sectional, Cluster-Design Examining Exposure and Compliance in Community Drinking Water Systems." *Environmental Health* 11 (1): 84.

Berwick, D., T. Nolan, and J. Whittington. 2008. "The Triple Aim: Care, Health and Cost." *Health Affairs* 27 (3): 759–69.

Bilello, L., A. Hall, J. Harman, C. Scuderi, N. Shah, J. Mills, and S. Samuels. 2018. "Key Attributes of Patient Centered Medical Homes Associated with Patient Activation of Diabetes Patients." *BMC Family Practice* 19 (1): 4.

Bodenheimer, T., and C. Sinsky. 2014. "From Triple to Quadruple Aim: Care of the Patient Requires Care of the Provider." *Annals of Family Medicine* 12 (6): 573–76.

Bresnick, J. 2015. "How Does an ACO Differ from the Patient-Centered Medical Home?" *Population Health News.* Published March 19. https://healthitanalytics.com/news/how-does-an-aco-differ-from-the-patient-centered-medical-home.

Brinkerhoff, N. 2014. "Leftovers from Afghanistan and Iraq Wars." AllGov.com. Published March 3. www.allgov.com/news/top-stories/leftovers-from-afghanistan-and-iraq-wars-1558-amputations-7224-severe-brain-injuries-118829-post-traumatic-stress-disorders-140303?news=852580.

Burke, M. 2012. "Advances in Prosthetics Pair Limbs with Robotics." Stars and Stripes. Published November 17. www.stripes.com/news/advances-in-prosthetics-pair-limbs-with-robotics-1.197530.

Callahan, D. 2008. "Health Care Costs and Medical Technology." In *From Birth to Death and Bench to Clinic: The Hastings Center Bioethics Briefing Book for Journalists, Policymakers, and Campaigns*, edited by M. Crowley, 79–82. Garrison, NY: The Hastings Center.

Centering Healthcare Institute. 2018. "About Us." Accessed July 10. www.centeringhealthcare.org/about.

Centers for Disease Control and Prevention (CDC). 2017a. "Cigarette Smoking and Tobacco Use Among People of Low Socioeconomic Status." Accessed January 15, 2018. www.cdc.gov/tobacco/disparities/low-ses/index.htm.

———. 2017b. "Preventive Health and Health Services Block Grant." Accessed January 15, 2018. www.cdc.gov/phhsblockgrant/.

———. 2017c. "Smoking and Tobacco Use." Accessed December 19. www.cdc.gov/tobacco/data_statistics/fact_sheets/youth_data/tobacco_use/index.htm.

———. 2016. "Current Cigarette Smoking Among Adults in the United States." Accessed December 19, 2017. www.cdc.gov/tobacco/data_statistics/fact_sheets/adult_data/cig_smoking/index.htm.

Centers for Medicare & Medicaid Services (CMS). 2017. "What is an ACO?" Accessed January 20, 2018. www.cms.gov/Medicare/Medicare-Fee-for-Service-Payment/ACO/.

Colby, S., and J. Ortman. 2014. "The Baby Boom Cohort in the United States: 2012 to 2060." *Current Population Reports*. Accessed December 29, 2017. www.census.gov/prod/2014pubs/p25-1141.pdf.

Congressional Budget Office. 2013. "Rising Demand for Long Term Services and Supports for Elderly People." Accessed December 29, 2017. www.cbo.gov/publication/44363.

CVS. 2017. "MinuteClinic History." Accessed December 29. www.cvs.com/minuteclinic/visit/about-us/history.

Gareau, S., A. Lopez-DeFede, B. Loudermilk, T. Cummings, J. Hardin, A. Picklesimer, E. Crouch, and S. Covington-Kolb. 2016. "Group Prenatal Care Results in Medicaid Savings with Better Outcomes: A Propensity Score Analysis of CenteringPregnancy Participation in South Carolina." *Maternal and Child Health Journal* 20 (7): 1384–93.

Hammick, M., D. Freeth, J. Copperman, and D. Goodsman. 2009. *Being Interprofessional.* Cambridge, UK: Polity Press.

HealthyPeople.gov. 2018. "Social Determinants of Health." Accessed January 15. www.healthypeople.gov/2020/topics-objectives/topic/social-determinants-health/interventions-resources.

Hollenbeck, B., R. Dunn, A. Suskind, Y. Zhang, J. Hollingsworth, and J. Birkmeyer. 2014. "Ambulatory Surgery Centers and Outpatient Procedure Use Among Medicare Beneficiaries." *Medical Care* 52 (10): 926–31.

Institute for Healthcare Improvement (IHI). 2009. "Triple Aim—Concept Design." Published June 29. www.ihi.org/Engage/Initiatives/TripleAim/Documents/ConceptDesign.pdf.

Institute of Medicine. 2003. *Health Professions Education: A Bridge to Quality.* Washington, DC: National Academies Press.

Kacik, A. 2017. "For the First Time Ever, Less Than Half of Physicians Are Independent." *Modern Healthcare.* Published May 31. www.modernhealthcare.com/article/20170531/NEWS/170539971.

Kaiser Family Foundation. 2015. "Hospitals by Ownership Type." Accessed December 20, 2017. www.kff.org/other/state-indicator/hospitals-by-ownership/.

Kaufman, B., S. Spivack, S. Stearns, P. Song, and E. O'Brien. 2017. "Impact of Accountable Care Organizations on Utilization, Care, and Outcomes: A Systematic Review." *Medical Care Research and Review.* Published December 12. doi.org/10.1177/1077558717745916.

Kennedy, M. 2016. "Lead-Laced Water in Flint: A Step-by-Step Look at the Makings of a Crisis." *The Two-Way: Breaking News from NPR.* Published April 20. www.npr.org/sections/

thetwo-way/2016/04/20/465545378/lead-laced-water-in-flint-a-step-by-step-look-at-the-makings-of-a-crisis.

Kindig, D., and G. Stoddart. 2003. "What Is Population Health?" *American Journal of Public Health* 93 (3): 380–83.

Lassman, D., M. Hartman, B. Washington, K. Andrews, and A. Catlin. 2014. "US Health Spending Trends by Age and Gender: Seclected Years 2002–2010." *Health Affairs* 33 (5): 815–22.

Luder, H., P. Shannon, J. Kirby, and S. Frede. 2018. "Community Pharmacist Collaboration with a Patient-Centered Medical Home: Establishment of a Patient-Centered Medical Neighborhood and Payment Model." *Journal of the American Pharmacists Association* 58 (1): 44–50.

MacDonald, I. 2016. "1 in 4 Physician Practices Now Hospital-Owned." *Fierce Healthcare.* Published September 7. www.fiercehealthcare.com/practices/1-4-physician-practices-now-hospital-owned.

Maryland Department of Health. 2017. "OFR Charter Template." Accessed December 18. https://bha.health.maryland.gov/OVERDOSE_PREVENTION/Documents/OFR%20Charter%20Template.docx

McClellan, M., A. McKethan, J. Lewis, J. Roski, and E. Fisher. 2010. "A National Strategy to Put Accountable Care into Practice." *Health Affairs* 29 (5): 982–90.

McNeil, D., M. Vekved, S. Dolan, J. Siever, S. Horn, and S. Tough. 2013. "A Qualitative Study of the Experience of CenteringPregnancy Group Prenatal Care for Physicians." *BMC Pregnancy and Childbirth* 13 (Suppl 1): S6–S13.

Munsey, C. 2008. "How to Help Your Clients Kick the Habit." *Monitor on Psychology* 39 (10): 38.

National Association of Community Health Centers (NACHC). 2014. *NACHC 2013–2014 Annual Report.* Accessed December 28, 2017. www.nachc.org/wp-content/uploads/2015/06/2013-2014-Annual-Report1-1.pdf.

National Center for Health Statistics. 2017. *Health, United States, 2016: With Chartbook on Long-Term Trends in Health.* Washington, DC: US Government Printing Office.

National Committee for Quality Assurance. 2018. "Latest Evidence: Benefits of the Patient-Centered Medical Home." Accessed January 20. www.ncqa.org/programs/recognition/practices/pcmh-evidence.

Potter, B. K., and C. R. Scoville. 2006. "Amputation Is Not Isolated: An Overview of the US Army Amputee Patient Care Program and Associated Amputee Injuries." *Journal of the American Academy of Orthopaedic Surgeons* 14 (10): S188–S190.

President's Advisory Commision. 1997a. "Consumer Bill of Rights and Responsibilities." Agency for Healthcare Research and Quality. Accessed December 20, 2017. https://archive.ahrq.gov/hcqual/final/append_a.html.

———. 1997b. "Statement of Responsibilities." Accessed December 20, 2017. https://archive.ahrq.gov/hcqual/final/append_a.html#chpt8.

Rebbert-Franklin, K., E. Haas, P. Singal, S. Cherico-Hsii, M. Baier, K. Collins, K. Webner, and J. Sharfstein. 2016. "Development of Maryland Local Overdose Fatality Review Teams: A Localized, Interdisciplinary Approach to Combat the Growing Problem of Drug Overdose Deaths." *Health Promotion Practice* 17 (4): 596–600.

Squires, D., and D. Blumenthal. 2016. "Do Small Physician Practices Have a Future?" The Commonwealth Fund. Accessed December 29, 2017. www.commonwealthfund.org/publications/blog/2016/may/do-small-physician-practices-have-a-future.

Strickland, C., S. Merrell, and J. Kirk. 2016. "CenteringPregnancy: Meeting the Quadruple Aim in Prenatal Care." *North Carolina Medical Journal* 77 (6): 394–97.

UCLA Health. 2017a. "About Us." Accessed December 20. www.uclahealth.org/about-us.

———. 2017b. "Patient Responsibilities." Accessed December 20. www.uclahealth.org/patient-experience/patient-responsibilities.

Vidant Health. 2017a. "Careers." Accessed December 20. http://careers.vidanthealth.com/About/Overview.

———. 2017b. "Patient Rights & Responsibilities." Accessed December 20. www.vidanthealth.com/Patients-Families/Patient-Rights-Responsibilities.

Vincent, G. K., and V. A. Velkoff. 2010. *The Next Four Decades: The Older Population in the United States: 2010 to 2050.* Washington, DC: US Census Bureau.

Whitman, E. 2017. "A Tale of Two Accountable Care Organizations." *Modern Healthcare.* Published February 4. www.modernhealthcare.com/article/20170204/MAGAZINE/302049983.

Wilensky, G. 2017. "Let's Not Forget About Medicare." *Milbank Quarterly* 95 (2): 249–52.

World Health Organization (WHO). 2018. "About Social Determinants of Health." Accessed January 15. www.who.int/social_determinants/sdh_definition/en/.

———. 2017a. "Hospitals." Accessed December 20. www.who.int/hospitals/en/.

———. 2017b. "Tobacco Fact Sheet." Accessed December 19. www.who.int/mediacentre/factsheets/fs339/en/.

———. 2015. "An Overview." Accessed December 19, 2017. www.who.int/fctc/WHO_FCTC_summary_January2015_EN.pdf.

PART II

INTERPERSONAL SKILLS

CASE STUDY

St. Luke's Health System: Transformational Leadership

This book addresses many of the conceptual, interpersonal, and business skills associated with healthcare management. Material covered in part II includes essential knowledge and skills related to the healthcare leader's interpersonal abilities, including leadership, communication, teamwork, emotional intelligence, conflict management, time management, and personal or professional management. In one way or another, the issues and strategies pursued by St. Luke's Health System leaders demonstrate a practical application of many of the concepts and concerns described in part II. The following case is based on Tracy Farnsworth's interviews with St. Luke's CEO David Pate (unless otherwise noted, quotations are from Pate 2017a, 2017b, 2018). Discussion questions at the end of the case facilitate additional insight and learning.

Introduction

David Pate, MD, JD, FACP, FACHE, began his new role as president and CEO of Boise, Idaho–based St. Luke's Health System in August 2009. At that time, Idaho's population was approximately 1.65 million. The greater Boise Valley—covering a population of 685,000 within a 45-minute drive—includes the cities of Boise, Meridian, Nampa, Kuna, Eagle, Star, Emmett, Garden City, Caldwell, and Mountain Home.

Since its founding as a six-bed cottage hospital in 1902, St. Luke's had grown to become the largest and one of the most respected healthcare organizations in the state. When Pate arrived, the system included two hospitals in Boise's Treasure Valley, one in Twin Falls, and one in the resort town of Sun Valley, 150 miles northeast of Boise. St. Luke's was poised to become a model healthcare organization that many hospital and healthcare leaders in Idaho and beyond sought to follow.

Background and Environment

At the time of Dr. Pate's arrival, the nation's fragmented, costly, and largely inefficient healthcare system was under assault. A 2005 report from the Institute of Medicine revealed that 40 to 50 percent of all medical expense is wasted; the *New England Journal of Medicine* reported half of all medical care is substandard; the Centers for Disease Control and Prevention affirmed 75 percent of medical costs are spent treating preventable disease; and a 2003 study reported by the *Wall Street Journal* revealed transaction costs consume up to 30 percent of every healthcare dollar (Hyde 2015).

In 2009, the US healthcare system, including hospital and physician providers across Idaho, was facing highly disruptive environmental forces that would severely test the viability and sustainability of how most healthcare organizations finance and deliver care. The Affordable Care Act, approved by Congress in March 2010, would fundamentally change the health insurance marketplace, facilitate a movement away from reimbursing providers on a "fee-for-service" basis and toward a "pay-for-value" system, and launch a nationwide movement toward population health. (Population health is defined as the health outcomes of a group, which may include geographic populations such as nations or communities, or groups such as employees, ethnic groups, disabled persons, or prisoners [IHI 2018].) Other changes and environmental forces included a challenging and precarious national economy, increasing difficulties in accessing capital, radical revisions to hospital–physician alignment models, unrelenting pressure on provider revenues and expenses, fast-moving updates to clinical and information technology, challenging workforce dynamics, and increasing merger and consolidation activity in virtually every market (see appendix A).

Call for Leadership

In response to these and other compelling forces, Dr. Pate understood that *transformational*, not incremental, leadership and change were needed. *Transformational change* may be defined as "a shift in the business culture of an organization resulting from a change in the underlying strategy and processes that the organization has used in the past. A transformational change is designed to be organization-wide and is enacted over a period of time" (BusinessDictionary.com 2018).

To facilitate the change process, Pate spoke of the need to lead St. Luke's on a journey, and employed Harvard professor John Kotter's model for leading change (Kotter 2012):

1. Establish a sense of urgency.
2. Create a guiding coalition.
3. Establish a vision and strategy.
4. Communicate the change vision.
5. Empower employees for broad-based action.
6. Generate short-term wins.
7. Consolidate gains and produce more change.
8. Anchor new approaches in the culture.

Managing the Process and Pace of Change

Dr. Pate understood that absent a real sense of urgency, St. Luke's leaders and employees would not embrace the attitudes, behaviors, and actions needed to fundamentally transform what they already regarded as a healthy, respected, and well-positioned healthcare organization. Pate keenly sensed it was best to start strategically repositioning the organization *now* rather than wait several years when draconian measures (notably radical changes in reimbursement models) would likely be thrust upon his unsuspecting organization. He knew his organization must move toward new financing and care delivery models quickly enough to gain needed experience and momentum—yet not so fast as to get too far ahead of key stakeholder groups, thus failing to gain their needed support. He also understood that although major changes to Medicare, Medicaid, and insurance reimbursement models were coming, no one really knew how quickly such changes would occur.

The challenge of leading a healthcare organization accustomed to generating revenues almost entirely from a traditional volume-driven, fee-for-service system—*but that was rapidly shifting toward a pay-for-value and population health–oriented system* (Nynon 2014)—was daunting. Like Cinderella knowing the stroke of midnight was coming, healthcare organizations needed to be dancing, or at least moving toward the door (Leavitt 2015). Yet moving too quickly from financial and care delivery models that still rewarded providers in a volume-based, fee-for-service manner would leave too much money on the table; moving too slowly would pose long-term financial and organizational risks of equal or greater consequence. In numerous formal and informal ways (notably through large and small group meetings, e-mails, letters, blog posts, social media, publications, and private conversations), Dr. Pate often emphasized to his board, staff, and community partners that St. Luke's needed to transition in a sure and steady way. As he stated in the St. Luke's 2017 annual report, "In an age of uncertainty in the world of health care, still we push on. Our strategy to evolve from 'fee-for-service' to 'pay-for-value' continues to advance, because regardless of what happens in Washington, DC, we know it's the right thing to do" (St. Luke's 2017, 3). By early 2017, St. Luke's Health System's total revenues came from roughly 66 percent fee-for-service payer sources, and 34 percent from some form of pay-for-value.

Selecting and Developing the Executive Team

Upon his arrival in 2009, Dr. Pate knew that assembling the right leadership team was job one. Most executives struggle with terminating other leaders or moving managers around. Undaunted, Pate took needed action, knowing that getting the right leaders in the right positions, doing the right things in the right way, was essential to long-term organizational success. Over time, he organized and developed a new senior leadership team that enthusiastically shared his vision and had the capacity to redirect and transform St. Luke's.

Getting the Message Right

Dr. Pate insisted that "the mindset of leaders and organizations who embrace transformational change must be right; people need to feel safe, willing to express their fears and concerns, and for leaders to address those issues in an open and candid way." Leaders and stakeholders, Pate continued, "must also anticipate rough spots—including both major and minor setbacks, and questions and challenges about their leadership." In dealing with the physician community, Pate adamantly insisted healthcare leaders "must lead with an absolute and unwavering focus on quality and patient safety. Doing so is essential to gaining both initial and sustained levels of trust and buy-in from the clinical community."

After St. Luke's gained that trust, then—*and only then*—did leaders talk about the so-called "value equation" and new business models related to "the total cost of care." There is a general consensus that the current level of healthcare spending is unsustainable. Hospitals and health systems are continuously striving to reduce costs and improve the efficiency of care. Historically, providers have focused on managing their own costs for a particular service, but new risk-based payment arrangements are making many hospitals and health systems accountable for a broader range of healthcare spending, including the cost of services delivered by other providers during an episode of care or for a defined population. It is, therefore, useful to consider the impact of measuring the "total cost of care" on hospitals and health systems, as well as to contemplate what steps healthcare leaders need to take. While a single definition of "total cost of care" does not exist, the phrase is generally used to refer to all direct and indirect costs associated with an episode of care for a period of healthcare coverage, such as a health plan benefit year (Smith and Keckley 2017).

Every decision made, Pate insisted, came down to two criteria: "Will it improve health and patient outcomes? Will it lower the overall cost of care?" He was both careful and emphatic about sending verbal and action-based signals indicating "we will not compromise or sacrifice patient safety or quality care." It was merely a baseline to conform to The Joint Commission's National Patient Safety Goals, which were established in 2002 to help accredited organizations address specific areas of concern regarding patient safety. By 2014, St. Luke's became widely recognized for its leadership and commitment to patient safety and quality care.

New Vision and Direction

Shortly after his arrival in 2009, Dr. Pate began what he often referred to as "our journey"—a journey that would substantively transform St. Luke's into its communities' most trusted partner in providing exceptional, patient-centered care, and to more fully realize a relatively new industrywide vision called the Triple Aim. Established by the Institute for Healthcare Improvement (IHI), the Triple Aim is a framework that describes an approach to optimizing health system performance. It is IHI's belief that new designs must be developed to simultaneously pursue three dimensions, which it calls the "Triple Aim":

- Improving the patient experience of care (including quality and satisfaction)
- Improving the health of populations
- Reducing the per capita cost of healthcare

By 2012, St. Luke's mission, vision, and values statements had evolved as follows:

- **Mission**: To improve the health of people in the communities we serve
- **Vision**: To be the communities' trusted partner in providing exceptional, patient-centered care
- **Values**: Integrity, compassion, accountability, respect, excellence

Growing and Integrating the Regional Healthcare System

In 2009, St. Luke's comprised four hospitals: 400-bed St. Luke's Boise; 250-bed St. Luke's Meridian (10 miles west of Boise); 225-bed St. Luke's Magic Valley Regional Medical Center in Twin Falls (117 miles east of Boise); and 25-bed St. Luke's Wood River located in Sun Valley (150 miles northeast of Boise). Trends toward hospital–provider consolidation increased significantly between 2009 and 2017, not only in response to the industry's need to drive greater efficiencies, but also to enable development of comprehensive and sophisticated clinically integrated networks. (The shift from volume- to value-based care, exploration of ways to manage population health, and the increasing influence of consumerism have challenged healthcare stakeholders to improve care delivery by reducing clinical variation while increasing access to capital. As a result, consolidation has become a defining factor in healthcare business models [Barker 2017].)

In this climate, Dr. Pate knew hospitals and healthcare systems had pursued various strategies to consolidate and to better align their strategic interests not only with one another, but especially with the physician community. Since his arrival, St. Luke's hospital–physician strategy favored alignment through physician employment or practice acquisition and the development of a wide network of wholly owned physician groups. (Other physician–hospital alignment models include accountable care organizations [ACOs], clinically integrated networks, patient-centered medical homes, physician–hospital organizations, quality collaboratives, clinical comanagement and service line arrangements, independent practice associations, joint ventures, and more [Cox 2018].) Pate was persuasive and largely successful in articulating the merits of the physician employment model.

His team also experienced important and difficult setbacks. In 2012, St. Luke's lost a costly, high-profile antitrust battle initiated by two cross-town rivals, requiring it to unwind its earlier purchase of a 40-person physician practice in Nampa, a town of roughly 100,000 people 20 miles west of Boise. The federal judge presiding over the case noted in his decision that the acquisition had been intended by St. Luke's and the Saltzer medical group primarily to improve patient outcomes, and "the court believes that it would have that effect if left intact, and St. Luke's is to be applauded for its efforts to improve the delivery of health care in the Treasure Valley." Still, he said there are other ways to achieve the same effect that do not run afoul of antitrust law and do not run such a risk of increased costs (Gamble 2014).

Pate was a dynamic communicator; every appropriate means and method of communicating and advancing the organization's vision and strategic imperatives, including Pate's own blog, was needed to gain the support of this organization of more than 14,000 people. One message read as follows (SLHP 2018b):

> SLHP [St. Luke's Health Partners] has a deep appreciation for the complexities that make up our healthcare system and is working actively to move from a volume-based model to a value-based model. This is why we are collaborating with partners, including like-minded providers, employers, payers, and members to develop a shared responsibility for healthcare costs, quality, and outcomes. By pooling our knowledge and resources, we can develop health plans that provide shared accountability, resulting in stabilized costs, increased savings, and satisfied employees. We are relentlessly focused on outcomes and costs and want to partner with employers over the long term to achieve these goals.

New Strategic Partners to Reflect a Changing World

In 2009, virtually 100 percent of St. Luke's Health System revenues were generated, in one form or another, from fee-for-service. By 2017, only 66 percent of total system revenues were generated via fee-for-service. One reason for this change was St. Luke's 2012 strategic alliance with Salt Lake City–based SelectHealth. In a blog post dated September 4, 2012, Dr. Pate explained the purpose and details behind that innovative partnership (Pate 2012):

> St. Luke's Health System will transform healthcare by aligning with physicians and other providers to deliver integrated, seamless, and patient-centered quality care across all St. Luke's settings. That's St. Luke's vision, and today, I'm excited to share news of a significant milestone in attainment of our vision and our Triple Aim: better health, better care, and lower cost.
>
> We've got an innovative new partner in SelectHealth, an insurance company based in Utah that shares our vision and our values, and has pledged to work with us toward achieving those much-needed goals. SelectHealth, a Salt Lake City-based not-for-profit health insurance company that serves more than 500,000 members in Utah and southern Idaho, is committed to helping its members stay healthy, offering superior service, and facilitating access to high-quality care. We believe our new relationship will help us align incentives for participating health care providers and their patients, and will help SelectHealth and its members achieve long-term improvements in health.
>
> SelectHealth is a subsidiary of Intermountain Healthcare, and while I'm aware of rumors that we're merging with Intermountain Healthcare, I can assure you that this is not true. Our alliance is one of collaboration with SelectHealth, an insurance company that has been a part of a provider organization for decades, and is not a merger of the two health systems or any other parts of our organizations.
>
> Our new alliance combines St. Luke's quality with SelectHealth's core competencies and expertise in supporting an integrated health care delivery system, and will be supported by BrightPath, an extensive network of St. Luke's physicians and facilities and independent physicians and facilities.
>
> Here's why this is so important: As regular readers of my blog know, the transformation of health care delivery calls for a completely different business model. Many insurance models only reward, and therefore health care providers have only focused on, improving the health of people who are already sick. Most efforts at wellness, health promotion, fitness, screenings, and preventative services have been poorly reimbursed, or not paid for at all, under many health plans. The current system promotes fragmentation of care, and there is currently little incentive for providers and payors to spend the extra time and effort to work together to coordinate care, ensure patients get the proper follow-up, and try to prevent the use of unnecessary or low-value services. That's

where SelectHealth comes in. St. Luke's alliance with SelectHealth is built upon trust, a commitment to collaboration and data-sharing, having each party perform the services they are best suited to perform without duplicating those same services, and by paying the insurance company for the services they perform and providing financial support to health care providers to invest in better health and to reward providers for eliminating low-value to no-value services according to evidence-based medicine.

That's a completely new and different paradigm. It's breakthrough thinking and a breakthrough relationship, and why I'm so inspired by this new alliance. It will take time to implement the necessary changes and to achieve the benefits and savings we are striving to return to SelectHealth members, but we are starting today. And while we're thrilled that this new relationship offers a very tangible and powerful opportunity to bend the cost curve and improve the health of the people we serve, we greatly value our current relationships with all the other insurance companies with which we do business. For example, we recently announced a new collaboration with Regence BlueShield of Idaho to improve the health of patients and their care experience by better coordinating their care within the health delivery system. In this new delivery model, physicians and nurses work closely with patients who have multiple health conditions to engage them more in their treatment plans, promote lifestyle adjustments, and improve their overall health. By delivering highly-personalized and coordinated care, the program aims to avoid unnecessary duplication and reduce overall costs.

Our new and innovative relationship with SelectHealth likewise may pave the way for other insurance companies to work with St. Luke's via new models, and we're keeping the door open and the conversation going to see what additional collaborations may be possible. This is a very exciting day for St. Luke's Health System and SelectHealth as we launch this new innovative alliance. Just as we set out to do in March of 2010, we are transforming health care!

Developing an Integrated Delivery System

Upon Pate's arrival in 2009, St. Luke's operated like a federation—each hospital with its own CEO and board of directors. In many ways these hospital leaders made plans and operated largely independently from one another. Consistent with the Triple Aim, Dr. Pate was determined to identify new efficiencies, reduce healthcare costs, improve clinical quality and patient safety, and improve the overall health of persons for whom St. Luke's had stewardship. He sensed the time was right to centralize and systemize what heretofore had been a loosely organized group of hospitals with one common owner. (St. Luke's Health System and its related subsidiary corporations are organized as tax-exempt, not-for-profit corporations.) Pate and his senior leaders also set about developing their own clinically integrated network—a collection of healthcare providers, such as physicians, hospitals, and post-acute care treatment providers, that comes together to improve patient care and reduce overall healthcare cost.

St. Luke's Health Partners

To facilitate realization of the Triple Aim and to develop a true clinically integrated healthcare system, Dr. Pate enlarged the vision and led the expansion of St. Luke's Health Partners (SLHP), an integrated network of approximately 2,200 employed and independent healthcare providers (see appendix B). Over time, SLHP engaged in contracts involving shared accountability arrangements between the providers and partner payers, including Blue Cross of Idaho, Mountain Health CO-OP, PacificSource Health Plans, and SelectHealth. Dr. Pate emphasized that SLHP was established as a separate albeit wholly owned subsidiary of St. Luke's, in part to enable it to delve into seemingly disruptive models of care (bundled payments; total cost of care; pay-for-value; and full risk/capitation) that were otherwise inconsistent with St. Luke's established and more traditional fee-for-service models for financing and delivering care. (The US healthcare system is the most expensive in the world, but disruptive innovations can improve both affordability and accessibility so more people get the care they need. To give these innovative models a chance to succeed, Dr. Clayton Christensen advised they be organized and operated as separate, freestanding entities so as not to compete with or be stifled from the business culture and practices of the parent organization; see Christensen [1997, 2013].)

Educating, orienting, and bringing along the team, including employees, physicians, governing boards, and other stakeholders, was an exhausting but critical endeavor in SLHP's quest for transformational change. Over the course of several years, Dr. Pate and his leadership team took many other bold steps to strengthen and improve St. Luke's culture, including the way it organized, financed, and delivered patient care. The organization introduced the following initiatives:

- *Implementation of evidence-based practices.* Early on, St. Luke's experts implemented new processes that research has proven effective, including bundling the steps for preventing sepsis infections and "Duke bundles" for warding off surgical site infections after colon surgery. St. Luke's also pursued disease specialty certifications, resulting in the new advanced primary stroke centers, for example.
- *Standardization.* St. Luke's relentless focus on trying to eliminate irrational variation in processes was key to the system's success. The implementation of the manufacturing industry's waste-fighting "Lean" methodology (known as TEAMwork within St. Luke's) was particularly helpful.
- *Physician engagement,* including identification of physician champions for numerous quality and safety initiatives.
- *Community board engagement.* Dr. Pate once observed, "I find those of us in healthcare make and accept excuses too readily. We will, for example, find a way to rationalize why handwashing might not happen all the time. It

is much harder to explain that to community board members. We might also understand why a patient with a hip fracture on a weekend might wait until Monday for surgical correction—it doesn't make a lot of sense to our community board members. St. Luke's boards have set the expectations for quality improvement and quickly dismiss excuses" (Pate 2016).

- *Use of data.* In its transformation journey, St. Luke's looked at all the publicly available data and rating reports to focus leaders' attention on the greatest areas of opportunity for improvement. The system consulted data from Healthgrades, Truven Health Analytics, and Centers for Medicare & Medicaid Services (CMS).
- *Establishment of multidisciplinary clinics.* These were opened to improve care coordination and reduce the costs of care, with notable examples including the Center for Spine Wellness, Pulmonary Nodule Clinic, and the Congestive Heart Failure Clinic. In 2016, Dr. Pate observed, "It is absolutely true that better quality of care results in lower costs." Outcomes from these clinics and other actions noted earlier offer further convincing evidence.
- *Electronic health records.* A systemwide electronic health record called EPIC went live in fall 2017—a staggering undertaking that connected all of St. Luke's from the smallest clinic to the largest hospital. It also connected St. Luke's patients and their healthcare providers in unprecedented ways.
- *Care coordination.* To break down silos and sharpen the organization's focus on patient-centered care, St. Luke's created the new position of "care coordinator," a professional found at more and more health systems whose job is to coordinate, monitor, and evaluate the team of interdisciplinary providers a single patient may need.
- *Lifestyle medicine.* To further the organization's readiness for the US healthcare system's shift toward wellness and population health, St. Luke's leaders embraced lifestyle medicine, which uses a collaborative care model that incorporates allied healthcare professionals to provide treatment through medication, coaching, and education. (According to the World Health Organization, 80 percent of the world's noninfectious diseases could be prevented if these four lifestyle practices were followed: eating a healthy diet, engaging in physical activity, avoiding tobacco, and drinking alcohol only in moderation.)

Recognition of a Job Well Done

By 2017, St. Luke's had grown into a fully integrated system comprising 9 hospitals (compared to 4 in 2009), more than 150 clinics, and more than 14,000 employees. It had also received numerous awards recognizing its transformative leadership. For four consecutive years, from 2014 to 2017, Truven Health Analytics deemed St. Luke's one of the "Top 15 Health Systems" in the United States, and CMS awarded its Five-Star Quality Rating to the Boise and Meridian campuses—the only five-star hospitals in Idaho—indicating they provide superior care.

Other awards, recognitions, and specialty certifications include the following:

- Magnet designation for nursing excellence, awarded four times by the American Nurses Credentialing Center
- Award of Excellence in Healthcare Quality from Qualis Health
- Top 50 Cardiovascular Hospital recognition for 12 years, awarded by Watson (Truven) Health
- Accreditations for the Chest Pain Center, blood and marrow transplant, and medical imaging
- St. Luke's Children's Hospital accreditation (since 1992), and Certifications for High-Quality Cancer Care, from the National Association of Children's Hospitals and Related Institutions

Despite these well-deserved accolades, Dr. Pate readily admitted his team made many leadership and management mistakes. Future healthcare managers can learn many important lessons by carefully noting St. Luke's leadership philosophy, decisions, processes, and actions over the past ten years.

Discussion Questions

1. What were the most pressing environmental forces causing Dr. Pate and his leadership team to pursue transformational change?
2. In what ways did Dr. Pate and his team demonstrate transformational leadership?
3. Explain and justify the change model St. Luke's leaders used to pursue transformational change.
4. What evidence demonstrates that St. Luke's stakeholders exemplified effective teamwork in pursuing transformational change?
5. What actions, including methods of organizational communication, did Dr. Pate employ to gain his stakeholders' trust and support?
6. Identify areas where conflict might have paralyzed St. Luke's progress in fulfilling its mission and realizing its vision to provide exceptional, patient-centered care.

Appendix A: The Future of Healthcare: Key Industry Trends

Healthcare is a dynamic and ever-changing industry, and its future has always been difficult to predict. The following list—written from the perspective of those years—summarizes the political and economic backdrop during the early portion of Pate's leadership at St. Luke's (Valentine and Masters 2013):

The economy. Although the current economy is slowly improving, it remains fragile, with significant exposure to unemployment and the economy in Europe. The national economy will continue to affect both demand and supply within the healthcare industry.

Healthcare reform. Various elements of the Affordable Care Act are being implemented on schedule, including ventures into bundled payment, ACOs, and value-based purchasing activities. State health insurance exchanges loom around the corner; many are in active development. This trend—with its focus on benefits and network development—must be monitored.

Hospital–physician alignment. Physician employment will remain the preferred approach to hospital–physician alignment. There will still be physician and medical groups that favor independence, and most hospitals and health systems will need to balance a dual approach to meeting the needs of both independent as well as employed physicians. The need to achieve clinical integration between and among both employed and independent physicians is critical if hospitals and health systems expect to respond effectively to healthcare reform.

Revenues and expenses. The next 12 to 24 months will likely see per-unit revenues increasing at a rate below cost trends. Medicare payments will increase less than 2 percent, and most states are likely to hold the line (if not decrease rates) on Medicaid. Commercial payers will likely hold rate increases to 4 to 6 percent. Some payers, including Medicare, are expected to tie certain rate increases to documented quality improvements. Value-based purchasing, bundled payment, readmission rate reductions, ACOs, and other risk-based arrangements present opportunities for greater financial reward to low-cost, high-quality providers. Reducing costs must remain a top priority in the coming fiscal years. Simultaneously, patient throughput and occupancy levels must increase in both acute care hospital-based and outpatient settings to maximize economies of scale and the use of resources.

Access to capital. Capital access will continue to be a key catalyst for mergers, sales, affiliations, and other alliances for many hospitals. Capital access will be more difficult in the immediate future due to the weak economy, soft volumes, and deteriorating payer mix. Most independent hospital boards continue to ask the questions, "Can we remain independent?" If so, "Should we?"

Information technology. Useful data that inform clinical and financial decisions in real time are becoming a key driver to increasing revenues and better managing expenses. Information technology systems and strategies must be sufficiently robust to capture large volumes of data that can be readily integrated into useful decision-making (clinical and financial) and marketing information.

Consolidations, closures, alliances, and mergers. The healthcare reform agenda will likely continue, and 5 percent of acute-care hospitals could close by 2020. Further consolidation and alignment of hospitals and medical groups is probable as these entities join together to improve access to capital, form ACOs, and achieve cost reductions through economies of scale.

Clinical integration and care-delivery redesign. Processes associated with clinical integration and care-delivery redesign are at the heart of the so-called "golden triangle" of cost containment, quality improvement, and financial performance. Achieving future success in clinical integration and care-delivery redesign will require paying attention to and coordinating all points of the care continuum: primary care, acute care, and post-acute care.

Workforce issues. Pressure to reduce operating costs from 10 to 20 percent over the next three to five years will continue. The enormity of this reduction will require making further reductions in nonclinical staffing, outsourcing functions to less costly vendors, reducing or holding wages flat, and adjusting benefit plans. Increased response from organized labor is expected.

Smart growth. Inpatient and selective outpatient use rates will decline in the immediate or intermediate future because of continued high unemployment, more cost-shifting from employers to employees for health-related benefits, and increased price shopping and postponing of nonessential medical care. Accordingly, healthcare leadership teams must identify ways to selectively grow market share in areas that improve profitability.

Appendix B: St. Luke's Health Partners

Part of the St. Luke's family is St. Luke's Health Partners (SLHP), a network of primary care clinics that is committed to improving outcomes and reducing care costs for the people of Idaho. To achieve its goals, SLHP (2018a) partners with clinicians as well as government and commercial health plans. St. Luke's aligns everyone's incentives so they can focus on providing cost-effective care and superior outcomes.

Who We Are

St. Luke's Health Partners

- is a financially and clinically integrated network of more than 2,200 employed and independent healthcare providers;
- is a wholly owned subsidiary of St. Luke's Health System, the only Idaho-based not-for-profit health system;

- is financially accountable for the health of a defined population of people as well as the clinical performance of the network;
- follows the practice of accountable care to manage or prevent serious health problems such as high blood pressure, obesity, prediabetes, and uncontrolled diabetes, thereby reducing hospital readmissions, emergency department visits, and additional physician visits;
- uses data gathered from clinic records to share best practices and follow the lead of providers achieving the best results for their patients; and
- features care coordinators who stay in close contact with patients to talk about concerns such as medication, diet, sleep, or their doctor's instructions.

St. Luke's Health Partners plays a large role in the health system's ability to deliver coordinated, affordable, accessible care. Through this network, clinicians and insurance providers work together to raise standards of care and lower overall costs. At the end of 2017, SLHP was accountable for the health of more than 161,000 people.

References

Barker, E. 2017. "How Consolidation Is Reshaping Healthcare." *HFMA Newsletter*. Published April 20. www.hfma.org/Leadership/E-Bulletins/2017/April/How_Consolidation_Is_Reshaping_Health_Care/.

BusinessDictionary.com. 2018. "Transformational Change." Accessed July 13. www.businessdictionary.com/definition/transformational-change.html.

Christensen, C. 2013. *The Innovator's Solution*. Brighton, MA: Harvard Business Publishing.

———. 1997. *The Innovator's Dilemma*. Brighton, MA: Harvard Business Publishing.

Cox, M. 2018. "Hospital–Physician Alignment Models: An Evolving Lexicon." *MGMA Insight Article*. Accessed March 7. www.mgma.com/resources/resources/business-strategy/physician-hospital-alignment-models-an-evolving-l.

Gamble, M. 2014. "The St. Luke's Antitrust Case: 10 Things You Should Know." *Becker's Hospital Review*. Published January 30. www.beckershospitalreview.com/legal-regulatory-issues/the-st-luke-s-antitrust-case-10-things-to-know.html.

Hyde, S. 2015. Keynote presentation at the Idaho Hospital Association Spring Meeting, June, McCall, Idaho.

Institute for Healthcare Improvement (IHI). 2018. "Leading Population Health Transformation." Accessed March 17. www.ihi.org/education/InPersonTraining/Leading-Population-Health-Transformation/Pages/default.aspx.

Kotter, J. 2012. *Leading Change*. Brighton, MA: Harvard Business Publishing.

Leavitt, M. 2015. Presentation at the Idaho Healthcare Summit, May 27, Fort Hall, Idaho.

Nynon, L. 2014. "Populations, Population Health, and the Evolution of Population Management: Making Sense of the Terminology in US Health Care Today." Institute for Healthcare Improvement. Published March 19. www.ihi.org/communities/blogs/population-health-population-management-terminology-in-us-health-care.

Pate, D. 2018. Interview with T. Farnsworth, March 22.

———. 2017a. Interview with T. Farnsworth, November 10.

———. 2017b. Interview with T. Farnsworth, September 27.

———. 2016. "St. Luke's CEO Dr. David Pate: The Journey to Becoming a 'Top 15 Health System.'" *Becker's Hospital Review*. Published April 27. www.beckershospitalreview.com/hospital-management-administration/st-luke-s-ceo-dr-david-pate-the-journey-to-becoming-a-top-15-health-system.html.

———. 2012. "St. Luke's Health System and SelectHealth Innovate with Breakthrough Strategic Alliance." St. Luke's blog. Published September 4. www.stlukesonline.org/blogs/st-lukes/news-and-community/2012/sep/st-lukes-health-system-and-selecthealth-innovate-with-breakthrough-strategic-alliance.

Smith, M., and P. Keckley. 2017. "Total Cost of Care: Key Considerations for Hospitals and Health Systems." *Hospitals and Health Networks*. Published September 13. www.hhnmag.com/articles/8528-total-cost-of-care-key-considerations-for-hospitals-and-health-systems.

St. Luke's. 2017. *2016–17 Health System Annual Report*. Accessed August 3, 2018. www.stlukesonline.org/about-st-lukes/annual-reports/annual-report-2016-2017.

St. Luke's Health Partners (SLHP). 2018a. "About Us." Accessed August 3. https://stlukeshealthpartners.org/about-us/.

———. 2018b. "For Employers." Accessed August 3. https://stlukeshealthpartners.org/for-employers/.

Valentine, S., and G. Masters. 2013. "For Board Members Only: Ten Trends That Will Drive Healthcare in 2013 (and Beyond)." *The Governance Institute's E-Briefings.* Published January. https://c.ymcdn.com/sites/www.governanceinstitute.com/resource/collection/14082583-FA83-45CD-9EFA-D9F250246B38/EBriefings_V10N1_Jan2013-AG.pdf.

CHAPTER 5

LEADERSHIP AND MANAGING CHANGE

Important Terms

- Change participants
- Change process
- Competencies
- Emotional intelligence
- Leadership
- Moving forward
- Refreezing
- Resistance to change
- Stakeholder
- Unfreezing

Learning Objectives

After reading this chapter, you will be able to do the following:

- ➤ Understand the evolution of leadership theory
- ➤ Identify leadership models
- ➤ Understand the reasons change is essential in leadership
- ➤ Understand the motivation behind resistance to change
- ➤ Apply a leadership model to a factual situation

Case Study: Resisting Change

Craig Lockhart needed to get Mariana Buchanan on board and "join the team." How could he convince this "old-timer" it was time to change?

Craig had been the practice manager at the High Country Primary Healthcare Clinics (HCPHC), a consortium of six clinics that serves five counties in Colorado, for three months. HCPHC had hired him because he had an MBA in health services management and because he had several years of experience with a practice in another state. The clinic physicians had encouraged him to make the practice more efficient, including changing the patient scheduling process. Currently, each practice location manages the schedules of the providers in their respective offices. Part of the interview process included an extended conversation about improved efficiencies for the practice, particularly the need for a centralized call center to schedule patient appointments. New reimbursement models and rising operating costs had sent the physician-owners in search of ways to cut costs and improve overall efficiency. All the physicians agreed that Craig's efficiency measures should align with their clinic mission: "Be responsible to the patient, be responsible to the staff, and provide excellent primary care for the people of Colorado." Craig had started his job with enthusiasm and confidence that he could help make the call center a reality and create efficiencies that achieved the physicians' vision of keeping pace with technology and meeting increased patient demand in the market.

Once Craig had set up his office, he personally met with the six clinic office managers. He told them he was there to improve the clinics, and he began to list the changes he would make to bring this about. For starters, at least one person from each office would be transferred to the new call center. And, because of efficiencies associated with centralizing the scheduling process, at least one and perhaps two members of the current staff would be laid off. However, one clinic manager would become the call center manager to avoid laying off any of the clinic office managers. In addition, two of the clinics would be consolidated, and computer networks would link the call center to the offices and produce the patient appointment schedule for each provider in their respective office. Craig concluded his meetings by instructing the managers on other efficiencies he wanted *them* to put into place. He was surprised the managers asked few questions, but he assumed they were on board and in agreement with him. He followed up with them via e-mail, instructing the managers to meet as a group every two weeks to move forward with his assignments. He told them he would provide a timeline for transferring the schedulers and consolidating the two offices after they identified who was to be transferred. Craig did not attend any of the clinic managers' follow-up meetings.

To date, some three months later, none of his recommendations related to improved efficiencies had been implemented, nor had the office managers identified any of the individuals to be transferred. Craig knew that one of the managers, Mariana Buchanan, had been negative about his ideas. In fact, she had often called the other office managers to complain about him and his efficiency plan. One of these office managers had met with Craig to express her concern about the situation. The office manager explained, "Mariana is starting to get on my nerves. Every time we office managers get together, she just complains all the time. I'm beginning to dread talking with her."

Mariana had earned an associate's degree in medical assisting 15 years ago, and she had been a clinic office manager for more than 20 years. She liked to run the office the way she had been taught at the local technical college. "If it isn't broken, don't fix it" was her motto. She knew that Craig's plan was designed to make the entire practice more efficient by improving how the clinics functioned, but she did not understand why he wanted to change everything she had been doing for so many years. He had never asked for her opinion, even though she had a lot of experience and on-the-job training. Furthermore, she knew what worked. She was exasperated by the decision that the practice needed a central patient database and central scheduling system. What was wrong with the current system, in which each clinic followed its own protocol regarding patient files and scheduling? Why change what works?

Introduction

The sine qua non of leadership is change. What is the purpose of leadership if not to move a group of people or organization toward a goal or objective? Most often, this arises in the context of something new, such as a new strategic direction, or as in Craig's situation in the case study, a new way of managing part of a business. Note that "leadership" can apply to a small part of a larger operation or to a whole mega system's strategic plan. The underlying concept is that the organization in question is about to change something about itself, and it is the function of leadership to make it happen. **Leadership** is critical to any endeavor that seeks to bring change to an organization.

Leadership
The act of engaging a group of people, often within an organization, to set and achieve goals.

Unplanned Change and Planned New Direction

Sometimes change is unexpected and, therefore, unplanned. For example, Hurricane Katrina slammed into New Orleans in August 2005. The Category 5 hurricane caused the city's levee system to fail, which spilled flood waters as high as 13 feet through various neighborhoods. The patients and remaining staff at Charity Hospital experienced a loss of electrical power and a lack of food and water, rising flood waters, and a dire shortage of medications. Physicians and nurses had to work in those conditions as they provided medical care to 200 patients while waiting for help to arrive (Fink 2009).

The situation at Charity Hospital is an example of unplanned change, triggered by a cataclysmic event that happened *to* a healthcare organization. It also is a story of the leadership necessary to adapt to dramatic new circumstances in order to care for patients. The aftermath of Hurricane Katrina was an extraordinary situation. Most of the change a healthcare manager experiences is change brought about because of a planned new direction—change that is contemplated. In this kind of change environment, employees of an organization work to implement changes that people in authority (or the team?) already determined fit with the organization's mission and purpose and will make the organization better.

The *how* we lead or advance organizational change has been the focus of practitioners and scholars for decades, if not centuries. There are many theoretical models intended to help guide managers in their efforts to lead change. The next section will provide a brief history of the evolution of leadership models.

Evolution of Leadership Theories

Leadership has a long history as a topic of study. Over time, the concept of leadership has evolved. Early thinking about leadership assumed that it was something into which one was born, when a member of the nobility or upper class was given both title and "leadership" by divine right. It has evolved into the contemporary thinking that leadership is relational, in the sense that it focuses on how the leader relates to others, as we shall see later in the chapter. The word *leadership* itself stems from fourteenth-century English, when it referred to political power (Greenwood 1993). Since then, the definition broadened, and in the early part of the twentieth century came to mean "the preeminence of one or a few individuals in a group in the process of control of societal phenomena" (Bass 1981, 7).

Today, leadership is primarily seen as a matter of fostering engaging relationships with peers. One of the leading scholars of leadership, John Gardner, defines the term this way: "The process of persuasion or example by which an individual (or leadership team) induces a group to pursue objectives held by the leader or shared by the leader and his or her followers" (Gardner 1990, 1). Rost says it is "an influence relationship among leaders and their collaborators who intend real changes that reflect their mutual purposes" (Rost 1993, 91).

Let us look more closely at how our view of leadership has evolved since the 1900s. Note that many of these theories overlapped as the prevailing theory of one era evolved into the next.

The *Great Man* theory, first proposed in the late nineteenth century and popular until the early parts of the twentieth, theorizes that leaders are born, not made; that leaders have natural abilities of power and influence. Next came the *Trait* theory, which was prevalent from early in the twentieth century through the mid-1940s; it suggests that a leader has superior qualities—different traits than his or her followers—which give him or her a natural ability to lead. This was followed by the *Behavioral* theory, which was popular from the mid-twentieth century until the 1980s and hypothesized that there was one best way to lead and defined leaders as people who expressed a high concern for others. The Behavioral theory was mostly contemporaneous with the *Situational Contingency* theory, which suggested leaders will act differently depending on the situation and that it is the situation that determines who will emerge as a leader. The *Influence* theory was popular from about the mid-1920s

Exhibit 5.1 Prominent Leadership Theories

Theory	Description
Great Man	• Mid-1800s to early 1900s • Leaders born, not made
Trait	• 1904–1947 • Leaders have special qualities
Behavioral	• 1950s to early 1980s • Effective leaders express concern for others
Situational Contingency	• 1950s to 1960s • Leadership behaviors are different for different situations
Influence	• Mid-1920s to 1977 • Leadership is a social exchange
Reciprocal	• 1978 to present • Leadership is relational, shared process
Chaos or Systems	• 1990 to present • Systems thinking is emphasis
Authentic Leadership	• 1990 to present • Leadership is valued and purpose driven

Source: Adapted from Komives, Lucas, and McMahon (2013).

until the late 1970s and observed that leadership is an influence or social exchange process. This was followed by the *Reciprocal* theory, which proposes that leadership is a relational process and an outcome of participants' interactions when striving toward a common goal. This theory remains significant today, along with *Authentic Leadership Approaches*, which state that leadership is genuine and transparent; that authenticity emerges between leaders and participants (Komives, Lucas, and McMahon 2013). Exhibit 5.1 provides a robust list of the theories, their major tenets, and scientific criticisms.

Today's predominant thought about leadership—that it is experienced through genuine and transparent relationships—is the product of these preceding models. Let us now discuss three contemporary perspectives on leadership in detail.

Three Contemporary Concepts of Leadership

Management research has revealed a number of different methods for leading, each of which has its own terminology. The following contemporary models were developed by scholars following extensive studies of leadership practices that the evidence indicates actually work and produce desired results.

The Leadership Challenge

Kouzes and Posner define leadership as "mobiliz[ing] others to want to struggle to get extraordinary things done in organizations" (Kouzes and Posner 2017, 24). Their study of leadership suggests that everyone can be a leader by following a model they call The Leadership Challenge. Through years of surveying leaders from all walks of life, they identified five exemplary leadership practices (Kouzes and Posner 2017, 24):

- Model the Way
- Inspire a Shared Vision
- Challenge the Process
- Enable Other to Act
- Encourage the Heart

Kouzes and Posner have suggested concrete behaviors that put their leadership concepts into practice. For each "Leadership Practice" point, they offer two specific behaviors that will help the leader develop positive relationships and become more effective. Those ten suggestions are as follows (Kouzes and Posner 2017, 24):

- Clarify values by finding your voice and affirming shared values.
- Set the example by aligning actions with shared values.
- Envision the future by imagining exciting and ennobling possibilities.
- Enlist others in a common vision by appealing to shared aspirations.
- Search for opportunities by seizing the initiative and looking outward for innovative ways to improve.
- Experiment and take risks by consistently generating small wins and learning from experience.
- Foster collaboration by building trust and facilitating relationships.
- Strengthen others by increasing self-determination and developing competence.
- Recognize contributions by showing appreciation for individual excellence.
- Celebrate the values and victories by creating a spirit of community.

Note that the Leadership Challenge falls squarely into the contemporary theory of relation-based leadership. Leaders are not the "commanders" of old, but rather peers who develop relationships based on their own character and integrity, which helps motivate others in the "struggle for shared aspirations."

The foundation to this model is credibility. The leader must "walk the talk" in making things happen. There is no substitute for genuineness in all aspects of life, but most particularly in leadership. You cannot expect others to follow your lead if you cannot model the appropriate behavior in front of colleagues and coworkers. The top characteristic people seek in their leaders is honesty (Kouzes and Posner 2017).

Another element of the Leadership Challenge is understanding the importance of "team." The leaders Kouzes and Posner interviewed during their research have, over time, consistently reported the importance of functioning as a group, rather than as an individual hero. Leaders mobilize others to achieve the tasks at hand (Kouzes and Posner 2017). This concept is found in nearly every leadership model used today: The essence of leadership is about motivating and inspiring others to achieve the objective, whether it be a new patient scheduling system or building a new hospital.

Goleman's Primal Leadership Model

Goleman's Model of Primal Leadership relies on the concept of **emotional intelligence**. Emotional intelligence is defined as "the ability to recognize, understand and manage our own emotions [and] recognize, understand and influence the emotions of others" (Institute for Health and Human Potential 2017). A more comprehensive definition comes from those who developed the term, Salovey and Mayer, whose research indicated emotional intelligence comes from five domains: self-awareness, managing emotions, motivating oneself, recognizing emotions in others, and building engaging relationships (Salovey and Mayer 1990).

Emotional intelligence
The ability to identify and manage your own emotions and the emotions of others.

In their book *Primal Leadership*, Goleman, Boyatzis, and McKee (2002) assert that emotional intelligence can (and should) be exercised by applying different leadership styles. The style of leadership to be applied would depend on the overall situation as assessed by the "emotionally intelligent" leader. The importance of self-awareness cannot be overstated in this context. One cannot adjust styles of leadership without first knowing fellow team members well and understanding how they interact with their surroundings. Leaders should, at varying times, be visionary, coaching, affiliative, democratic, and, on occasion, pacesetting and commanding (Goleman, Boyatzis, and McKee 2002). This might be considered something of a theoretical hybrid, as the leader varies his or her relationship with peers based on the situation in which the group finds itself.

A *visionary* leader moves people toward shared dreams when change requires a new direction. A *coaching* leader connects an employee's own aspiration with organizational goals by helping the employee improve performance. An *affiliative* leader creates harmony in a team by connecting team members with each other. A *democratic* leader builds consensus by obtaining input, and ultimately commitment, from employees.

Less frequently, one might be a *pacesetting* leader who sets challenging goals of high-quality results from a motivated team. Likewise, on rare occasions the leader might be called upon to employ a *commanding* style, which gives clear direction to calm fears in a crisis or in a turnaround situation (Goleman, Boyatzis, and McKee 2002).

Applying any of these leadership methodologies requires understanding one's own emotions and the emotions of others, harnessing those emotions, and linking them to motivating team members to engage in meeting a common challenge. Just the act of thinking about the application of leadership models gives rise to the question of how to approach and engage others in moving the organization forward (Goleman 2014).

One view of how this might work is depicted in exhibit 5.2, which offers a framework of emotional competencies. Note how the concepts of "recognition" and "regulation" are assessed in a dichotomous framework referencing "self" and "others." This is a handy reference tool to assess what kind of leadership style to employ. It also serves as a guide for

Exhibit 5.2 A Framework of Competencies

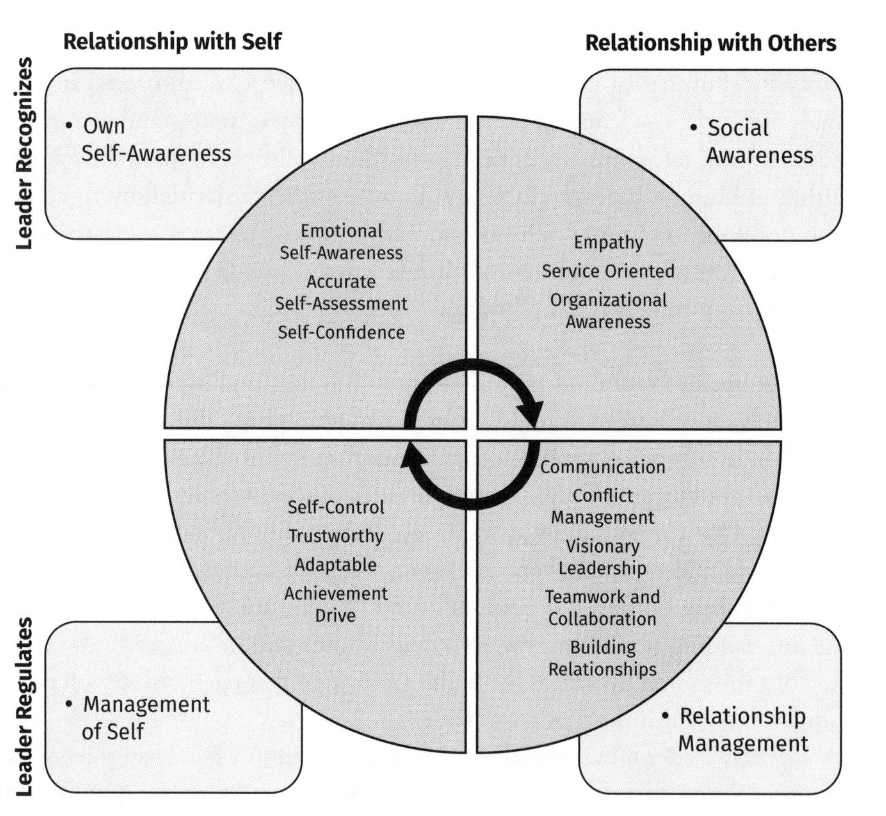

Source: Adapted from Charniss and Goleman (2001, 29).

assessing one's level of self-awareness and ability to manage one's feelings (Charniss and Goleman 2001).

Healthcare Services Competency Models

Focusing on the notion that leadership is about behavior and interaction with other people, many healthcare management experts promote leadership models based on **competencies**. This approach stems from the belief that knowledge about the healthcare industry alone is not sufficient to be a successful healthcare manager. Further, a "competency" by itself is not the same as leadership. It is one thing to know how to perform certain discrete acts that qualify one as "competent," such as creating a return-on-investment analysis. But the skill to develop genuine, transparent relationships that empower colleagues to contribute to the success of a shared organizational vision is a different type of competency altogether. That explains why many graduate and undergraduate health administration programs have adopted competency models that include multiple dimensions of assessment as a way of measuring skill development in their students. In addition, several professional groups and scholars have developed a handful of "competency models" specifically for healthcare.

Competencies
A set of professional and personal skills, knowledge, values, and traits that guide a leader's performance, behavior, interactions, and decisions.

The HLA Leadership Model

The Healthcare Leadership Alliance (HLA), composed of major healthcare-related associations in the United States, promulgates a model referred to as the "HLA Leadership Competency Directory." Initially completed in 2005, it focuses on the following domains:

1. Communication and relationship management
2. Leadership
3. Professionalism
4. Knowledge of the healthcare environment
5. Business skills and knowledge

Each of the HLA domains contains several "clusters" that may be considered subsets of the domain. For example, the "communication and relationship management domain" has a cluster for "relationship management," one for "communication skills," and another for "facilitation and negotiation." Then, within each of those clusters is a group of competencies that aims to measure an individual's level of competence in that area (HLA 2017; Stefl 2008).

The IHF Leadership Model

Similarly, the International Hospital Federation (IHF), working with the American College of Healthcare Executives and other hospital associations from around the world, published *Leadership Competencies for Healthcare Services Managers* (IHF 2015). The IHF model focuses on the following domains, which are similar to the HLA directory model:

1. Communication and relationship management
2. Professional and social responsibility
3. Health and the healthcare environment
4. Business
5. Leadership

Within each of these domains are skills and behaviors that an effective healthcare services leader would be expected to master (IHF 2015).

These leading models are both widely used for leadership development in healthcare. While one can see the overlap in the domains, there are nuanced differences between them at the individual competency level. Those competencies, however, remain more alike than different. The important characteristic in any competency model is how a given competency can be assessed. The choice of a competency model is a judgment call, and while people can—and do—disagree about them, each model is a useful guide that can help leaders be more effective. These scientific underpinnings of any model relies on informed, but subjective, judgments that do not come together as an exact science. Models can help provide structure enabling the leader to be more effective, but the science of human relations is amorphous and thus we lack perfection, but attain progress.

The NCHL Leadership Model

The third major leadership competency model takes a different tack from the HLA and IHF models. The National Center for Healthcare Leadership (NCHL) Leadership Competency Model consists of three domains and 26 behavioral and technical competencies. "The three domains—transformation, execution, people—capture the complexity and dynamic quality of the health leader's role" (NCHL 2006, 14), as shown in exhibit 5.3.

By focusing on the three domains, the NCHL model attempts to recognize both intellectual and social skills. Some individuals are better at "soft" skills, also referred to as "people" skills, while others are more oriented toward quantitative thinking. Note that "execution" sometimes blends elements from the other two domains; thus, "collaboration" can be considered an amalgamation of "team leadership" from the "people" domain and "achievement orientation" from "transformation." The NCHL model goes beyond suggesting that one should attain some minimum level of proficiency in each competency.

Exhibit 5.3
NCHL Competency Model 3.0

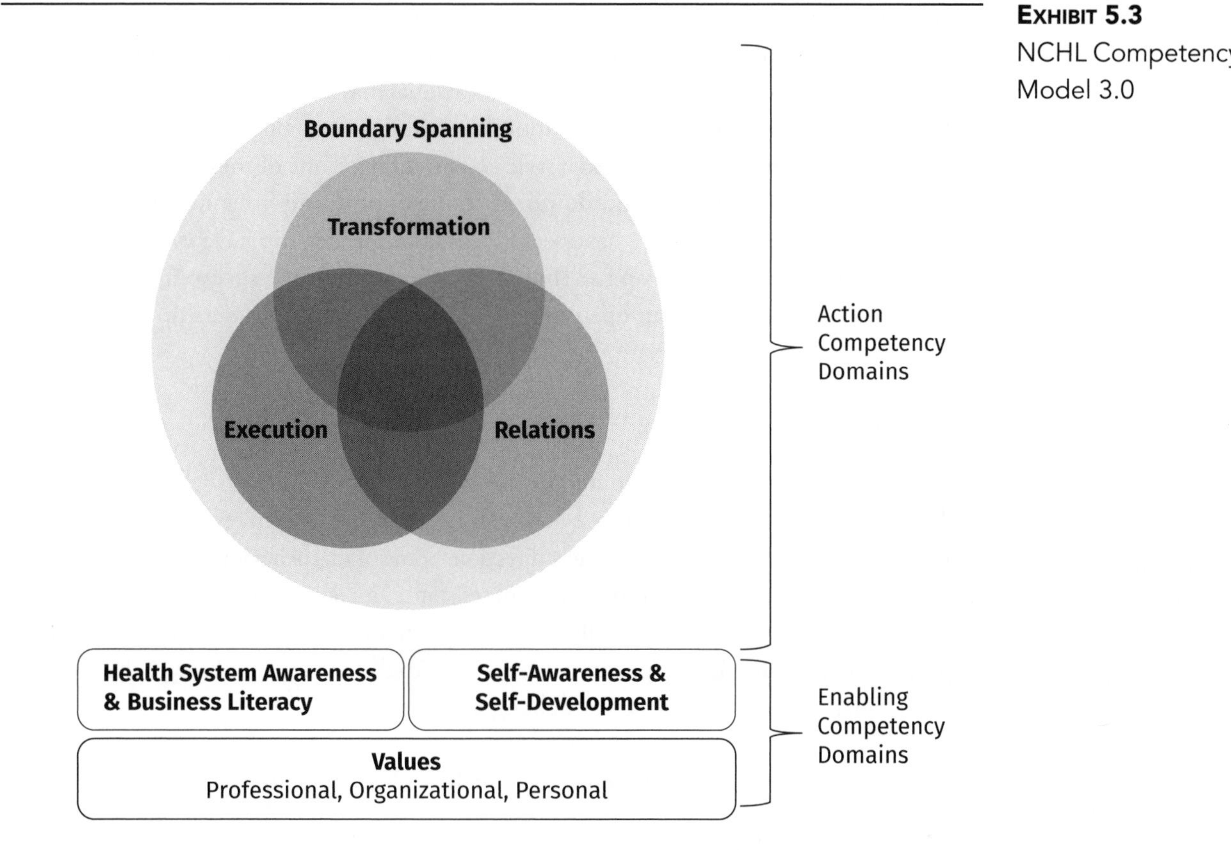

Source: Reprinted with permission from National Center for Healthcare Leadership.

In 2018, the NCHL updated its model as shown in exhibit 5.3. Note that several domain categories have been added under "Enabling Competency Domains," and a new one called Boundary Spanning in the "Action Competency Domains." The concept of "enabling" competencies points out the fundamental need for managers (and other leaders) to be value-centered and highly self-aware. And a competent person, from this model, would be looking across the boundaries searching for ways to expand their contribution to the enterprise.

The NCHL model establishes identifiable competencies to assess leaders at all levels of their career development (NCHL 2006). Although the Leadership Challenge and Primal Leadership models implicitly expect varying degrees of proficiencies based on career status, the NCHL model is explicit in identifying levels of competency at various career levels.

Using the Models

Beyond abstract leadership models, whatever their foundation, leaders who aspire to be effective in bringing change to an organization need to understand the "how" of engaging in effective and meaningful relationships, which all the leadership models describe. The benefit of understanding one or more leadership models is that they serve as a guide to inform and amplify leadership efforts. Thus, whatever leadership "model" an individual may consciously choose to embrace, he or she will still need to bring those relationship-building concepts to life in the workplace.

Even after you have developed a style consistent with one of these models and effectively integrated it into your work, do not miss the opportunity to continue reading and learning about leadership. As we have seen, ideas about leadership have evolved over time and no doubt will continue to do so. Thus, it is imperative for the successful leader to stay abreast of new thinking with an open mind to new ideas on how leadership works.

Resistance to Change

Change participants The staff members whose work behaviors may be affected by any implemented changes.

Resistance to change Change participants' hesitation or refusal to comply with the vision for the future and management's attempts at carrying out that vision.

Unfreezing Reducing the forces that are keeping an organization in its current state.

Moving forward Implementing the managed change.

Refreezing Stabilizing the forces that have brought about a newly implemented change so they become part of the organization.

As we saw with Mariana in the case study, there will always be those who resist change. While leaders are busy attempting to improve an organization, some employees will lag behind—or worse, actively work to undermine the new direction. Some of this behavior is just human nature. This section will examine some of the sources of resistance. It takes multiple people in an organization to implement change successfully. How leaders envision change, how managers and staff implement it, and how **change participants** respond to the change all influence the outcome.

Leaders initiate and implement changes that may be

- procedures designed for efficiency, such as Craig's plan in the case study;
- responses to problems in the workplace;
- actions to improve healthcare delivery;
- adaptations to environmental or technical changes outside the organization; or
- responses to ensure a good fit with the organizational mission.

Craig has a problem to address at the Colorado health clinics, and it goes beyond getting Mariana "on board." Craig is responsible for implementing the efficiency changes successfully, and he is not succeeding. None of his ideas have been implemented in the clinics. Mariana's **resistance to change** has successfully delayed Craig's plans.

Lewin (1947) introduced the concept of resistance to change in social science. He proposed that successful change requires three conditions: **unfreezing**, **moving forward**, and **refreezing**. Unfreezing refers to reducing the forces keeping an organization in its current state. Moving forward refers to implementing the change (e.g., Craig's implementation of the new patient database). Refreezing refers to stabilizing the forces again and making the newly implemented change part of the organization (Lewin 1947). Craig is caught in the unfreezing stage; Mariana's resistance shows that Craig's pressure for change has not significantly altered her desire to maintain the current condition.

According to Lewin (1947), our understanding of an employee's behavior rests upon our understanding of that person and the environment in which he or she operates. Although the **change process** may affect the person and the work environment, the manager has more control over the environment and can set the stage for effective change by assessing and altering the environment. Lewin introduced the term "resistance to change" to describe a condition that affects managers and employees (Burnes 2007). Change occurs when the driving forces for change increase and the resistance forces against change decrease. A manager may be able to create an effective change implementation plan by properly identifying the driving and restraining forces for change.

Change process
The process whereby managed change is envisioned and implemented (successfully or unsuccessfully) in an organization.

The successful implementation of change depends on a manager's ability to reduce the resistance to change. Questions to ask to assess the success of an implemented change include: "How did we introduce the change ideas?" "What has been the response of those affected by the change?" "What, if anything, should we do differently?" A lack of effective communication is apparent between Craig and the office managers in the three clinics. In addition, he has not considered the reasons for the resistance to his efficiency plan. Did he introduce his ideas well? Has he identified the driving and restraining forces for change? Did he involve **stakeholders** when he developed the plans for change in the first place?

Stakeholder
An individual, group, or entity that has an interest in organizational success.

Several of the reasons in the following box may explain Mariana's resistance to Craig's plan. She has worked at the primary care clinic for more than 20 years, and this tenure affords her a place of honor. Craig has introduced changes without consulting her, which may cause Mariana to fear losing that place of honor, or *losing face*, reason one in Kanter's (2001) list. In addition, Mariana was not part of the decision-making process and may fear a loss of control (reason two), and the change plan involves performing work in a different way than it is currently being performed (reason five).

⊛ TEN CLASSIC REASONS PEOPLE RESIST CHANGE

The following is Kanter's (2001) list of classic reasons people resist change. When confronting change, some people may be concerned about some or all of these factors:

1. **Loss of face:** concern that they will lose their place of honor and a degree of dignity.
2. **Loss of control:** concern that they are not part of the decision-making process and are losing power.
3. **Excess uncertainty:** concern they may not know what is going on or what will happen next, and they may feel unsure of what this change means.
4. **Surprise, surprise:** no advance warning and little to no chance to prepare themselves for the change.

(continued)

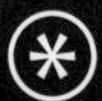

TEN CLASSIC REASONS PEOPLE RESIST CHANGE *(CONTINUED)*

5. **The "difference" effect:** change does not fit with the current way of doing work. The change presents unfamiliar challenges to the way work is currently performed.
6. **"Can I do it":** concern about their competence once the change is implemented.
7. **Ripple effects:** changes and disruptions to their other work activities and the negative effect the change may have on these tasks.
8. **More work:** concern they do not have the time to learn new procedures or tasks, and the change may increase their workloads.
9. **Past resentments:** memories of unresolved negative experiences with those involved in implementing the change. They resist the change because of their resentments toward the people involved in the process.
10. **Real threats:** Individuals may perceive the change to be a real threat that will result in real losses to them as the participants of change.

Source: Kanter (2001, 256–57).

The Leadership Challenge: Applying Kouzes and Posner's Lessons to the Colorado Clinics

The outcome of the case at the beginning of the chapter would have been vastly different had Craig actively engaged in leading the managers instead of merely giving them a series of directives and expecting something to happen. Note how using Kouzes and Posner's (2017) leadership model would help Craig overcome Mariana's resistance to change and would positively affect events at HCPHC.

The owners of the clinics (i.e., the physicians) wanted to respond effectively to several changes in the healthcare environment: new reimbursement methods, market demands, and technological opportunities. They directed Craig to implement efficient office management protocols. However, Mariana's comments that she did not understand why Craig wanted to change everything indicate that the physicians and Craig may be the only ones in the clinics who understand why the changes are needed. The physicians wanted to purchase new equipment to, in effect, keep the practice current and competitive. Simply put, a vision motivated the change at the higher administrative levels. This is managed change; a contemplated new direction or, in this case, a contemplated new way of doing things. Craig is trying to initiate change designed to help the clinics become better and more efficient. However, he is experiencing resistance.

Communication Style and Relationship Building

First, note that Craig's initial communication with the office managers had nothing to do with HCPHC's mission or vision. He *told them* he was there to improve the clinics and informed them of changes that would bring this about. He did not indicate *why* the changes were necessary, nor *how* they would improve HCPHC's ability to fulfill its mission of providing high-quality primary care.

Craig's first step here should not have been so directive, but more consultative. His task in this scenario is not to give direction, but to establish a positive relationship with the office managers predicated on genuineness and transparency. Inviting the office managers to help him contemplate *how* to achieve the ends contemplated by the physician-owners of the clinic by focusing on the HCPHC mission would have gone a long way toward building a positive working relationship with the managers and engaged them in the process of change. Perhaps more importantly, such a dialogue might have generated creative ideas helpful to bringing about the change sought by the physician-owners of the clinics.

Failure to Create Shared Vision

Craig's second mistake was failing to create a shared vision by imagining ennobling possibilities or enlisting the office managers in a common objective. He merely said, in effect, "Here are some changes we are going to make." In approaching the conversation in that way, Craig denied the opportunity for the office managers to claim any ownership in the new direction; he did not let them share in the excitement the changes would bring. Collins and Porras (1991) also discuss the importance of creating a shared organizational vision. They recommend a vision framework that encompasses a firm's guiding philosophy (i.e., its values, beliefs, and purpose) and a tangible image (i.e., a vivid description of the outcome). The final product of the firm's vision is therefore clear and shared. Craig's current problem has resulted from the absence of a clear, shared objective. A critical factor for successful change is consistent and clear communication of the vision to everyone responsible for making the change happen. Engaging the managers to help plan the clinic's changes would have helped them share the vision by cultivating their ownership of a new call center and centralized scheduling system.

Build Confidence Through Small Wins

Third, in challenging the process Craig certainly had some ideas to improve efficiencies in the organization, and he took the initiative to move them forward. However, as a new leader he had not yet earned the confidence of the office managers; participating in their routine meetings and showing support would have earned him small victories with them, which would then have helped move his project along. He should have helped the managers learn about the technology required for a central call center. This small win would have engendered their confidence in Craig as well as their own self-confidence. This would then have helped the managers successfully implement, and continue sharing, the plan to create a new scheduling system through the central call center.

Failure to Understand Managers' Competencies

Fourth, while one could argue Craig enabled others to act because he gave them instructions and then got out of their way, by not attending the managers' regular meetings, he did not *foster collaboration* among them. Indeed, his absence enabled Mariana to complain openly about the new direction and foster seeds of discontent. Further, Craig was unaware that he was asking office managers to do things they might not have done before, such as re-assign staff or teach others new scheduling templates. He did not consider what competencies they needed to transfer people, lay people off, and perhaps assume new responsibilities, such as training staff members on a new scheduling system or evaluating their performance using a new system. Although Craig's absence from the managers' meetings might have been perceived as empowering them to act, in fact he also created an expectation that they move ahead with the changes even though they were not certain about *how* to do some of the things he wanted. Again, Craig's role should have been more like that of a coach or teacher: Assess what the managers need to learn to be successful and then help them develop those competencies. By leading in this fashion, not only would the managers learn the tools needed and become less fearful of change, they would also evolve into a higher-functioning team.

Failure to Create Sense of Commitment

Finally, Craig never got far along or close enough to *encourage the heart.* Because he omitted so many crucial leadership steps, he never had the opportunity to recognize individual achievement or celebrate community values. Had Craig engaged in a meaningful and authentic way with the office managers he would have had the opportunity to help them understand the shared mission and vision of the physician owners; he would have had the chance to engage them in a common aspiration; and he would have helped them overcome fear by helping them take risks to learn new tools and in the process strengthened their mutual confidence in him and in one another. If he had done these things, he would now be in the position to recognize the managers' contributions and reward excellence in performance. In short, he would have created a common bond and a positive community spirit that would have been uplifting for the managers.

The Alternative Approach

So what should Craig have done? First, he should have been more consultative when he initially met with the office managers. He should have explained the realities of the current healthcare market, including how technology was an emerging tool in physician practice management. He should have explained how a new central call center would improve patients' access to care by maximizing provider time in the clinic. He could also have pointed out that the new model would spare office managers from having to respond to physician preferences about their individual schedules. But most important, Craig should have asked the office managers their opinions on how to accomplish the goals set by the physicians; he should have given them the chance to ask questions about the need for change. He should have begun the process of coaching the managers about the "why" and given them a chance to fully understand the vision.

Having done that, then Craig should have invited the office managers' ideas on how best to staff the new central call center and manage the relationship between the center and the provider offices. This would have given the managers ownership of "how" the plan would be implemented. Once that plan became theirs, then Craig's job would be to encourage and provide the managers the competencies they would need to succeed.

If he had followed this approach, Craig would have been in a far superior position to demonstrate the new call center's advantages. There would, of course, still be changes that some employees would find difficult, but overall the clinic managers would more readily accept the process if the benefits had been made clear to them. In this way, they all would have a *shared vision* within an empowering culture that rewards initiative and produces small wins along the way.

Similarity of Leadership Models

You probably noticed some overlap or similarity among the three leadership models. Although some of their terminology differs, the skills they describe are the same. For example, had Craig followed the principles developed in the Leadership Challenge, he would also have demonstrated several of the competencies from the NCHL model, such as engaging in a higher level of communication (under "execution") and relationship building (under "relations"). He also would have engaged his team to focus on achievement orientation (under "transformation"). Had he actively empowered the managers to act, he would have provided them with lessons in self-development (under "relations") and helped them achieve greater levels of self-confidence (also under "relations").

Similarly, had Craig followed Leadership Challenge principles, he would have been demonstrating several similar competencies from the HLA model. In establishing an initial relationship with the managers, Craig would have been demonstrating "Communication and Relationship Management" from the HLA model. Helping the managers understand *why* the change was necessary comes from the "Knowledge of the healthcare environment" component of the HLA model, while engaging the managers in a shared aspiration by inviting their participation would fall under the "Leadership" component of HLA.

The larger point here is that the leadership models have several of the same basic elements. One may vary in emphasis and style of development from another, but transparency and integrity are at the root of all the models.

A leader's effectiveness is largely measured in terms of behaviors, not charisma (Kouzes and Posner 2017). Again, these behaviors may be classified several ways. But regardless of the model a leader embraces, he needs, for example, to be competent in communication skills to inspire a shared vision. In examining Craig's case, we used the Leadership Challenge philosophy to demonstrate a better way of handling the situation. One might easily have used either of the other two models to make the same demonstration.

Adapting any of these well-established, research-based models will help future leaders develop a style of their own. Aspiring leaders might be well advised to learn one of the approaches well and cultivate their own sense of how to lead based on the research. In addition, one should emulate good leaders by cultivating a sense of lifelong learning to continually discover new ideas about how leadership works, thereby achieving exceptional results for the organization as well as the people we hope to lead.

Leadership is a fine-tuned balance of skills, behavior, and art (Battistella et al. 2007). While no leadership model is perfect for every manager in every situation, together the models can serve as guides for healthcare managers. Healthcare is in great need of effective leaders. If not you, who?

Solidifying the Changes

Let us assume that Craig, in fact, followed one of the change models previously discussed. He sought and obtained buy-in from the managers by asking questions; he solicited advice about how to proceed; and he created a shared vision and got the managers to collaborate with him and with each other in making the call center a reality. Then what happens? Does everyone celebrate the successful change and return to work? How should Craig go about consolidating the gains they have made while creating a more efficient medical practice?

At this point, Craig will need to understand that resistance to change is always waiting to reassert itself (Kotter 1996). Mariana has not changed her spots; the new process has altered her way of doing things and she may remain unhappy about it. She may mute her vocal complaints, but she can be expected to drag her feet and remain uncooperative with things like new weekly reports that need to be generated as part of the new system.

So what should Craig do to ensure the new call center and the new way of scheduling appointments is a success? He should start by recognizing that this change is the first step in a transformation that will affect everyone in the organization. The doctors and physician assistants likely will be pressured to see more patients in light of the new scheduling model. That means the nurses will also be busier tracking test results and patients. Likewise, the medical assistants will be busier taking patient histories at check-in. Some of these people will be celebrating the change because they value the improvement, but they also will be tired from all the work associated with completely changing the scheduling model. They may say things like, "Whew, I'm glad that's done; we can take a breather." Others, like Mariana, will celebrate the change because it can be the moment to say, "Okay, we can slow down now." The difference is, of course, that Mariana will most likely do everything she can to undermine the changes because her version of "slowing down" is to induce atrophy to the new way of doing things.

At this point, Craig will need to seize the moment and take advantage of the credibility he has gained by successfully implementing the new scheduling system (Kotter 1995). In doing that, he can look ahead to even more changes: Does the practice have an electronic medical record? Does the scheduling system prompt appointment reminder calls? Does the system prompt follow-up calls and appointments for those patients with chronic ailments whose conditions and symptoms need to be managed? Is there a website? Does it include a patient portal that lets patients access their own records or make appointments?

Craig's job is less about implementing a new central call center and scheduling system and much more about transforming the practice into an organization prepared to care for patients in the most modern, convenient, efficient, and effective way possible. Remember that his interview conversation was about bringing efficiencies to the practice. The physician-owners merely wanted to begin with the centralized call center. To accomplish this and any additional changes, Craig will need help in the form of leadership from the physician-owners (Kotter 1996). And in order to continue his success, he will need to remind all the staff that the mission of the practice is to "be responsible to the patient . . . [and] provide excellent primary care for the people of Colorado."

Conclusion

This chapter presented three contemporary models of leadership. Kouzes and Posner (2017) demonstrate how a leader can be effective by empowering their colleagues to support a shared vision and creating a culture that rewards successes. Goleman (2014) identifies a foundation of shared emotive and intellectual strengths outlining how emotional intelligence can be employed to effectively bring change to organizations through relationships with others. Finally, the NCHL (2006) model and the HLA (2017) model provide healthcare-specific definitions of competencies, the proficiency of which should improve over time with career advancement. These competencies, in turn, will help move organizations in new, more effective directions.

Students are encouraged to learn about these and other leadership models in order to identify one that may be most beneficial to them given their individual styles and their organizations. The overlap among the models, in terms of how relationships are built and why, suggests that human behavior defies precise characterization. Though the terminology and emphasis vary from model to model, each offers valid points—supported by rigorous research—for how to effectively lead organizations to implement necessary and positive change.

Resistance to change has many forms and many causes. Kanter's (2001) ten classic reasons people resist change will be useful to any leader seeking to apply one of the models discussed in this chapter. Understanding the source of the resistance is key to reducing its intensity and the toxic influence it can have on an organization.

Finally, Kotter (1996) emphasizes that once having achieved a modicum of change, the leader's job is *not* to celebrate the success and then relax. Consolidating the gains made by successful change can be safeguarded only by anchoring that change in the organization's culture—often by creating an environment of constant change, always seeking to improve and ensure the organization fulfills its mission. In short, the goal of a leader is to help the organization seek continuous improvement in its processes. That, in turn, will enable the organization to serve patients in a way that is safe and effective, which is the goal of any healthcare services organization.

Mini Case Study: Ego and Resistance to Change

Hank Collins is the director of the Medical / Surgical Unit at St. Anthony's Catholic Hospital in Rhode Island. Hank wants to implement a program to help prevent medical errors. Specifically, he wants the staff to adopt the Agency for Healthcare Research and Quality's "20 Tips to Help Prevent Medical Errors" (see box). He has already posted the tips in the pediatric waiting room and at the nurses' station, and now he wants the staff to sign the postings to show they agree with the tips. Furthermore, he wants the staff to wear buttons that read, "Ask me if I have washed my hands."

He has been having trouble with one of his best employees. Anne Gordon is 55 years old and has been with the hospital for 35 years. She started out as a new graduate from the local university's licensed practical nurse program, and she rarely misses a day of work. She is helpful, friendly, and smart. She knows the departmental procedures—such as making the patients and their families feel cared for, ensuring quality in patient delivery—better than anyone, and she prides herself on the fact that many of the younger employees come to her for help. She takes particular pride in being their mentor.

However, Anne will not sign the postings and has adamantly refused to wear the button that reads, "Ask me if I have washed my hands." She is vocal about her disapproval, saying, "How demeaning is it to be asked to wear a button on my uniform? Buttons are for political candidates to wear during political campaigns; they are not for us to wear as we take care of patients! And signing the posting would be like admitting that I had committed medical errors. No way am I going to be involved with this cockamamie idea!"

20 TIPS TO HELP PREVENT MEDICAL ERRORS: A PATIENT FACT SHEET

Medicines

1. **Make sure that all of your doctors know about every medicine you are taking.**
   This includes prescription and over-the-counter medicines and dietary supplements, such as vitamins and herbs.
2. **Bring all of your medicines and supplements to your doctor visits.**
   "Brown bagging" your medicines can help you and your doctor talk about them and find out if there are any problems. It can also help your doctor keep your records up-to-date and help you get better quality care.
3. **Make sure your doctor knows about any allergies and adverse reactions you have had to medicines.**
   This can help you to avoid getting a medicine that could harm you.
4. **When your doctor writes a prescription for you, make sure you can read it.**
   If you cannot read your doctor's handwriting, your pharmacist might not be able to either.
5. **Ask for information about your medicines in terms you can understand—both when your medicines are prescribed and when you get them:**
   - What is the medicine for?
   - How am I supposed to take it and for how long?
   - What side effects are likely? What do I do if they occur?
   - Is this medicine safe to take with other medicines or dietary supplements I am taking?
   - What food, drink, or activities should I avoid while taking this medicine?
6. **When you pick up your medicine from the pharmacy, ask: Is this the medicine that my doctor prescribed?**
7. **If you have any questions about the directions on your medicine labels, ask.**
   Medicine labels can be hard to understand. For example, ask if "four times daily" means taking a dose every 6 hours around the clock or just during regular waking hours.
8. **Ask your pharmacist for the best device to measure your liquid medicine.**
   For example, many people use household teaspoons, which often do not hold a true teaspoon of liquid. Special devices, like marked syringes, help people measure the right dose.
9. **Ask for written information about the side effects your medicine could cause.**
   If you know what might happen, you will be better prepared if it does or if something unexpected happens.

Hospital Stays

10. **If you are in a hospital, consider asking all health care workers who will touch you whether they have washed their hands.**
    Handwashing can prevent the spread of infections in hospitals.

(continued)

20 TIPS TO HELP PREVENT MEDICAL ERRORS: A PATIENT FACT SHEET *(CONTINUED)*

11. **When you are being discharged from the hospital, ask your doctor to explain the treatment plan you will follow at home.**
    This includes learning about your new medicines, making sure you know when to schedule follow-up appointments, and finding out when you can get back to your regular activities. It is important to know whether or not you should keep taking the medicines you were taking before your hospital stay. Getting clear instructions may help prevent an unexpected return trip to the hospital.

Surgery

12. **If you are having surgery, make sure that you, your doctor, and your surgeon all agree on exactly what will be done.**
    Having surgery at the wrong site (for example, operating on the left knee instead of the right) is rare. But even once is too often. The good news is that wrong-site surgery is 100 percent preventable. Surgeons are expected to sign their initials directly on the site to be operated on before the surgery.
13. **If you have a choice, choose a hospital where many patients have had the procedure or surgery you need.**
    Research shows that patients tend to have better results when they are treated in hospitals that have a great deal of experience with their condition.

Other Steps

14. **Speak up if you have questions or concerns.**
    You have a right to question anyone who is involved with your care.
15. **Make sure that someone, such as your primary care doctor, coordinates your care.**
    This is especially important if you have many health problems or are in the hospital.
16. **Make sure that all your doctors have your important health information.**
    Do not assume that everyone has all the information they need.
17. **Ask a family member or friend to go to appointments with you.**
    Even if you do not need help now, you might need it later.
18. **Know that "more" is not always better.**
    It is a good idea to find out why a test or treatment is needed and how it can help you. You could be better off without it.
19. **If you have a test, do not assume that no news is good news.**
    Ask how and when you will get the results.
20. **Learn about your condition and treatments by asking your doctor and nurse and by using other reliable sources.**
    For example, treatment options based on the latest scientific evidence are available from the Effective Health Care Web site. Ask your doctor if your treatment is based on the latest evidence.

Source: Reprinted from Agency for Healthcare Research and Quality (2018).

Mini Case Study Questions

1. What is the problem, and what is causing it?
2. What should Hank do to gain Anne's endorsement? What recommendations do Kanter (2001), Kouzes and Posner (2017), and Goleman (2014) make that might help Hank?
3. Recommend a solution to the problem. Why do you think your solution will work?

Points to Remember

- Leadership is critical to the process of changing the way an organization conducts itself.
- Change is essential to the future of any organization. Organizations must be prepared to deal with new circumstances.
- Leadership has evolved from "divine right" to "great man" to "trait" theories and more.
- Current leadership theories focus on the concepts of genuine relationships and transparency.

Challenge Yourself

1. What are some of the similarities among the leadership models discussed in the chapter? Is there one model that is better than the others? Why?
2. How would you describe your leadership style? Justify your conclusion. Does it fit closely with one of the models discussed here?

For Your Consideration

1. Research one of your favorite heroes in history—someone like Abraham Lincoln, Martin Luther King Jr., or Harriet Tubman. How would you describe their leadership style?
2. Research one of history's villains. How would you describe their leadership style? Contrast that to your conclusions about the style you observed in question 1.

References

Agency for Healthcare Research and Quality. 2018. "20 Tips to Help Prevent Medical Errors: Patient Fact Sheet." Reviewed August. www.ahrq.gov/patients-consumers/care-planning/errors/20tips/index.html.

Bass, B. 1981. *Stodgill's Handbook of Leadership*, 2nd ed. New York: Free Press.

Battistella, R., J. Hill, S. Levey, and T. Weil. 2007. "Leadership Development in MHA Programs: A Response and Commentary." *Journal of Health Administration Education* 22 (3): 241–50.

Burnes, B. 2007. "Kurt Lewin and the Harwood Studies: The Foundations of OD." *Journal of Applied Behavioral Science* 43 (2): 213–31.

Charniss, C., and D. Goleman. 2001. *The Emotionally Intelligent Workplace*. San Francisco: Jossey-Bass.

Collins, J. C., and J. I. Porras. 1991. "Organizational Vision and Visionary Organizations." *California Management Review* 34 (1): 30–52.

Fink, S. 2009. "The Deadly Choices at Memorial." *New York Times Magazine*. Published August 30. www.nytimes.com/2009/08/30/magazine/30doctors.html.

Gardner, J. 1990. *On Leadership*. New York: Free Press.

Goleman, D. 2014. "What Makes a Leader." *Harvard Business Review* 81 (1): 82–91.

Goleman, D., R. Boyatzis, and A. McKee. 2002. *Primal Leadership: Realizing the Power of Emotional Intelligence*. Boston: Harvard Business School Press.

Greenwood, R. G. 1993. "Leadership Theory: A Historical Look at Its Evolution." *Journal of Leadership Studies* 1 (1): 4–19.

Healthcare Leadership Alliance (HLA). 2017. "About the HLA Competency Directory." Accessed May 9, 2018. www.healthcareleadershipalliance.org/directory.htm.

Institute for Health and Human Potential. 2017. "What Is Emotional Intelligence?" Accessed July 11. www.ihhp.com/meaning-of-emotional-intelligence.

International Hospital Federation (IHF). 2015. *Leadership Competencies for Healthcare Services Managers*. Bern, Switzerland: IHF.

Kanter, R. M. 2001. *Evolve: Succeeding in the Digital Culture of Tomorrow*. Boston: Harvard Business Press.

Komives, S., N. Lucas, and T. McMahon. 2013. *Exploring Leadership*, 3rd ed. San Francisco: Jossey-Bass.

Kotter, J. 1996. *Leading Change*. Boston: Harvard Business School Press.

———. 1995. "Why Transformation Efforts Fail." *Harvard Business Review* 73 (2): 59–67.

Kouzes, J. M., and B. Z. Posner. 2017. *The Leadership Challenge*, 6th ed. Hoboken, NJ: John Wiley & Sons.

Lewin, K. 1947. "Frontiers in Group Dynamics." *Human Relations* 1 (1): 5–41.

National Center for Healthcare Leadership (NCHL). 2006. *Competency Integration in Health Management Education*. Accessed August 18, 2018. www.nchl.org/Documents/Ctrl_Hyperlink/doccopy5755_uid892012228502.pdf.

Rost, J. 1993. "Leadership Development in the New Millennium." *Journal of Leadership Studies* 1 (1): 91–110.

Salovey, P., and J. Mayer. 1990. "Emotional Intelligence." *Imagination, Cognition and Personality* 9 (3): 185–211.

Stefl, M. 2008. "Common Competencies for All Healthcare Managers: The Healthcare Leadership Alliance Model." *Journal of Healthcare Management* 53 (6): 360–74.

CHAPTER 6

A MEMBER OF THE PROFESSION

Important Terms

- American College of Healthcare Executives (ACHE)
- Association of University Programs in Health Administration (AUPHA)
- Competencies
- Control
- Cultural adaptability
- Cultural relativism
- Diversity
- Ethnocentrism
- Functions of management
- Industrial revolution
- Integrity
- Lead
- Medical Group Management Association (MGMA)
- Organize
- Plan
- Profession
- Professional
- Professionalism
- Scientific management
- Scientific method of inquiry

Learning Objectives

After reading this chapter, you will be able to do the following:

- ➤ Explain what it means to be a member of a profession
- ➤ Explain the concept of professionalism
- ➤ Describe the foundations of scientific management and its application to healthcare management research and theory
- ➤ Understand the function and value of professional associations
- ➤ Understand the significance of diversity in the workplace

Case Study: First Day

Mark Barton entered his new office at the Health West Clinic in Pocatello, Idaho. He had been recently hired as the community's program coordinator. In this position, he would be responsible for managing public relations and marketing communications, volunteer work, and grant-writing efforts on behalf of six clinics located in different rural towns in southeastern Idaho. Health West, a federally funded healthcare facility, focuses on the delivery of primary care regardless of patients' ability to pay. Mark was excited to start his job and was thankful that his healthcare management education had prepared him to work in a field that mattered to him personally. He would be able to help other Idahoans like himself. The patients who went to the clinics paid for healthcare based on their income and ability to pay. When Mark was growing up in rural Idaho, his family was not able to afford health insurance. Clinics like Health West ensured that he and his family received the primary care they needed to stay healthy. Now he would be able to help other families.

Kimberly Lauren entered her new office at Kohler Company in Kohler, Wisconsin. She had been recently hired as a Wellness Program Coordinator. In this position, she would be responsible for a comprehensive and integrated wellness program aimed at improving the health habits and wellness of Kohler Company associates and their dependents. Kohler Co. develops innovative products, such as plumbing fixtures, furniture, tile and stone, and backup power systems. Kohler Co. also develops services through its two luxury resort properties in the United States and Scotland. Kimberly was excited to start her job and thankful that her undergraduate degree in health education with a minor in business management, along with her master's degree in public health, had prepared her to work in a field that mattered to her personally. She would be able to help workers and their dependents learn about and engage in healthy lifestyles. When Kimberly was growing up, her family encouraged healthy nutrition and exercise habits. She remembered preparing meals together, playing softball and basketball together, and attending exercise classes together. She looked back on those times with great fondness. Now she would be able to help other families.

Mark and Kimberly are part of a formal discipline that focuses on the delivery of products and services to improve the business performance of an organization. While Mark and Kimberly will work in different environments, both have developed skills and will learn new skills that will help them integrate the work of others to meet the missions and achieve the goals of their respective organizations and ensure the work is done right and is on target.

Mark sat down at his desk in his office in Idaho; Kimberly sat down at her desk in Wisconsin. Both looked forward to their new management positions, and both knew they possessed skills that would help them in these new roles. However, this was their first day of work, and both said to themselves, "Help!"

Introduction

We see in this example what motivated both Mark and Kimberly to become managers in their respective healthcare-related fields. Moreover, they illustrate managers who are at the entry level of their careers, excited and a little anxious about their ability to be an effective professional. Mark and Kimberly have acquired a foundation of management knowledge from their education (his in healthcare management and hers in health education, business, and public health). Throughout their careers, their knowledge, skills, ability, and conduct will develop as they accumulate firsthand experience in the workplace. Both are beginning their careers and both are poised to model **competencies** that will enable them to be **professionals** at each career stage.

Competencies
A set of professional and personal skills, knowledge, values, and traits that guide a leader's performance, behavior, interactions, and decisions.

Professional
A person who has received specialized education and training and has qualified to serve in a specific occupation.

In the last chapter, we discussed the criticality of managers' mastering leadership and change management skills to ensure that the healthcare organization may serve patients effectively, efficiently, and safely. In this chapter, we address the healthcare management profession and what competencies you should focus on as you prepare to join and advance in the profession. You will learn about the profession of management that is based on theory and research. On a more personal level, you will read about the importance of your exhibiting professionalism during work and outside of work; this includes managing your time and dealing with stress successfully, understanding the significance of cultural competency and diversity in the workplace, and working well with others as you contribute to the field of healthcare management.

The Profession

Profession
A body of knowledge shared by people who have received specialized education and training and share common values.

What does it mean to belong to a **profession**? Sociologists propose that members of a profession have similar education and work backgrounds, rely on a network of formal and informal relationships to do their work, and ascribe to shared norms (Caplow 1954; Greenwood 1957; Parsons 1954). In particular, sociologist Greenwood (1957) notes that professions share five attributes: systematic theory, authority, community sanction, ethical codes, and a culture. Gayle L. Capozzalo, executive vice president, chief operating officer, and chief strategy officer of the Yale–New Haven Health System, illustrated these attributes when she noted in an interview (Meacham 2015, 116) that

> there is something incredibly special about health care that draws uniquely focused, determined, and passionate people to the field. . . . Working in health care administration is an avocation driven by exceptional commitment and an underlying sense of purpose. It is a mission driven profession that relies upon a solid foundation of integrity and lifelong learning.

Capozzalo also served as 2012–2013 chairman of the **American College of Healthcare Executives (ACHE)**—the professional organization for healthcare executives. Members of ACHE enjoy opportunities to network with one another, to advocate for issues pertinent to the profession, and to access resources that help them grow professionally. Thus, professional organizations, such as ACHE, provide a place driven by management theory and possessing the authority to exert community sanctions, establish and enforce ethical codes, and provide a culture based on integrity and lifelong learning.

American College of Healthcare Executives (ACHE)
An international professional society of 48,000 healthcare executives who lead hospitals, healthcare systems, and other healthcare organizations. ACHE has 78 chapters that provide access to networking, education, and career development at the local level. ACHE publishes *Healthcare Executive, Journal of Healthcare Management*, and *Frontiers of Health Services Management*. It also has its own publishing division, Health Administration Press, which published this book.

Healthcare management is a formal discipline based on theory and research. Managers acquire knowledge and tools to do their jobs well from theoretical perspectives and research findings. A manager may work in an organization that provides consumer products, consumer services, or both. Regardless of the organization's purpose, a manager works to improve business performance. This is true for manufacturing, service, and healthcare businesses.

In the introductory case study, Kimberly's overall role as a manager at Kohler Co. was in the delivery of innovative and creative products and services. Kohler's (2014) mission reads:

> The corporation and each associate have the mission of contributing to a higher level of gracious living for those who are touched by our products and services.
>
> Gracious living is marked by qualities of charm, good taste and generosity of spirit. It is further characterized by self-fulfillment and the enhancement of nature.
>
> We reflect this mission in our work, in our team approach to meeting objectives and in each of the products and services we provide our customers.

Kimberly's management activities center on worker wellness programs that will in turn improve business performance regarding the *products and services* and help the company prosper in a complex and competitive business environment.

Managers in health service organizations create an environment in which high-quality care can be provided. Wherever care is available, someone needs to attend to the business side of the practice so caregivers can spend their time providing care. Management activities need to focus on quality to ensure that departments and offices run as well as possible. Healthcare managers integrate the work of others throughout the organization to ensure the mission is met, the goals are achieved, and the work is done right and is on target.

The managers of MD Anderson Cancer Center focus on the delivery of innovative cancer treatment, research, and teaching. Its mission reads (MD Anderson 2018):

> The mission of The University of Texas MD Anderson Cancer Center is to eliminate cancer in Texas, the nation, and the world through outstanding programs that integrate patient care, research and prevention, and through education for undergraduate and graduate students, trainees, professionals, employees and the public.

The managers of the University of Virginia Health Center focus on the delivery of innovative patient care, research, and teaching. Its mission is (University of Virginia 2018)

> to provide excellence, innovation, and superlative quality in the care of patients, the training of health professionals and the creation and sharing of health knowledge within a culture that promotes equity, diversity and inclusiveness.

Medical Group Management Association (MGMA)
A professional association of medical group practice professionals with more than 40,000 members who lead and manage more than 12,500 organizations. Members includes administrators, CEOs, physicians in management, board members, and office managers.

Association of University Programs in Health Administration (AUPHA)
An international association of more than 400 colleges and universities dedicated to improving health by promoting excellence in healthcare management education. AUPHA provides opportunities for member programs to learn from each other by influencing practice and by promoting the value of healthcare management education. AUPHA publishes *Journal of Health Administration Education.*

In the introductory case study, Mark's overall role as a manager at Health West is to focus on the delivery of primary healthcare. Health West's (2018) mission reads as follows:

> Empowering our patients and communities by proactively providing quality, affordable patient-centered healthcare.

Whether their organization's services are focused on specific healthcare issues or general healthcare concerns, healthcare managers' activities center on improving business performance regarding health services and prospering in a complex and competitive business environment.

Management associations encourage and facilitate the professional development of healthcare managers. Like ACHE, organizations such as the **Medical Group Management Association (MGMA)** and the **Association of University Programs in Health Administration (AUPHA)** state that they work to enhance the profession and promote excellence. The values statements of all three organizations also refer to the importance of integrity, continuous learning, and leadership in professional development. MGMA further states that teamwork is important for medical group practice managers.

All these organizations have a code of ethics that holds members to a high standard of behavior. While codes vary by discipline, they share basic ethical principles, which will be discussed in more detail in chapter 10. Briefly, these principles focus on managers' acting in the best interests of others (beneficence); taking actions only if they do not bring harm (nonmaleficence); being honest, telling the truth, and treating others with respect (autonomy); and being fair in the distribution of resources and treatment of patients (justice). The code for healthcare organizations will specifically address how healthcare professionals should behave and identify their responsibilities to the patient, the organization, the larger community, and their profession. Along with a code of ethics, ACHE offers a self-assessment that healthcare executives can take to help them evaluate their ethical strengths and note where they might want to improve (ACHE 2018).

Theory and research confirm that high standards of behavior influence management performance. When managers act with integrity, maintain flexibility and willingness to learn, provide effective leadership, and work with interdisciplinary healthcare teams, employee performance and clinical outcomes tend to be better (Amos, Hu, and Herrick 2005; Black 2016; Flaherty 1999; Lee and Doran 2017; Lemieux-Charles and McGuire 2006). Therefore, an understanding of the theoretical foundations of management in general and of healthcare management specifically, combined with an understanding of research methods and findings, helps managers to do their jobs well. And, as Mark's and Kimberly's situations illustrate, it helps to answer their call for help as they begin their management careers.

Foundations of Scientific Management

People practiced effective management skills long before **scientific management** emerged as a formal discipline. Julius Caesar kept records of employment and equipment procurements and marked the progress of war campaigns (Caesar 1999). We can consider the events he wrote about 2,000 years ago as management activities because his focus was on improving performance (the expansion of Roman rule) and achieving goals to ensure the work was done right and was on target (e.g., transporting equipment, paying soldiers' salaries).

Scientific management
The study of management activities based on theory and research.

Dunn (2016) traces scientific management back even further in her discussion of the construction of the Great Wall of China and the Egyptian pyramids. Chinese and Egyptian "managers" planned the projects, she says; they organized the workers, and ensured that the work was done right and was on target.

Social, political, and economic events spurred the development of scientific inquiry and the establishment of a formal discipline of management. It is not within the scope of this book to describe in detail the changes in Western civilization that encouraged this development. The following sections provide a brief summary of events from the seventeenth century to the present that shaped our method of intellectual inquiry and management theory.

Early Influences on the Development of Management Theory and Research

The scientific and industrial revolutions shaped the way research is conducted. The development of the scientific method is central to our understanding of management research. MGMA asserts that teamwork is important for medical group practice managers, and research supports this emphasis. As we will discuss in chapter 8, teamwork and collaboration among healthcare team members is positively associated with improved healthcare delivery to patients. The scientific revolution influenced the method of research—how the researchers conducted the studies on teamwork. The steps of the **scientific method of inquiry** are as follows:

Scientific method of inquiry
The formal process of research. Steps include observation and description, hypothesis formulation, data gathering, data analysis, discussion of the findings, and conclusion.

- *Idea generation*: Researchers ask a question, such as "Do healthcare teams affect patient care?"
- *Hypothesis formulation*: Researchers propose a possible answer, such as that the presence of effective teamwork positively affects length of stay for geriatric

patients following congestive heart failure, or that good teamwork lowers the probability an infant may contract a healthcare-associated infection.

- *Methodology formulation*: Researchers determine how the research will be conducted. In this case, they could survey team members for subjective opinions regarding teamwork effectiveness and determine a method for measuring length of patient stay, or review patient records and note the presence of a healthcare-associated infection.
- *Data gathering*: Researchers conduct a survey of healthcare workers to measure their perceptions of their teamwork; they also review patient records.
- *Data analysis and interpretation*: Researchers analyze the data and debate applications of the findings.
- *Data and outcomes reporting*: Researchers present the findings.
- *Implications for future research*: The same researchers or others may study this phenomenon again, this time considering a different aspect or implication.

To note a few research studies, Profit et al. (2017) found that good teamwork in the neonatal intensive care unit (NICU) brought about better outcomes for the infants. With each 10 percent rise in the number of NICU staff members who reported that teamwork was "good," infants were 18 percent less likely to contract a healthcare-associated infection. Similarly, Ettinger (2001) assessed the impact of teams on an older population and found that effective teamwork yielded benefits to patients who had experienced congestive heart failure.

This scientific model evolved from the fields of philosophy, sociology, psychology, science, economics, and mathematics. French philosopher and mathematician René Descartes (1596–1650) wrote "*cogito, ergo sum*," which translates to "I think, therefore I am" (Descartes 1637). Descartes's revolutionary approach underscores the importance of addressing questions via scientifically based methods. Italian scientist Galileo Galilei (1564–1642) used experiments to conduct research. One of his experiments compared the speed of two objects of different weights released from the same height at the same time. Galileo hypothesized that the two objects would fall at the same speed no matter what their individual weights were, and by following the method of scientific inquiry, he found evidence to support his proposition. Later, French philosopher Voltaire (1694–1778) proposed the rejection of theories that do not withstand the test of facts, stressing the importance of looking "*aux faits*" ("to the facts") for explanations (Voltaire 1762).

Industrial revolution
The shift from an agrarian economy to an industrial economy in Western countries in the eighteenth and nineteenth centuries. This shift resulted in changes to social and economic organization.

Other changes that helped spur the adoption of the scientific method of inquiry include the social and economic changes provoked by the **industrial revolution**. The rise of industry originated in Britain in the eighteenth and nineteenth centuries and moved to other Western nations, such as the United States, in the 1800s, as the agrarian economy shifted to an industrial economy. In 1840, about 11 percent of the US population lived in urban areas (Shi and Singh 2001); by 1900, about 40 percent did (Stevens 1971). This demographic shift was accompanied by technological advances enabling the mass production of goods (e.g., the Ford Motor Company assembly line, established in the early 1900s), transportation gains made with the construction of railroads, and little government intervention regarding workers' rights. With people working in central locations and goods and services being mass produced, businesses turned their attention to finding rational principles that would make production more efficient and help them to prosper in a growing, competitive environment.

Dunn (2016) summarizes the theoretical frameworks for organizational management that emerged from these changes, while Zuckerman, Dowling, and Richardson (2000) discuss current theoretical perspectives (from the 1980s to the present) that address managers' roles. Readers are encouraged to refer to these works for a more detailed discussion. Their main points regarding the rise of management theory are as follows.

Frederick Winslow Taylor (1856–1915)

Taylor, an American mechanical engineer, studied efficiencies and applied scientific inquiry to the workplace. According to Peter Drucker (1909–2005), known as the father of modern corporate management, Taylor was "the first man in recorded history who deemed work deserving of systematic observation and study" (Drucker 1974, 181). Taylor introduced time and management studies, during which he would observe and record what the worker did and how long it took the worker to complete each task. Then he would redesign the work so that time and effort were conserved and production efficiency was maximized. Taylor (1911) also proposed four principles of management:

- Develop a science for each element of an individual's work. (This applied scientific methods of study to the workplace.)
- Scientifically select and then train, teach, and develop the worker. (This introduced the concepts of recruitment, retention, and professional development.)
- Cooperate with workers to make certain that work guidelines are followed. (This developed the notion of worker incentives, such as pay increases, to improve productivity.)
- Divide work and responsibilities between management and workers. Managers plan the work and workers carry out the plan by doing the work.

Taylor's proposals resulted in an increased focus on establishing efficiencies. For example, Ford Motor Company adopted his time-and-effort approach to hone its assembly lines.

In addition, Taylor's work laid the foundation for further ideas about efficiency, recruitment, retention, rewards, and specialization of tasks at the workplace. Drucker concluded that Taylor's hope was that laborers could earn a "decent livelihood" through increasing productivity (Drucker 1974, 24).

Henri Fayol (1841–1925)

Fayol, a Frenchman who had managed a large coal mining company, proposed that workers be supervised by a single person charged with managing employees' tasks. This helped establish a functional organizational structure for business. Fayol (1916) proposed that the five functions of managers were to plan, organize, command, coordinate activities, and control performance. Over time, these **functions of management** have evolved into managers' responsibilities to **plan**, **organize**, **lead**, and **control**. Managers plan as they define the goals of treatment and education and coordinate staffing, scheduling, marketing, and education to achieve these goals. Managers organize as they make a schedule, delegate tasks to specific staff members, and follow the established hierarchy and division of labor. In addition, their position affords them the authority to organize the activities needed to accomplish goals. Managers lead as they exhibit competence and **integrity**, and as they motivate others. Finally, managers control as they monitor and evaluate the plan as it unfolds and determine how to get their efforts back on track if needed. How well they plan, organize, lead, and control influences how effective they are in their position.

Functions of management
The basic responsibilities of a manager, which include planning, organizing, leading, and controlling.

Plan
To devise or create a way to accomplish a defined task.

Organize
To coordinate and carry out tasks.

Lead
To be in charge of or responsible for people or tasks.

Control
To guide or check; the act of accountability.

Integrity
Firm adherence to a code of ethics or to a moral code of behavior.

Frank Gilbreth (1868–1924) and Lillian Gilbreth (1878–1972)

Frank Gilbreth worked as a bricklayer, contractor, and management engineer. He knew from experience that money was not the only incentive for laborers. Rather, cooperation from workers was key to bringing about efficiencies in the workplace. Lillian Gilbreth earned her PhD in applied management from Brown University. She integrated psychological perspectives into her consideration of the importance of worker satisfaction in efficiency. The Gilbreths would film the work under study and then offer recommendations for reducing the time and effort spent on tasks. For example, they filmed surgeries and recommended that nurses hand the surgeons the tools they needed as opposed to the surgeons retrieving the tools themselves (Gilbreth 1914, 1916). This change reduced operation time and benefited both caregivers and patients. A key difference between the Gilbreth analyses and Taylor's efforts is that the Gilbreths focused on the workers and the efforts they exerted doing the work. Their motion studies offered recommendations that would reduce worker fatigue and increase efficiency.

Henry Gantt (1861–1919)

Gantt, an American contemporary of Taylor and the Gilbreths, was a mechanical engineer and management consultant. He created the Gantt Chart, a tool that facilitates the planning and control of specific work projects. Drucker (1974, 182) elaborates:

> The Gantt Chart, in which the steps necessary to obtain a final work result are worked out by projecting backward, step by step from end result to actions, their timing and their sequence, though developed during World War I, is still the one tool we have to identify the process needed to accomplish a task, whether making a pair of shoes, landing a man on the moon, or producing an opera.

Versions of the Gantt Chart are still used today. Managers have employed the chart to build the Hoover Dam (1931) and plan the US interstate highway project (1956). Gantt's approach allowed for the development of specific tools to help managers get tasks accomplished. In the case study that opened this chapter, Mark Barton's responsibilities include managing volunteer efforts. To do this, Mark might design a Gantt Chart like the one depicted in exhibit 6.1.

Exhibit 6.1 Health West Volunteer Recruitment Plan

	Timeline (2019)				
Task	**January**	**February**	**March**	**April**	**Responsible Party**
Announcements made and placed in all Health West clinics and local newspapers	Start 1-5-2019 End 1-30-2019				Mark
Present volunteer announcement on community calendar on local television stations	Start 1-12-2019			End 4-3-2019	Mark
Appear on Community Channel's noon local talk show		Booked 2-18-2019			CEO of Health West and Mark
Inquire about church and school newsletters		Start 2-2-2019	End 3-6-2019		Jennifer (student intern)
Take current volunteers to lunch; continue regular contact and establish Bring a Friend to Volunteer Initiative	Start 1-23-2019			Ongoing	Mark and Jennifer
Report and assess recruitment efforts with board				4-22-2019	Mark

Max Weber (1864–1920)

Weber, a German sociologist, proposed that bureaucratic coordination of activities was one of the distinguishing features of the industrial revolution. Rational principles guide the organization of bureaucracies (Coser 1971). Activity is based on the relationship between people in varying positions of authority, which are characterized by a division of labor, a defined hierarchy, and rules and regulations. Weber also proposed that jobs consist of well-defined tasks, authority is based on workers' positions in the organization (e.g., manager, laborer), and people work for salaries and pursue careers within organizations. Still, he was concerned about the depersonalization that could result from rationalization and the growth of bureaucracies.

Mary Parker Follett (1868–1933)

Follett, an American social worker and management consultant, addressed the issue of worker and management relations. Negotiation, conflict resolution, and collaboration between worker and manager were central to her writings (Follett 1941). She addressed the significance of the individual in the workplace and the value of individuals working together in an environment of democratic authority (Eylon 1998).

Chester Barnard (1886–1961)

Barnard, president of New Jersey Bell Telephone Company, focused on the role of the person in an organization. He proposed that the manager's role was to communicate with workers and encourage them to recognize the common goals of the organization and the workers' performance to attain those common goals (Barnard 1938).

These contributors to the development of the management field came from various disciplines. Some offered proposals that concerned the structure and function of theory and research (e.g., Descartes, Galileo, Voltaire), others focused on scientific management (e.g., Taylor, the Gilbreths, Gantt), and still others focused on the role of people and their interactions with one another at the workplace (e.g., Follett, Barnard). What they have in common is that their efforts helped lay the foundation for good management and for other contributions to the development of the professional.

Professionalism

Management research today is built on the foundation established by these early contributors, who set the stage for subsequent efforts that offer substantive information and guidance to new managers such as Mark and Kimberly, from this chapter's case study, so they may perform well and improve quality, performance, and outcomes at their workplaces. Simply put, Kimberly and Mark are developing the tools of **professionalism**, which refers to "the ability to align personal and organizational conduct with ethical and professional standards that include a responsibility to the patient and the community, a service orientation, and a commitment to lifelong learning and improvement" (Garman et al. 2006, 219).

Professionalism
Knowledge and understanding of beliefs and behaviors expected of a professional.

At each career level, you will learn more and develop more as a professional. For instance, at the entry level of your career, you will learn how to improve your ability to collaborate by listening to feedback and engaging in networking opportunities both within and outside your department. During the senior level of your career, you will help to provide and encourage others to seek ways to improve their abilities. Over time, you will hone and sharpen your perspective on how to do the work well, both on behalf of your stakeholders and for your own personal goals. Developing the following four areas will enable you to learn and exhibit professionalism (Garman et al. 2006, 219–20):

- *Understanding professional roles and norms.* What behaviors are expected of you as a healthcare manager? How will you learn about the expectations and receive training to learn about them?
- *Working with others.* How should you establish working relationships and manage these relationships well and in an ethical and respectful manner?
- *Managing yourself.* How do your ethical standards align with the profession? What is your personal responsibility for your work standards? What lifelong learning are you engaged in to continue to grow and learn throughout your career?
- *Contributing.* How do you give back to your profession, the healthcare field, and your community?

Your mastery of professionalism includes working well with others and helping other people in your field learn and develop as members of the profession. Actively learning by joining your healthcare professional association (e.g., MGMA for physician practices, ACHE for hospitals and health systems, AUPHA for health administration education); networking and allowing yourself to be a mentee to learn from more senior healthcare managers; and contributing where you can to bring about better outcomes in your workplace as well as your community will help you develop professionally. When you have reached the senior career level, serving as a mentor, preparing successors to move up in healthcare management, and encouraging professionalism in others will help ensure the continuous improvement of healthcare managers and the field of management so the delivery of healthcare in your institution is better, is of higher quality, and improves the patient experience.

Specific skills such as how to communicate more effectively or how to manage your time better will be covered in later chapters. For now, our discussion of professionalism will focus on what you need to consider as you align your personal and organizational conduct with ethical and professional standards. As a healthcare administrator, you will find yourself in situations that may be unfamiliar, but you will have guidance from your profession and your colleagues to help you navigate them.

Diversity Issues

Diversity
A list of characteristics, including gender, race, ethnicity, educational level, socioeconomic status, culture, language, religion, disabilities, sexual orientation, and age, that indicates an individual's background.

One unfamiliar situation you may find yourself in as a healthcare manager concerns **diversity** in the workplace. We typically understand that we should all treat each other well and with respect. This corresponds to the ethical principle of autonomy. But, how do you react when you learn that a coworker has been sexually harassed? What do you do if you see it is your boss who is the harasser? What should you do if you experience harassment in your workplace? The "#MeToo" movement that gained national attention in 2017 illustrates the significance of our understanding of the importance of diversity and how we treat others in the workplace. While the "#MeToo" movement gained this recognition from entertainment performers who reported publicly about sexual harassment and, in many instances, sexual violence, the reports also grew to include men from the entertainment profession as well as men and women from other professions. The "MeToo" movement began in 2006 from the actions of Tarana Burke, a civil rights activist (Parker 2017). The "#MeToo" hashtag later became a way for persons who have experienced sexual harassment to go public with their stories, to join others and state that this happened to them as well (Zacharek, Dockterman, and Edwards 2017).

Sexual harassment is not new to the workplace. What has changed is the unwillingness of women and men to remain silent. Actor Ashley Judd told the *New York Times* of her harassment by the head of the Miramax studio, Harvey Weinstein (Zacharek, Dockterman, and Edwards 2017). Engineer Susan Fowler wrote about her sexual harassment by her manager at the ridesharing company Uber (Fowler 2017). California lobbyist Adama Iwu spoke of her harassment in the state capital (Kravarik 2017). All reported they had not received support or positive action by others to help them resolve the situation. And all were women working in an environment in which power was largely controlled by men. Hence, while the actions were unprofessional at the very least and illegal in some instances, they also illustrate how critical it is that we understand diversity issues. (We will return to #MeToo in chapter 12 in our discussion of how human resources should be involved when workers are harassed in the workplace.)

Although to date there have been no publicized examples of the #MeToo movement involving healthcare professionals, that does not mean sexual harassment is absent in the field. A 2014 survey of assistant professor–level clinician-scientists who had received career development awards from the National Institutes of Health between 2006 and 2009 found that 30 percent of the women and 4 percent of the men reported experiencing sexual harassment (Jagsi et al. 2016). And in 2017, Boston Fenway Community Health Center's CEO did not abide by legal advice that he remove a physician from practicing at the clinic because of his sexual harassment of employees (Healy and Pfeiffer 2017); the CEO's resignation came about precisely because he did not act to stop the harasser, demonstrating an absence of professionalism (Finnegan 2017). Healthcare professionals in leadership positions must investigate complaints of sexual harassment, even if there is a physician involved.

Considering the sexual harassment at Fenway in more detail you might ask, "What actions could the health center's CEO have taken to support the victimized employees?" Or, "What training, if any, could have helped administrators and clinicians to understand appropriate behavior so employees could work together, without harassment, to provide quality healthcare?" In the Fenway case, a male physician was accused of sexually harassing a male employee and bullying female employees. The outside law firm that recommended the physician's dismissal had been called in twice over a four-year period to investigate. The CEO eventually resigned his position, but only after the harassed employee was paid $75,000 to settle allegations against the physician (Healy and Pfeiffer 2017). As you think about the facts of this case, consider the CEO's actions in light of the four components of professionalism: understanding professional roles and norms, working with others, managing oneself, and contributing. The CEO did not, for example, understand his responsibility to stand up for his employees when they were harassed, he did not provide training to educate workers about harassment, and he failed to manage working relationships. What should he have done that would have led you to believe he exhibited professionalism? What training could have helped in this situation? What communications should the CEO have initiated, and with whom, to address the issue? To whom should he have listened during the four-year period to help him take proper action?

Such questions address the management of gender and sexual differences and sexual harassment as well as bullying. As a professional, the notion that employees are on the receiving end of such behavior is egregious. Actions must be taken not only to stop such occurrences but also to ensure professionals work to create and sustain an environment in which such actions are unacceptable. Understanding diversity and why it matters in the workplace is key to developing professionalism.

Diversity is defined as differences in a long list of background characteristics that include gender, race, ethnicity, education level, socioeconomic status, culture, language, religion, disabilities, sexual orientation, and age (Shi 2007). While these differences are omnipresent in US culture, they have historically separated peoples into different work and social circles. Such separation led to disparities in access to advancement opportunities (e.g., segregated schools), healthcare (e.g., segregated hospitals), and the workplace (e.g., glass ceilings). Because of demographic, socioeconomic, and political changes, people from different genders and cultures are now going to school together, working together, and providing and receiving healthcare from one another.

In addition to gender differences affecting workplace interactions, consider cultural differences among Americans. Except for the Native Americans, we are a nation of immigrants. Sociologist William Sumner (1840–1910) proposed that people may judge aspects of other cultures based on the standards of their own. Further, they may assume that their own culture and way of life are superior to those of another culture (Sumner 1906). Sumner used the term "**ethnocentrism**" to refer to this way of thinking. Ethnocentrism is functional for groups in that believing one's culture is superior reinforces its belief systems and practices, promoting solidarity. Consider, for example, international sports and the Olympics, where nationalism and patriotism are promoted via athletic competitions among the United States and other countries.

Ethnocentrism
The tendency to judge aspects of other cultures based upon the standards, beliefs, and traditions of one's own culture.

Obviously, ethnocentrism may also have negative effects. The opinion that "mine is better than yours" can lead to social isolation of groups, which in turn leads to different levels of access to resources, rights, and privileges. The Tuskegee Syphilis Study illustrates differential healthcare treatment (Jones 1981). In 1933, the United States Public Health Service in Alabama conducted a clinical trial to assess how syphilis would naturally progress if it were untreated medically. For 40 years, 399 African-American men who had contracted syphilis received no clinical treatment, even as healthcare providers followed and documented their deteriorating health. The men were not told about their health condition, nor were they informed that they were participants in a research study. Instead, the researchers told them they were being treated for bad blood. *New York Times* reporter Jean Heller noted that the Tuskegee study was the longest-running nontherapeutic experiment on human beings (Heller 1972). The research was assessed by John Heller, director of venereal diseases at the Public Health Service. James Jones interviewed Heller for a book on the Tuskagee study and quoted him as saying, "The men's status did not warrant ethical debate. They were subjects, not patients; clinical material, not sick people" (Jones 1981, 179).

The Tuskegee Syphilis Study spurred ethical debates regarding health research protocol and the treatment of segregated groups in medical research. In 1997, President Clinton formally apologized for the study, discussed the nature of the work, and remarked on how researchers should behave when working in a diverse culture (Clinton 1997):

> We are constantly working on making breakthroughs in protecting the health of our people and in vanquishing diseases. But all our people must be assured that their rights and dignity will be respected as new drugs, treatments and therapies are tested and used. So I am directing Secretary Shalala to work in partnership with higher education to prepare training materials for medical researchers. . . . They will help researchers build on core ethical principles of respect for individuals, justice and informed consent, and advise them on how to use these principles effectively in diverse populations.

Healthcare managers and providers working in diverse environments need to understand the concepts, and importance, of cultural relativism and cultural adaptability. **Cultural relativism** refers to our understanding of another culture by its own standards—the opposite of ethnocentrism. Healthcare providers' adoption of cultural relativism could improve awareness of the customs of their coworkers and their patients. **Cultural adaptability** refers to the willingness and ability to not only understand cultural differences, but also to work effectively across cultures to enhance the quality of care. Thus, providers and patients from diverse backgrounds may be able to interact more positively to achieve access to care and improve healthcare outcomes (Council on Graduate Medical Education 1998).

Cultural relativism
Understanding another culture based on its own standards, beliefs, and traditions.

Cultural adaptability
The willingness and ability to understand cultural differences and act upon that understanding to yield cooperative outcomes.

Professional associations for clinicians and administrators, including ACHE, AUPHA, MGMA, the American Medical Association, and the American Academy of Pediatrics (AAP), support efforts to adopt cultural relativity and adaptability. The AAP noted that by the year 2020, about 40 percent of school-aged children will be nonwhite. The sheer numbers of ethnic minorities, and the resulting cultural diversity in the United States, have implications for pediatric healthcare providers, prompting the AAP to state the following (Committee on Pediatric Workforce 2000, 129):

> The health care needs of the pediatric population are influenced by factors relating to culture and ethnicity. Pediatricians must acquire the knowledge and practice skills that will allow them to: recognize and address culture and ethnicity; make valid assessments of clinical findings; and, provide effective patient management.

To provide high-quality healthcare, it is essential for administrators and providers to understand cultural differences and work across cultures to minimize potential barriers, such as prejudice or negative predetermined beliefs. Mott (2003) described initiatives taken by a 210-bed, acute-care, not-for-profit hospital to address diversity issues in its patient population. These initiatives included employee training by various cultural experts, interfaith unity programs to promote better understanding of different religions, public relations efforts to highlight and celebrate diversity internally (e.g., serving ethnic foods in the hospital cafeteria, celebrating Black History Month), and surveying patients directly about the hospital's ability to meet their cultural needs during their stay. Diversity initiatives inform all aspects of workplace management, culture, and patient experiences.

Wentling and Palma-Rivas (1999) evaluated the qualities of effective diversity training programs. They interviewed 12 diversity experts—researchers who conducted studies about diversity, served as business consultants regarding diversity issues, or were involved with diversity work efforts. All the experts agreed that endorsement and support from top management—the organizational leadership—was essential to training program success. Other key factors include the following (Wentling and Palma-Rivas 1999):

- Making diversity training part of the organizational strategic plan
- Ensuring the training meets the specific needs of the organization in terms of employees' cultural makeup and the population served
- Using qualified trainers
- Combining the training with other diversity initiatives

More recent research also supports the view that organizational commitment and support by top management are essential components of successful diversity training (Gardenswartz and Rowe 2009; Pendry, Driscoll, and Field 2007; Von Bergen, Soper, and Foster 2002). Dessler (2009) summarized significant components of diversity management initiatives; as with previous studies, he found that leadership support and endorsement of the importance of cultural adaptability and diversity issues are primary factors in positive outcomes. Dessler's list of factors includes the following:

- Strong leadership that champions diversity efforts
- Methods to measure success of diversity initiatives, including employee surveys, employee retention, hiring practices, and focus group discussions
- The presence of employee education and training that addresses diversity issues
- Integration of employee education and training with other organizational initiatives and practices, such as supervisor appraisal measurement regarding diversity issues
- Overall evaluation of diversity management initiatives, including assessment of positive or negative effects of initiatives on, for example, employee attitudes

Diversity training initiatives give healthcare professionals the opportunity to learn what diversity is and why it matters. Whitman and Davis (2008) propose that the healthcare management curriculum should promote cultural and linguistic competencies. Exposure to diversity information would better prepare healthcare management students at the undergraduate and graduate levels to develop and maintain a culturally competent organization. Healthcare professionals manage and work with diverse employees and colleagues. Coworkers, supervisors, and subordinates come from diverse backgrounds. Estimates predict that more than half of all US citizens will be nonwhite by midcentury (US Census Bureau 2001). As a result, the healthcare workforce is becoming more culturally diverse. Diversity training not only improves patient care, but also increases understanding among coworkers.

Organizations for healthcare management professionals, such as the American Hospital Association (AHA) and ACHE, recognize the growing diversity in the workplace and its effect on the healthcare management field. The AHA (2018) launched the #123forEquity campaign in 2015 and asked for increased diversity in leadership and governance at healthcare centers (Livingston 2018). ACHE (2012) also endorses such efforts:

> ACHE values diversity and initiatives that promote diversity because they can improve the quality of the organization's workforce. ACHE also values and actively promotes diversity in its leaders, members, and staff because diverse participation can serve as a catalyst for improved decision making, increased productivity, and a competitive advantage.

Simply put, diversity refers to the differences among people and their cultural backgrounds. Only 10 percent of countries in the world today have a homogeneous culture (Harris, Moran, and Moran 2004). Consequently, most people, including those living in the United States, interact with people of other cultures on a daily basis. Providers, patients, stakeholders, and customers are more likely to work with and treat people with dissimilar backgrounds from their own. The idea that diversity matters is based on the following principles:

- *Demographics*: Peoples from different cultures and backgrounds are present in our multicultural society.
- *Ideology*: The lack of representation of people from different backgrounds results in exclusion, lowers access to healthcare, and presents ethical dilemmas stemming from disparate treatment.
- *Business practice*: The lack of representation is costly in terms of time and effort, and it reduces healthcare quality.

Diversity is real. Being effective as a healthcare manager requires considering diversity worthy of attention. Efforts must be supported by top management, middle-rank executives, and early careerists. It is the first step to mastering professionalism.

Conclusion

At the beginning of this chapter, we met Mark and Kimberly, who were at the entry level of their careers. Both had been prepared for their positions through education and experience, and both exhibited enthusiasm to begin work in the field. Throughout this chapter, we illustrated how their continued growth as professionals at every career state (entry, middle, and senior) will help them continue to be effective healthcare managers. Their growth will depend on their mastery of certain competencies (e.g., understanding professional roles and norms, working well with others, managing themselves, contributing). Management theory and research continue to offer substantive information and guidance to help them perform well to the benefit of patients, coworkers, the institutions in which they work, and the communities in which they live. In addition, to help prepare them—and you—to do the work well, we have underscored the significance of diversity issues.

Mini Case Study: Mr. Khil and the Hospital

Mr. Khil was an elderly gentleman who arrived at St. Teresa's Hospital with pneumonia and breathing difficulties. Admission personnel determined Mr. Khil could not speak English and offered to arrange for a translator. Mr. Khil's family members refused this offer. His daughter, Seomoon Khil, did speak English, and all communications between the medical staff and Mr. Khil were conducted through her. The language barrier was not the only difficulty. More than a dozen relatives visited Mr. Khil at the same time. Mr. Khil was in a semiprivate room, and his relatives' presence was disruptive to the staff and to the patient in the room's other bed. Further disruption occurred when Mrs. Khil brought in a rice steamer and hot plate and cooked for Mr. Khil and the visiting family members.

One evening, the hospital floor staff was very busy, as all private and semiprivate rooms were occupied. Mrs. Khil and some relatives were setting up dinner in Mr. Khil's room, and about six other relatives were standing in the hallway. While the nurses could enter other patients' rooms, there was concern about the number of people in and near Mr. Khil's room. Moreover, his roommate's wife could not visit with her husband quietly because of the presence of Mr. Khil's extended family.

On the second night of Mr. Khil's stay, a patient down the hall experienced a cardiopulmonary arrest, requiring a team of providers to rush to her room and begin immediate resuscitative efforts. The code blue team was able to revive the patient but complained to the nursing supervisor that even though their efforts were not hampered by the visitors in the hallway, they were concerned about the number of people in that location. The code blue team captain told the supervisor, "They could have slowed us down, and you know every second counts on a code blue." The nursing supervisor called hospital security to remove the family members from the floor.

Mini Case Study Questions

1. What is the problem in this mini case?
2. Explain how a lack of actions that would have demonstrated cultural adaptability helped to create the problem.
3. What would you have recommended the nursing supervisor do instead of calling security?

Points to Remember

- Mastering professionalism continues throughout your career.
- Belonging to a profession means that members share similar education and work backgrounds, rely on a network of formal and informal relationships to do their work, and ascribe to shared norms.
- Belonging to healthcare professional organizations may facilitate professional development.
- Learning about management theory and research may help healthcare managers better perform tasks, which in turn improves quality and outcomes.
- Developing professionalism includes understanding professional roles and norms, working well with others, managing yourself, and contributing.
- Understanding diversity matters.

Challenge Yourself

1. Reflect on Mark Barton's and Kimberly Lauren's stories described in the opening case study, "First Day." Both have chosen career paths that fit with their skill set and professional goals. What is your career goal? What skills have you developed to help meet the missions and achieve the goals of your future employer? What else should you be doing currently to prepare yourself better for the profession?
2. In the professions, the notion that employees are on the receiving end of sexual harassment is egregious. Consider the #MeToo movement that has become a way for people who have experienced sexual harassment to go public with their stories. As a healthcare manager, how should you respond if a coworker shares with you that they have been sexually harassed in the workplace? Would your answer be different if they were supervised by you? Why or why not?
3. Elaborate upon the point to remember, "Mastering professionalism continues throughout your career." Think about people you know who are at a different level of their career and who also exhibit professionalism. Give an example of their mastering professionalism during the entry, middle, and senior levels of their careers. How have they demonstrated mastery of professional roles and norms, working well with others, managing themselves, and contributing back? Explain how these examples may influence your professional growth.

For Your Consideration

1. Healthcare leaders such as Jack Bovender, retired CEO of the Nashville-based Hospital Corporation of America (HCA), demonstrated his understanding of diversity when he launched HCA's chief operating officer (COO) development program, which paired new administrator recruits with mentors and allowed them corporate-level experience so they were prepared and ready to be future COOs (Rubenfire 2015). Moreover, he demonstrated his understanding of the importance of diversity by ensuring that the program focus on hiring more women and other minorities. He even took on the title of chief diversity officer to underscore its importance (Rubenfire 2015). Why do you think it was effective for Bovender to identify himself as the "chief diversity officer?" What professionalism components would you be mastering if you were to participate in such a program?
2. Bovender's efforts represent one step forward regarding support for diversity in healthcare settings. Conversely, findings from a 2017 management study indicate we may also be taking one step back. Surveying 1,000 top management executives from large and mid-sized US companies with sales of more than $50 million, researchers found that more top white male executives provided less task-related help to their executive colleagues and reduced recommendations for them for career-advancing positions after a woman or person of color was appointed CEO (McDonald, Keeves, and Westphal 2017). In addition, the presence of a woman or racial minority as CEO was found to discourage white male executives from serving as mentors or giving work-related help to female and racial-minority colleagues (McDonald, Keeves, and Westphal 2017). Researcher James Westphal, a finance professor at the University of Michigan, proposed that the " . . . theory is that the appointment of minority CEOs triggers biases" (Berman 2018). Discuss this study in light of what you have learned about the concept of cultural adaptability. How do the studies' findings sync (or not) with positions taken by organizations such as ACHE regarding diversity?

References

American College of Healthcare Executives (ACHE). 2018. "Ethics Self-Assessment." Accessed January 4 , 2019. www.ache.org/about-ache/our-story/our-commitments/ethics/ethics-self-assessment.

———. 2012. "Statement on Diversity." Revised March. www.ache.org/about-ache/our-story/our-commitments/policy-statements/statement-on-diversity.

American Hospital Association (AHA). 2018. "American Hospital Asociation #123forEquity Campaign to Eliminate Health Care Disparities." Accessed July 17. www.equityofcare.org/.

Amos, M., J. Hu, and C. Herrick. 2005. "The Impact of Team Building on Communication and Job Satisfaction of Nursing Staff." *Journal for Nurses in Staff Development* 21 (1): 10–16.

Barnard, C. 1938. *The Functions of the Executive*. Cambridge, MA: Harvard University Press.

Berman, J. 2018. "When a Woman or Person of Color Becomes CEO, White Men Have a Strange Reaction." *MarketWatch*. Published March 3. www.marketwatch.com/story/when-a-woman-or-person-of-color-becomes-ceo-white-men-have-a-strange-reaction-2018-02-23.

Black, J. 2016. *The Toyota Way to Healthcare Excellence: Increase Efficiency and Improve Quality with Lean*, 2nd ed. Chicago: Health Administration Press.

Caesar, J. 1999. *The Gallic War*. Trans. C. Hammond. Oxford, UK: Oxford University Press.

Caplow, T. 1954. *The Sociology of Work*. Minneapolis, MN: University of Minnesota Press.

Clinton, W. J. 1997. "Presidential Apology." Accessed July 23, 2018. www.cdc.gov/tuskegee/clintonp.htm.

Committee on Pediatric Workforce. 2000. "Enhancing the Racial and Ethnic Diversity of the Pediatric Workforce." *Pediatrics* 105 (1): 129–31.

Coser, L. 1971. *Masters of Sociological Thought*. New York: Harcourt Brace Jovanovich, Inc.

Council on Graduate Medical Education. 1998. "The Health Status of Minority Populations." In *Minorities in Medicine*, edited by US Department of Health and Human Services, Health Resources and Services Administration, 7–13. Washington, DC: US Department of Health and Human Services.

Decartes, R. 1637. *Discourse on Method and Meditations*. Trans. F. E. Sutcliffe. London: Penguin, 1995.

Dessler, G. 2009. *Fundamentals of Human Resource Management*. Upper Saddle River, NJ: Prentice Hall.

Drucker, P. 1974. *Management: Tasks, Responsibilities, Practices*. New York: Harper & Row.

Dunn, R. 2016. *Dunn & Haimann's Healthcare Management*, 10th ed. Chicago: Health Administration Press.

Ettinger, W. 2001. "Six Sigma: Adapting GE's Lessons to Healthcare." *Trustee* 54 (8): 10–16.

Eylon, D. 1998. "Understanding Empowerment and Resolving Its Paradox: Lessons from Mary Parker Follett." *Journal of Management History* 4 (1): 16–28.

Fayol, H. 1916. *Industrial and General Administration*. Paris, France: Dunod.

Finnegan, J. 2017. "It Happens Here, Too: Sexual Harassment Occurs in Healthcare Field." *FierceHealthcare*. Published December 14. www.fiercehealthcare.com/practices/sexual-harassment-healthcare-reshma-jagsi-new-england-journal-medicine.

Flaherty, J. 1999. *Peter Drucker: Shaping the Managerial Mind*. San Francisco: Jossey-Bass.

Follett, M. 1941. *Dynamic Administration: The Collected Papers of Mary Parker Follett*, edited by H. Metcalf and L. Urwick. New York: Harper's.

Fowler, S. 2017. "Reflecting on One Very, Very Strange Year at Uber." Published February 19. www.susanjfowler.com/blog/2017/2/19/reflecting-on-one-very-strange-year-at-uber.

Gardenswartz, L., and A. Rowe. 2009. "The Effective Management of Cultural Diversity." In *Contemporary Leadership and Intercultural Competence*, edited by M. A. Moodian, 35–43. Los Angeles: Sage.

Garman, A., R. Evans, M. Krause, and J. Anfossi. 2006. "Professionalism." *Journal of Healthcare Management* 51 (4): 219–22.

Gilbreth, F. 1916. "Motion Study in Surgery." *Canadian Journal of Medicine and Surgery* 40: 22–31.

———. 1914. "Scientific Management in the Hospital." *Modern Hospital* 3: 321–24.

Greenwood, E. 1957. "Attributes of a Profession." *Social Work* 2 (3): 45–55.

Harris, P. R., R. T. Moran, and S. V. Moran. 2004. *Managing Cultural Differences: Global Leadership for the Twenty-First Century*, 6th ed. Oxford, UK: Elsevier-Butterworth-Heinemann.

Health West. 2018. "About Us." Accessed July 17. www.healthwestinc.org/?page_id=17.

Healy, B., and S. Pfeiffer. 2017. "For Years, Fenway Health Center Kept Prominent Doctor Accused of Harassment, Bullying." *Boston Globe*. Published December 8. www.bostonglobe.com/metro/2017/12/08/for-years-fenway-health-center-kept-prominent-doctor-accused-harassment-bullying/djZugTTaxy1upIJfThMQZK/story.html.

Heller, J. 1972. "Syphilis Victims in the U.S. Study Went Untreated for 40 Years." *New York Times*. Published July 26. www.nytimes.com/1972/07/26/archives/syphilis-victims-in-us-study-went-untreated-for-40-years-syphilis.html.

Jagsi, R., K. Griffith, R. Jones, C. Perumalswami, P. Ubel, and A. Stewart. 2016. "Sexual Harassment and Discrimination Experiences of Academic Medical Faculty." *Journal of the American Medical Association* 315 (19): 2120–21.

Jones, J. H. 1981. *Bad Blood: The Tuskegee Syphilis Experiment—a Tragedy of Race and Medicine*. New York: Free Press.

Kohler. 2014. "Mission Statement." Accessed January 4, 2018. www.corporate.kohler.com/mission/.

Kravarik, J. 2017. "Sexual Harassment Claims by Women Rattle California Capital." CNN News. Published October 19. www.cnn.com/2017/10/19/us/california-legislature-sexual-harassment-allegations/index.html.

Lee, C., and D. Doran. 2017. "The Role of Interpersonal Relations in Healthcare Team Communication and Patient Safety: A Proposed Model of Interpersonal Process in Teamwork." *Canadian Journal of Nursing Research* 49 (2): 75–93.

Lemieux-Charles, L., and W. McGuire. 2006. "What Do We Know About Health Care Team Effectiveness? A Review of the Literature." *Medical Care Research and Review* 63 (3): 263–300.

Livingston, S. 2018. "Racism Still a Problem in Healthcare's C-Suite." *Modern Healthcare*. Published February 24. www.modernhealthcare.com/article/20180224/NEWS/180229948/racism-still-a-problem-in-healthcares-c-suite.

McDonald, M., G. Keeves, and J. Westphal. 2017. "One Step Forward, One Step Back: White Male Top Manager Organizational Identification and Helping Behavior Toward Other Executives Following the Appointment of a Female or Racial Minority CEO." *Academy of Management Journal* 61 (2) : 405–39.

MD Anderson. 2018. "Mission Statement." Accessed January 4. www.mdanderson.org/about-md-anderson.html.

Meacham, M. 2015. *From Backpack to Briefcase: Professional Development in Health Care Administration*. Boston, MA: Cengage Learning.

Mott, W. J. 2003. "Developing a Culturally Competent Workforce: A Diversity Program in Progress." *Journal of Healthcare Management* 48 (5): 337–42.

Parker, N. 2017. "Who Is Tarana Burke? Meet the Woman Who Started the Me Too Movement a Decade Ago." *Atlanta Journal-Constitution*. Published December 6. www.ajc.com/news/world/who-tarana-burke-meet-the-woman-who-started-the-too-movement-decade-ago/i8NEiuFHKalvBh9ucukidK/.

Parsons, T. 1954. *Essays in Sociological Theory*, revised ed. Glencoe, IL: The Free Press.

Pendry, L. F., D. M. Driscoll, and S. C. Field. 2007. "Diversity Training: Putting Theory into Practice." *Journal of Occupational and Organizational Psychology* 80 (1): 27–50.

Profit, J., P. Sharek, P. Kan, J. Rigdon, M. Desai, C. Nisbet, D. Tawfik, E. Thomas, H. Lee, and J. Sexton. 2017. "Teamwork in the NICU Setting and Its Association with Health Care–Associated Infections in Very Low-Birth-Weight Infants." *American Journal of Perinatology* 34 (10): 1032–40.

Rubenfire, A. 2015. "Jack Bovender: Rebuilding a Quality Culture at HCA." *Modern Healthcare*. Published March 14. www.modernhealthcare.com/article/20150314/MAGAZINE/303149982.

Shi, L. 2007. *Managing Human Resources in Health Care Organizations*. Sudbury, MA: Jones & Bartlett.

Shi, L., and D. Singh. 2001. *Delivering Health Care in America*. Gaithersburg, MD: Aspen.

Stevens, R. 1971. *American Medicine and the Public Interest*. New Haven, CT: Yale University Press.

Sumner, W. G. 1906. *Folkways*. New York: Dover, 1959.

Taylor, F. 1911. *The Principles of Scientific Management*. New York: Harper Bros.

University of Virginia. 2018. "Mission Statement." Accessed January 4. https://uvahealth.com/about/health-system-info/mission-vision-and-values.

US Census Bureau. 2001. *Statistical Abstract of the United States 2001*. Washington, DC: US Census Bureau.

Voltaire. 1762. *Candide*. Trans. T. Cuffe. New York: Penguin, 2005.

Von Bergen, C. W., B. Soper, and T. Foster. 2002. "Unintended Negative Effects of Diversity Management." *Public Personnel Management* 31 (2): 239–51.

Wentling, R. M., and N. Palma-Rivas. 1999. "Components of Effective Diversity Training Programs." *International Journal of Training and Development* 3 (3): 215–26.

Whitman, M. V., and J. A. Davis. 2008. "Implementing Cultural and Linguistic Competence in Healthcare Management Curriculum." *Journal of Health Administration Education* 25 (1): 109–25.

Zacharek, S., E. Dockterman, and H. Edwards. 2017. "Person of the Year 2017." *Time Magazine*. Accessed February 5, 2018. http://time.com/time-person-of-the-year-2017-silence-breakers/.

Zuckerman, H., W. Dowling, and M. Richardson. 2000. "The Managerial Role." In *Health Care Management: Organization Design and Behavior*, 4th ed., edited by S. Shortell and A. Kaluzny, 34–60. Albany, NY: Delmar.

CHAPTER 7

COMMUNICATION AND RELATIONSHIP MANAGEMENT

Important Terms

- Accommodating style
- Active listening
- Aggressiveness
- Assertiveness
- Avoidance style
- Compromising style
- Criticality
- Dominating style
- Downward communication
- Effective communication
- Emotional intelligence
- Feedback
- Lateral communication
- Nonverbal cues
- Power
- Problem-solving style
- Receiver
- Relationship conflict
- Relationship management
- Sender
- Situationally appropriate
- Task conflict
- Upward communication
- Verbal cues

Learning Objectives

After reading this chapter, you will be able to do the following:

- ➤ Explain the importance of effective verbal and nonverbal communication
- ➤ Identify clear and concise communication
- ➤ Identify the components of communication: sender, receiver, and message
- ➤ Recognize the value of attentive listening

- Provide and receive constructive feedback
- Explain ways to manage conflict
- Explain relationship management
- Explain the significance of emotional intelligence for effective communicating

Case Study: An Absentminded Professor

Susan Morrison excitedly approached Dr. Hans Lackenski's office. She had scheduled this appointment with her human resources (HR) in healthcare professor two weeks earlier. Susan was working toward a BS in healthcare administration, and she had a great idea for her senior paper. Each student was to present an idea to a professor and ask that professor to serve as the adviser for the paper. Susan enjoyed studying healthcare administration. Her GPA was 3.75 on a 4.0 scale, and she had taken Dr. Lackenski's course the previous semester.

Susan was interested in working in HR, particularly on recruitment and retention issues for healthcare professionals. In Dr. Lackenski's HR class, Susan had learned that hospitals, nursing homes, and clinics were engaging in nontraditional methods to recruit nurses. She had an associate's degree in nursing and had earned her RN degree five years earlier. She had been working at the university hospital ever since, and she had maintained her work schedule even after she returned to school to earn her BS. She had firsthand experience with the nursing shortage. It was not uncommon for her to be called back to the hospital to work extra shifts. She also knew that her RN experience would add value to her future work as a hospital administrator. She had been researching the nursing shortage in the United States and wanted to ask Dr. Lackenski to serve as her adviser and to guide her with his expertise on recruitment and retention issues.

The department secretary ushered Susan into Dr. Lackenski's office. Dr. Lackenski was sitting at his desk, looking at the computer screen. He waved for Susan to sit down and said, without moving his eyes from the computer screen, "What can I do for you?"

Susan began to talk about her research efforts: "Dr. Lackenski, I wanted to ask you what you thought about the current US hospital recruitment practice of hiring US traveling nurses, as well as nurses from other countries such as Canada, English-speaking Caribbean and African countries, Great Britain, India, and the Philippines. Don't you think that this is really a short-term solution to the nursing shortage?" Susan leaned forward in her chair and awaited Dr. Lackenski's response.

Dr. Lackenski hit a few keys on his computer and shifted in his chair. He stopped typing for a moment and looked at his wristwatch. "Yes, there is a nursing shortage," he said. He stood up and walked over to a file cabinet. On top of the cabinet was a tray labeled "In Box." He selected a few of the letters from the box and proceeded to open them.

Susan repeated her interest in learning his opinion on the recruiting practice. The professor kept his eyes focused on his mail. He did not appear to be interested in the topic or in her as a student at that moment. Susan asked, "Is this a bad time for you? Should I reschedule our appointment?" Dr. Lackenski looked at Susan. "Can you hold on for a minute?" He then left his office to give the letter he had been reading to the secretary.

Susan mumbled, "I see you are busy at the moment. Thank you for your time, Dr. Lackenski." She followed Dr. Lackenski out of the office. Nonplussed, she walked down the hall wondering if her professor was as smart as she had thought. What was she going to do about her senior paper?

Communication Matters

Effective communication Communication in which the receiver receives and understands the message as the sender intended it.

Sender The producer of a message.

Receiver One who is given the message produced by the sender.

Professor–student collaboration creates an educational exchange of value that benefits the students, the professors, and the university learning community. A collaborative relationship depends on **effective communication**. In the case study, Dr. Lackenski does not appear to be engaged in this collaboration, leaving Susan to ponder what to do about her paper. However, the professor and the student may gain from effective communication and meaningful discussion. Unfortunately, this did not happen for Susan and Dr. Lackenski.

Communication is a process whereby information is conveyed between a **sender** and a **receiver**. We know that when we communicate with our family, friends, and colleagues, the information is not always understood the way we intended. Consider the game of Gossip, or Broken Telephone. One person whispers a phrase to another person; that person whispers the information to the next person, and so on. By the time the last person receives the message, it may have changed considerably.

A recent healthcare management class of 45 students played Gossip as a classroom exercise. They started with the following communication: "The final exam will be held on Tuesday from 1:00 p.m. to 4:00 p.m. It will have four essay questions; the student will select three of them to answer. There are also 75 multiple-choice and true/false questions." When the forty-fifth student received the information, he announced the following to the class: "The exam is on Thursday from 2:00 p.m. to 4:00 p.m. It has three essay questions and 75 multiple-choice questions. No true/false questions." If this were the way the professor had communicated final exam information, many of the students would have had a stressful end to the semester. As the game of Gossip illustrates, effective communication matters.

Shannon and Weaver (1949) developed a communication model to address Bell Telephone's need for efficient phone cables and radio waves. While Shannon and Weaver were both engineers, their communication model became the basis for human communication research: The information source (the sender) produces the message. The transmitter (nonverbal and verbal communication) translates the message into signals. The channel refers to adaptation of voice signals to be sent over telephone cables. The channel is influenced by noise sources (any interference with the message). (Shannon and Weaver [1949] were referring to phone line static; human communication research considers any distraction that may interfere with the message to be a noise source.) The receiver receives the information and decodes the message that is sent. In human communication research, the destination and the receiver are the same.

The Shannon and Weaver (1949) communication model has been simplified and adapted for human communication research (see exhibit 7.1). Parsons's model stresses the role of communication to inform and to persuade (Parsons 2001, 13):

> In the context of your job as a healthcare manager, one of the most important reasons to consider the quality of your communication is because the relationships that you have with other individuals—and that your organization has with other groups and organizations—often originate directly from the quality of the communication that has flowed between you and others.

In the case study, Susan attempted to communicate with Dr. Lackenski about a topic for her senior paper. But was her communication clear? She neglected to explain her reason for being there, even though her nonverbal communication supported her interest in the meeting. Dr. Lackenski's **feedback** seemed to indicate his lack of interest. Whether he was not interested in Susan's topic or in her senior paper is unclear. What is clear is that his nonverbal communication effectively told Susan that he was not listening to her and thus was not interested in the meeting. His attention to his computer screen and his mail represents the noise that may interfere with effective communication, as Shannon and Weaver (1949) indicate; this same activity represents the feedback factor illustrated in Parsons's (2001) model. The end result is that the noise and feedback Dr. Lackenski sent to Susan affected their relationship as professor and student. Susan probably will go to another professor who is willing to *listen* to her ideas, and her opinion of Dr. Lackenski will have suffered from their exchange.

Feedback
Critical assessment of information or action.

EXHIBIT 7.1
Communication Model for Healthcare Managers

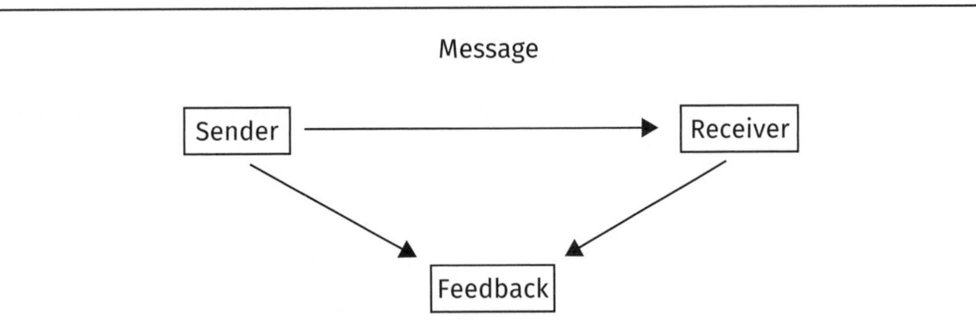

Source: Adapted from Parsons (2001).

Active Listening

Active listening
The process of paying close attention to a message so that it is received accurately.

A key component of communication is the receiver's ability to hear accurately what the sender is saying. This depends on whether the receiver is practicing **active listening**, which is essential for managers to communicate effectively (Durutta 2006; Weger et al. 2014). The manager (sender) should check with the receiver to make certain the message is accurately received. One method is to summarize the information and ask if this summary is accurate. Furthermore, the manager needs to let the receiver respond. Both parties—sender and receiver—should be willing to listen.

Nonverbal cues
In communication theory, the behaviors of persons who are interacting with one another. Body language, posture, and facial expressions may elaborate the message that is being sent or received.

Verbal cues
In communication theory, the tone and manner of the message sent and received.

There are costs for parties who do not listen, in terms of lost information and damaged relationships. Clark (1999), a professor at Xavier University, asked management students to recall a time when someone was actively listening to them. Students noted that they had perceived the other person was actively listening through **nonverbal cues** (e.g., eye contact, nodding) and **verbal cues** (e.g., repeating the information back to the speaker, asking relevant questions). They reported that they liked speaking to active listeners. The interaction indicated respect and conveyed that the receiver thought the speaker was intelligent. Further, they held the active listener in high esteem.

The opposite was found regarding student perceptions of inattentive listeners (such as the behavior exhibited by Dr. Lackenski). They knew they were not communicating with an active listener because of nonverbal (e.g., walking away) and verbal cues (e.g., irrelevant interruptions). The inattention caused the students anxiety, and they attributed negative qualities (e.g., arrogance, condescension) to inactive listeners.

Greenleaf (1977) proposed that learning to listen helps a manager become a servant leader, one who serves first and aspires to lead. Through active listening, servant leaders not only receive insights for effective management but also build strengths in those with whom they are speaking. Greenleaf recommends that managers ask themselves, "Am I really listening?" when engaged in conversation. Perhaps if Dr. Lackenski had asked that question, his meeting with Susan would have been different.

Suggestions for improving listening skills include the following:

1. Stop talking. Allow the sender and receiver to speak.
2. Focus on the speaker. Use nonverbal and verbal cues to indicate your interest in what the speaker is saying.
3. Respect the other person. Take time to listen.
4. Be careful with interpretations. Avoid making assumptions. Ask questions to clarify what the speaker is saying.
5. Avoid distracting actions, such as looking at mail or shuffling papers. These behaviors give the impression that the receiver is not interested.

6. Do not interrupt. Let the speaker finish the thought before responding.
7. Do not talk while the other is talking. You cannot listen while speaking.

The challenge of an effective communication process is understanding how to speak and listen well. Dye (2017) proposed that effective listening skills are a critical competency for healthcare executives. Healthcare managers who listen well are not merely waiting for their turn to speak in the conversation. According to Dye (2017, 123), they

1. ask a lot of questions,
2. ask clarifying questions,
3. restate the answers,
4. keep an open mind,
5. are receptive to bad news,
6. minimize interruptions,
7. seek suggestions, and
8. involve others in the conversation.

Active listening may not always create effective rapport or provide the answer to a problem, but adopting active listening skills will certainly secure an advantage. Moreover, the additional showing of respect for each other is key for effective outcomes from the conversation. As Dye (2017, 124) wrote,

> Respect is the value that multiplies the desire of both the leader and follower to work harder and deliver consistently excellent performance.

Dr. Lackenski only engaged in one of Dye's (2017) recommendations: He restated an answer. However, he did not listen as though he meant it. He may have been interested in directing Susan's paper on the nursing shortage, but his lack of attention effectively ended his opportunity to do so. Effective communication requires that the sender send a clear message to the receiver and receive clear feedback from the receiver. In an ideal situation, Dr. Lackenski would have listened closely, acknowledged his understanding of the messages Susan presented to him, and sent his own messages back clearly. If he had been unable to attend to the conversation for some reason, he should have rescheduled the meeting. One of a manager's responsibilities is to assess and respond to a situation as appropriately as one can. If Dr. Lackenski had rescheduled and listened attentively to Susan's next attempt to discuss her paper, the outcome could have been better.

Internal and External Communications

Managers communicate with a variety of groups and individuals. Within the organization, managers interact with their bosses, their colleagues, and their staff. Staff expect their managers to share pertinent organizational information and to explain how that information will affect their work efforts (Men 2014; Whitworth 2006). Communication flows may be downward (e.g., CEO to department head), upward (e.g., nurse to nurse manager), or lateral (e.g., radiology technologist discussing work matters with another radiology technologist). **Downward communication** is primarily informational and initiated by the superior in the organization. Such communications are not solely face-to-face interaction. An e-mail or text message that explains a clinic's vacation policy guidelines is an example of this form. **Upward communication** primarily lets managers know about staff issues. Face-to-face communication in the form of open meetings to discuss employees' concerns, open-door policies, and walking the halls help create effective forums for this type of communication (Katz 1974; Men 2014). Moreover, e-communication methods may also be effective, such as employee responses to a survey via SurveyMonkey or Qualtrics (Naresh 2017).

Downward communication Communication that is primarily informational and initiated by the superior in the organization.

Upward communication Communication that allows supervisors to know about staff members' concerns, issues, or recommendations.

Lateral communication Communication between staff members of the same status.

Lateral communication usually focuses on work processes. A frequent topic among colleagues of the same status is how to provide care that is more efficient, more customer-friendly, and more patient-centered. When lateral communication pertains to work functions, it may lead to positive outcomes in workload and efficiencies. However, lateral communication may also have negative consequences. Staff members who manipulate information for their own advantage or who offer misinformation may cause conflicts among other staff members. Managers should identify and deal with these conflicts to address such negative outcomes, which we will address later in this chapter regarding conflict at the workplace.

Such interpersonal skills are also important for healthcare managers in an external setting, such as when interacting with members of the media. Health and healthcare are newsworthy, and having a manager serve as media liaison helps the public understand any healthcare issues under scrutiny. Plain language and honesty are essential. Successful communication efforts with the media build relationships that can help a healthcare organization broadcast its messages and solidify its role in the community.

Consider, for example, managers in not-for-profit hospitals who are trying to communicate budget expenses for community benefits. A community benefit is a program developed by a not-for-profit hospital to serve its surrounding community and to increase health awareness among local residents. Common community benefit programs include community health education programs, screenings, immunizations, and education of healthcare professionals. Hospitals may also donate free bicycle helmets or offer childbirth classes. Not-for-profit hospitals receive tax-exempt status because of their community benefit efforts—but the community benefit messages must be communicated clearly for the hospital to maintain this status. Regular, clear, consistent, and honest communication with media representatives about community benefit efforts allow for future communication efforts between the hospital and the public via members of the media.

Written Communication

Letters, memos, reports, and PowerPoint presentations are central to the healthcare business. Effective written communication is important, as it is relatively permanent, retrievable, and, at times, legally binding. Parsons (2001) and Meacham (2015) offer direct writing advice to aspiring and new healthcare managers. Accuracy, truthfulness, and purposefulness convey the facts and provide the reader with truthful and useful information. Clear, organized, complete, and appropriately targeted writing helps the reader understand the information.

Effective communication includes accepting the responsibility to hone one's writing skills. Managers should be able to write well, and they can improve via proper training. Gratto Liebler and McConnell (2008) offer a series of guidelines to help managers improve their writing skills. Like Parsons (2001), Meacham (2015) stresses the importance of targeted writing; he also stresses the importance of targeted marketing. Writers should know who the reader is and how well the reader knows the subject matter. This helps the manager select a writing style and determine which information to include. If the audience is the manager's primary team, an informal style may be appropriate. The amount of background material and level of detail will vary according to the audience; for example, the general community's need to know will differ from an internal department's need to know. Gratto Liebler and McConnell (2008) and Meacham (2015) encourage managers to use only the words necessary to make the point—to be clear and concise. Last, to develop writing skills, they encourage managers to edit, rewrite, and review.

Many of you have taken a writing-intensive course as part of your college curriculum. The importance of the writing-intensive experience cannot be overstated. Clear, concise writing represents clear, concise thinking. The way in which you make and support your assertions, and elaborate with a discussion, conveys your points to the reader and demonstrates your ability as a healthcare manager to communicate effectively and with purpose.

Relationship Management

Sometimes, no matter how hard you try to communicate effectively, you cannot completely avoid conflict. In theory, **relationship management** focuses on the ongoing connection between you, your workplace, and its stakeholders. Employing effective communication and understanding that when we are communicating, we should treat others with respect and **civility**, are important for positive relationship management. To illustrate, let us consider the situation of a student internship placement. Shaun, a senior student in the health services management program, has requested that his internship experience for college credit be earned in the public relations and marketing division at the regional healthcare center. He has spoken with the health services management program director, Bob, who has approved that he pursue this option with Jane, the center's director of public relations and marketing. All three are stakeholders of their respective place of employment or study. Shaun represents

Relationship management
The connections between you and your workplace with stakeholders. These connections depend on how you and the stakeholders treat each other in the context of work. Acting with integrity and treating each other with civility helps lead to positive relationship management.

Civility
Positive interpersonal behavior that includes kind, courteous treatment of others.

the students (stakeholders at the university) and future interns (stakeholders at the university and healthcare center). Bob represents the university (stakeholder at the healthcare center) as well as current and future student interns (stakeholders at the university and healthcare center); and Jane represents the healthcare center (stakeholder at the university). All want the relationship between the two organizations to be a positive experience—for Shaun, the university, and the healthcare center. To that end, Shaun arrives at the center prepared and ready to work. His positive work ethic and professionalism will affect how he and the health services management program at the university are viewed by the healthcare center. Jane's mentoring and work assignments for Shaun will affect how the placement site at the healthcare center is viewed by Shaun and the health services management program director. Both the university and the regional healthcare center want to support internship experiences, and it is positive experiences given and received, with everyone acting with integrity and treating each other with civility, that help to yield continued positive relationship management. The internship relationship continues, and Jane tells Bob to "send more like Shaun to intern." And Shaun tells Bob that Jane is an excellent mentor and the site is one that other students should experience if they are interested in healthcare public relations and marketing.

The concept of civility refers to our behavior while we communicate with others. Research supports the assertion that treating others with respect and establishing a civil climate positively influences healthcare workers' perceptions of patient care performance (Oppel, Mohr, and Benzer 2017). This assertion is probably not news to you, but the value of civility should not be downplayed, as effective communication and relationship management help you to form and maintain good working relationships. Garman, Fitz, and Fraser (2006) noted that communication and relationship management are about demonstrating integrity and gaining trust. You may be respected simply because of the position you hold within your healthcare organization, but you have to earn the trust of your colleagues and other stakeholders by behaving with integrity.

Still, rude and uncivil behavior are often present in the workplace, and they negatively affect how we manage relationships. For example, let us turn to the Baltimore Workplace Civility Study, which examined civility and incivility in the workplace (Forni et al. 2003). Sampling Baltimore-area employees from various industries (nonprofit, manufacturing, business services, and bio-sciences), Forni and colleagues (2003) found that more than one-third of survey respondents had experienced incivility at the workplace and about two-thirds reported they had witnessed incivility.

While civil communication in face-to-face environments is important, so is civil communication in writing. Francis, Holmvall, and O'Brien (2015) defined uncivil behavior via e-mail communication at work to include writing belittling or condescending comments and sharing personal private e-mails with others. Part of their 2015 research on e-mail and civility assessed whether uncivil behavior encouraged more uncivil behavior over e-mail. The authors found that when people received an uncivil e-mail they were more likely to write back with a similar, uncivil tone. Thus, incivility may lead to conflict and poor relationship management.

Conflict and Relationship Management

Conflict is everywhere: at home, in the government, in your community, and at work. While conflict may be unpleasant, it is not always bad. It can be a positive force in organizations. Conflict fuels creativity and innovation (Anderson, Potocnik, and Zhou 2014), maintains stimulation and activation, contributes to adaptation and innovation (Anderson, Potocnik, and Zhou 2014), and can call attention to problem areas, thereby leading to a search for solutions and improvements (Rubino, Esparza, and Chassiakos 2014).

Still, conflict is something most of us avoid when possible. It is stressful and time-consuming. It can be perceived as destructive, a hindrance to performance, disruptive to teamwork, irrelevant to tasks, and harmful to relationships among coworkers (Chou and Yeh 2007; Cochran and Elder 2015; Wombacher and Felfe 2017).

Whether conflict is good or evil, it is bound to happen in organizations, and managers spend a significant amount of their time dealing with it. It is important to understand conflict and your instincts in dealing with it, and to have a framework for the better management of conflicts at work.

There are two primary sources of conflict in the workplace: relationship and task. **Relationship conflict** refers to "tension, animosity, and annoyance" among coworkers (Chou and Yeh 2007, 1037); it is often unrelated to work and is interpersonal in nature. **Task conflict** describes disagreement among coworkers about the tasks being performed (Chou and Yeh 2007). Aspects of task conflict include disagreements regarding goals, and competition or dependencies among coworkers, departments, or workers assigned to a team (Kuypers, Guenter, and Emmerik 2018). Task conflict in healthcare often centers on differences in approaches to work, philosophies of care, or priorities and desired outcomes. Task and relationship conflict are easily intertwined: When working with a coworker whom one does not like, it is often hard to agree on what needs to be done and how to accomplish it. Conversely, when one disagrees with a coworker about a task or desired goal, it is easy to see annoying habits and negative characteristics in that coworker.

Regardless of the source of conflict, the options for responding to it can be categorized into five general styles (Ayoko 2016; Chou and Yeh 2007; Prause and Mujtaba 2015). The names of the five styles vary, but they are characterized by depth of concern for one's stance in the conflict and for the other party's stance.

1. The **dominating style** has high concern for self and low concern for others. *Dominating* refers to demanding and imposing one's will on others with little or no concern about the impact on the other party.
2. The **accommodating style** demonstrates low concern for one's own position in the conflict and high concern for those of others. One example of accommodating is a situation in which you have no strong feelings one way or the other, but because the situation is important to the other party, you simply

Relationship conflict
Disagreement and antagonism unrelated to the specific situation and interpersonal in nature.

Task conflict
Disagreement about tasks, goals, methods, or desired outcomes.

Dominating style
A conflict style involving high concern for self and low concern for others; demanding and imposing one's will on others with little or no concern about the impact on the other party.

Accommodating style
A conflict style involving low concern for one's own position and high concern for that of others.

go along with the other party's wishes. Or, it could be a situation in which you do not wish to assert yourself, even though you do care about the conflict situation, and you simply submit to the other party's wishes.

Avoidance style
A conflict style involving low concern for self and low concern for others; often presents itself as withdrawal or lack of cooperation.

3. The **avoidance style** has low concern for self *and* low concern for others, and often presents itself as withdrawal or lack of cooperation. One example of this style is when the conflict is of so little importance to you, and you have so little concern about the other party, that you choose to ignore it. Avoidance, however, can be more malicious than just ignoring a problem; it can be passive-aggressive and highly uncooperative. It can be an attempt to control others not by what you do, but by what you don't do.

Compromising style
A conflict style involving a reasonable level of concern for self and for others; aims to keep both sides equal and actively searches for the middle ground, ensuring that one side does not give in more than the other.

4. The **compromising style** demonstrates a reasonable level of concern for self and for others. This orientation is concerned about keeping both sides equal and will attempt to match concessions, make conditional promises or threats, and actively search for the middle ground. The goal in compromising is to ensure that one side doesn't give in more than the other. Both sides do their part and give equally to resolve the conflict.

Problem-solving style
A conflict style involving high concern for self and high concern for others; searches for more than the middle ground and actively works toward finding the best possible outcome for all parties.

5. The **problem-solving style** demonstrates high concern for self and high concern for others. It does more than search for the middle ground; it actively works toward finding the best possible outcome for all parties. It is assertive and cooperative.

Most managers have a particular, preferred style for responding to conflict. You might assume that the problem-solving orientation is always best. However, it is important to realize that "if all you have in your toolbox is a hammer, all issues start to look like nails" (Harris 2007, 93). For example, you would not use a collaborative, give-and-take approach with a young child playing with matches; you would simply say "no, don't do that—you can hurt yourself" and take away the matches. Thus, an alternative way to think about handling conflict is to consider the situation and make a decision regarding which style is more likely to help you resolve *that* conflict (Raines 2012).

Power
The ability to enact one's own will based on status, rank, knowledge, level of education, reputation, or a combination of these and other factors.

When handling a conflict, you should take into account and balance the dimensions of **power**, criticality, and confrontation (Callanan and Perri 2006; Chang, Chen, and Chen 2017). Perhaps the most obvious of these dimensions in handling conflicts is power (Harris 2007). In the workplace, power can be based on status, rank, knowledge, level of education, reputation, or a combination of these and other factors. When the two parties have similar power, the compromising style, where each side gives equally, and the problem-solving style are often most effective.

Position and rank in the workplace affect which conflict-management style you should select. The more power you have, the more you are able to use a conflict-management style that is highly centered on self and unconcerned about the effect on others, such as the dominating style. However, you should also consider that while dominating may be effective, it does not mean you should also be uncivil.

Another factor to consider when choosing a conflict-management style is the **criticality** of the issue—the material effect upon the individuals and the time pressure involved in resolving the conflict. The more critical and urgent the issue is to the individual, the more assertive that individual's style should be. The less critical the issue is to the individual, the more cooperative and accommodating the individual can be. You may ask yourself how high the stakes are regarding the conflict at hand. If the issue is so critical that you may lose your position at work, take a moment to consider if you really want to risk your job to win the conflict.

Criticality
The ultimate importance of an issue and its material effect on the individuals and time pressure involved in resolving the conflict.

When considering the criticality of the issue, be certain the issue is accurately defined. This is not as easy as it sounds, particularly when you are caught up in the emotion of a conflict. If the issue is complex, the stakes and criticality are higher, and both parties are more likely to choose assertive conflict styles. If the issue is solvable and the parties agree on a solution that works, be gracious and take the solution offered. It is more important to find a suitable outcome than to win a conflict for the sake of winning.

A final dimension of conflict is each party's willingness to engage in confrontation. Some people are naturally shy and reticent and will almost always choose accommodation or avoidance over a confrontation or argument. Others are outgoing and assertive and love to argue and force the issue. Our society often confuses **assertiveness** (positivity and self-confidence) with **aggressiveness** (hostility and combativeness). In the midst of a conflict, it is easy to cross the line from assertive into aggressive behavior. Some basic guidelines from Rue and Byars (2004, 323) can help those who struggle to be assertive demonstrate greater confidence, and to prevent those who are naturally assertive from crossing over into aggressiveness.

Assertiveness
Behavior that is positive and self-confident.

Aggressiveness
Behavior that is hostile and combative.

1. Don't try to place blame. This only polarizes the participants.
2. Don't surprise either party with confrontations for which they are not prepared.
3. Don't attack sensitive areas that have nothing to do with the conflict at hand.
4. Don't argue aimlessly.
5. Identify areas of mutual agreement.
6. Emphasize mutual benefits to both parties.
7. Don't jump to conclusions or solutions too quickly.
8. Encourage both sides to examine their own biases and feelings.

Situationally appropriate
In a conflict, taking into account the power and criticality of the issue and each party's willingness to confront the other.

The beginning of this chapter focused on communication, and accurate, clear communication is essential to conflict management. The eight points just stated are part of good communication techniques that can be used not only in business, but in your personal life as well.

Conflict can be complex, emotional, and intense. It might seem natural to avoid conflict or to respond with anger, but you should consider taking a step back, clearly defining the issues, and thinking about the relative power of the parties, the criticality of the issue, and each party's willingness to confront the other. Once these contingent dimensions have been considered, a **situationally appropriate** style for handling the conflict can be chosen.

Emotional Intelligence and Relationship Management

Emotional intelligence
The ability to identify and manage your own emotions and the emotions of others.

The concept of **emotional intelligence** was introduced by psychologist and journalist Daniel Goleman (1998), who proposed that you should learn how to master not only the ability to manage relationships with others, but also to manage yourself. Your future success as a healthcare manager depends on this. You can hone these abilities by developing your self-awareness, self-regulation, motivation, empathy, and social skills. While it is imperative that you learn all the materials and tools associated with the healthcare industry, such as how to construct budgets, it also is essential that you learn emotional intelligence, which will help you to better respect others and earn respect for yourself—all factors that will help you perform well as a healthcare manager.

For example, consider the case of a senior healthcare executive who insists on having lunch with a prospective job candidate. By the time the lunch has been arranged, the candidate has interviewed with other healthcare managers and been approved as someone they are ready to hire. The lunch offers time for the senior executive to observe how the candidate interacts not only with him but also with others who work in the restaurant. The executive will note if the candidate remembers to thank the waiter for bringing water to the table; if she stays calm and dignified if something out of the ordinary occurs, such as a passerby accidentally brushing her chair; or if she shows respect and keeps a positive attitude not only to him but also to the restaurant staff. The executive wants to see how she might treat others and how she manages herself, for while he knows she is likely to be positive and kind to him, a potential supervisor, this gives him a sense of how she will treat others with a lower status at the healthcare facility, such as the medical assistants, secretaries, or the older, more vulnerable patients. It is a simple lunch, but not so simple. The executive is assessing the candidate's emotional intelligence.

Goleman and Boyatzis (2017) discuss 12 elements of emotional intelligence. As you review their list, ask yourself how competent you are in each of the following areas (Goleman and Boyatzis 2017, 3):

- Emotional self-awareness
- Emotional self-control
- Adaptability

- Achievement orientation
- Positive outlook
- Empathy
- Organizational awareness
- Influence
- Coach and mentor
- Conflict management
- Teamwork
- Inspirational leadership

Emotional self-awareness addresses how much you know about yourself. Are you a morning person and accomplish your best work at that time of day, and knowing this, do you schedule your day so you can work more diligently at that time? How do you behave if you cannot schedule that time for productivity? Or, do you find you complete projects early because a deadline is your anathema? If you are aware of these aspects of yourself, you understand your strengths and what behaviors you may exhibit that will affect others. That is high emotional self-awareness.

The next four elements of emotional intelligence include aspects of how you manage yourself. Do you control your emotions? Do you possess and have you demonstrated that you have a positive outlook regarding work? Regarding others? How adaptable are you to new situations? Are you achievement-oriented? Do you work well with others to accomplish a task? If you are aware of these aspects, then you understand your ability to self-regulate. You know how not to lose your temper or hold a grudge. That is high self-regulation.

Two more elements of emotional intelligence address your ability to be empathetic and your understanding of how things work at your organization. Empathy refers to your ability to consider others' emotions and behave accordingly. Organizational awareness is the ability to understand the unwritten rules of an organization, its power relationships, and the values that drive it. In chapter 6, we discussed how an organization's mission statement demonstrates its values. For example, consider the mission of Health West (2018):

> Empowering our patients and communities by proactively providing quality, affordable patient-centered healthcare.

Read this mission statement carefully. What do you think are the values that drive Health West? Noting that the goal is to provide high-quality healthcare to all, and to do so in a manner that the patient can afford, demonstrates organizational awareness.

The final five elements of emotional intelligence are influence, coaching and mentoring skills, conflict management, teamwork, and inspirational leadership. In addition to behaving with respect, civility, and integrity, all of these elements are associated with effective relationship management and concern how you interact with and treat others with whom you communicate. Do you choose your words carefully when speaking in an emotionally charged atmosphere? Are you known to encourage others to succeed and then be happy for them when they do? Do you make introductions and help junior managers network with other professionals? Are you a good team player? Do you find you energize and help others see direction and sense of purpose with the task at hand as well as future tasks you and they could accomplish? If you answer "yes" to these questions, you are exhibiting excellent relationship management potential.

Conclusion

At the beginning of this chapter, we were introduced to Susan, who was excited to meet with her professor about a topic she was considering for her senior paper. She left the meeting puzzled by what had happened. The poor communication and relationship management skills exhibited by her professor resulted in his failure to inspire and her failure to experience appropriate, professional mentoring. Throughout this chapter, we proposed that communication and relationship management are essential skills for becoming effective healthcare managers. Susan's growth depends on her willingness to remain positive and be resilient even though she experienced a negative interaction with someone who could have and should have been more supportive. For Susan—and you—to flourish in the field, it is essential to learn emotional intelligence skills, to manage relationships with others in addition to managing yourself.

Mini Case Study: Emotional Intelligence and the Interview

The committee for the HR director search had been working hard these past three months. Of the 21 applicants, 5 candidates had been interviewed by phone and 2 candidates had been brought to the Hot Springs, Arkansas, hospital campus for face-to-face interviews. The two finalists' references had been called, and the purpose of today's meeting was to decide which candidate should receive the job offer. The committee members reviewed the two finalists:

Evan Scott, an assistant HR director at a hospital in Oregon, was interested in the position because she had experience in the field and wanted to move back to her home state of Arkansas. Evan still had family in the Hot Springs area and wanted to raise her children there. Evan demonstrated great poise throughout the interview, listening to each committee member and answering their questions well. The committee members liked Evan's credentials and the way she had conducted herself. She exhibited self-assurance and confidence. The chair of the search committee reported that her references had been called, and all had said Evan would be a good fit for the HR director position. A common statement made by the references was, "Evan is smart and just knows how to read people."

Catherine Curlington, an assistant HR director at a hospital in Texas, was interested in the position because she had experience in the field and was seeking an opportunity to serve as an HR director. Catherine answered all the interview questions well. She was smart, and her record showed she had done a lot to help increase retention of the healthcare personnel at her hospital in Texas. The committee members respected Catherine's credentials and past performance, but were concerned about the way she had conducted herself during the interview. She had had an altercation with the waitress at the restaurant where they all had dinner, and the behavior had seemed odd. The chair of the search committee reported that her references had been called, and all of them said Catherine was great at achieving the CEO's goal of increased retention. A common statement made by the references was, "Catherine is smart and focused on what she wants."

Mini Case Study Questions

1. With reference to the concept of emotional intelligence, whom do you think will receive the position?
2. Why do you think Evan will or will not receive the position?
3. Why do you think Catherine will or will not receive the position?

Points to Remember

- Communicating with others requires constant attention to the present interaction.
- Active listening is an important component for effective communication.
- Written communication is important, as it is relatively permanent, retrievable, and, at times, legally binding.
- Relationship management focuses on the ongoing connection between you and your workplace and its stakeholders. Employing effective communications, and understanding that when we are communicating we should treat others with respect and civility, are important factors for positive relationship management.
- When handling conflict, consider the dimensions of power, criticality, and confrontation.
- Understand that how you treat people—at work and outside of work—matters.

Challenge Yourself

1. Emotional intelligence was presented as an important concept regarding relationship management. Describe how the areas of self-awareness, self-management, social awareness, and relationship management might enhance your ability to be an effective healthcare manager.
2. Give some examples of verbal and nonverbal clues. How do they help or hinder effective communication?
3. Offer an example of conflict that you have experienced that was a positive force. Why do you consider it to be so?

For Your Consideration

1. Communication flows downward, laterally, and upward. Offer an example of lateral communication and discuss how managers might use it to their benefit.
2. Explain how power, criticality, and confrontation are important factors to consider when addressing conflict.
3. Explain why active listening is key to effective communication. Offer two examples to illustrate.

Exercise 7.1 Trouble in Billing

The billing office at Mt. Holyoke Regional Hospital is a converted inpatient room that has been divided into cubicles for the billing personnel. Wardlaw Martinez and Harriet Lockwood sit in adjacent cubicles and have shared the small working space peacefully for more than a year. However, Harriet has started a diet plan that encourages her to eat a lot of vegetables. Wardlaw is supportive of Harriet's effort to lose weight. It is important to her, and since she was diagnosed recently with type 2 diabetes, he knows her success with losing weight is important to her overall health.

However, Harriet constantly crunches raw carrots, raw celery, and just about any raw vegetable throughout the day. The *crunch, crunch, crunch* noise she makes when she eats is irritating to Wardlaw, and it is interrupting his work. The *crunch, crunch, crunch* has started again this morning, and it is only 9:00 a.m. Wardlaw sighs and stops working on billing. How can he do his work well with the *crunch, crunch, crunch* constantly coming at him? Wardlaw decides he must confront Harriet now.

Exercise 7.1 Questions

1. What is the problem in this scenario?
2. Indicate how the five conflict-management styles may help or hinder conflict resolution between Wardlaw and Harriet.
3. Which conflict-management style(s) would you recommend that Wardlaw use when he confronts Harriet?

Exercise 7.2 A Matter of Degree

Alaska Sound Family Clinic operates with two physicians, two nurses, one clinic manager, and three office assistants. Everyone knows everyone else; everyone is friends with everyone else. The office serves families in rural Alaska, and doctors and nurses treat patients in the clinic or fly to rural sites to provide annual checkups and follow-up care to patients who cannot travel to the clinic. The two physicians have earned MD degrees, and both are held in high regard by the communities they serve. Their diplomas are framed and hang on the wall in the clinic waiting room.

The clinic's two nurses—Sarah, hired six years ago, and Christy, hired almost a year ago—had reported on their application forms that they had earned BS degrees in nursing, even though the requirement was that applicants have only an associate's degree in nursing. Sarah hung her framed diploma on the wall by the receptionist desk. Christy has not brought her diploma in to be displayed. When she was asked to bring it in to hang by Sarah's diploma, Christy said she had lost it in the move from Washington State to Alaska and just has not gotten around to replacing it.

Next month, Christy will have been employed at the clinic for one year. She is a good nurse; the doctors like her work, the patients like her compassionate manner, and everyone likes her pleasant personality. The office assistants have decided that a nice way to recognize Christy's one-year anniversary would be to contact her alma mater, purchase a duplicate diploma, frame it, and hang it for all to see. When the clinic manager contacts the university, she is informed that it has no record of Christy having graduated from their BS in nursing program. It does, however, have a graduate by that name who received an associate's degree in nursing.

Exercise 7.2 Questions

1. Assume you are the clinic manager. Identify the problem in this case. What action, if any, should you take? What should you say, if anything, and to whom?
2. Assume you are Sarah, the other nurse in the clinic. Identify the problem in this case. What action, if any, should you take? What should you say, if anything, and to whom?
3. Assume you are one of the office assistants. Identify the problem in this case. What action, if any, should you take? What should you say, if anything, and to whom?

References

Anderson, N., K. Potocnik, and J. Zhou. 2014. "Innovation and Creativity in Organizations: A State-of-the-Science Review, Prospective Commentary, and Guiding Framework." *Journal of Management* 40 (5): 1297–1333.

Ayoko, O. 2016. "Workplace Conflict and Willingness to Cooperate: The Importance of Apology and Forgiveness." *International Journal of Conflict Management* 27 (2): 172–98.

Callanan, G., and D. F. Perri. 2006. "Teaching Conflict Management Using a Scenario-Based Approach." *Journal of Education for Business* 81 (3): 131–39.

Chang, T., C. Chen, and M. Chen. 2017. "A Study of Interpersonal Conflict Among Operating Room Nurses." *Journal of Nursing Research* 25 (6): 400–410.

Chou, H. W., and Y. J. Yeh. 2007. "Conflict, Conflict Management, and Performance in ERP Teams." *Social Behavior and Personality* 35 (8): 1035–48.

Clark, T. 1999. "Sharing the Importance of Attentive Listening Skills." *Journal of Management Education* 23 (2): 216–23.

Cochran, A., and W. Elder. 2015. "Effects of Disruptive Surgeon Behavior in the Operating Room." *American Journal of Surgery* 209 (1): 65–70.

Durutta, N. 2006. "The Corporate Communicator: A Senior-Level Strategist." In *The IABC Handbook of Organizational Communication*, edited by T. L. Gillis, 19–30. San Francisco, CA: Jossey-Bass.

Dye, C. 2017. *Leadership in Healthcare*, 3rd ed. Chicago: Health Administration Press.

Forni, P., D. Buccino, R. Greene, N. Freedman, D. Stevens, and T. Stack. 2003. "The Baltimore Workplace Civility Study." Published January. www.ubalt.edu/jfi/jfi/reports/civility.pdf.

Francis, L., M. C. Holmvall, and E. L. O'Brien. 2015. "The Influence of Workload and Civility of Treatment on the Perpetration of Email Incivility." *Computers in Human Behavior* 46: 191–201.

Garman, A., K. Fitz, and M. Fraser. 2006. "Communication and Relationship Management." *Journal of Healthcare Management* 51 (5): 291–94.

Goleman, D. 1998. "What Makes a Leader?" *Harvard Business Review* 76 (6): 93–102.

Goleman, D., and R. Boyatzis. 2017. "Emotional Intelligence Has 12 Elements. Which Do You Need to Work On?" *Harvard Business Review*. Published February 6. www.proveritas.com.au/downloads/Emotional-Intelligence-12-Elements.PDF.

Gratto Liebler, J., and C. R. McConnell. 2008. *Management Skills for the New Health Care Supervisor*, 5th ed. Boston: Jones & Bartlett Publishers.

Greenleaf, R. K. 1977. *Servant Leadership: A Journey into the Nature of Legitimate Power and Greatness*. New York: Paulist Press.

Harris, G. 2007. "If Your Only Tool Is a Hammer, Any Issue Will Look Like a Nail: Building Conflict Resolution and Mediation Capacity in South African Universities." *Higher Education* 55 (1): 93–101.

Health West. 2018. "About Us." Accessed April 10. www.healthwestinc.org/?page_id=17.

Katz, R. 1974. "Skills of an Effective Administrator." *Harvard Business Review* 52 (5): 90–102.

Kuypers, T., H. Guenter, and H. Emmerik. 2018. "Team Turnover and Task Conflict: A Longitudinal Study on the Moderating Effects of Collective Experience." *Journal of Management* 44 (4): 1287–311.

Meacham, M. 2015. *From Backpack to Briefcase: Professional Development in Health Care Administration*. Boston, MA: Cengage Learning.

Men, L. 2014. "Strategic Internal Communication: Transformational Leadership, Communication Channels, and Employee Satisfaction." *Management Communication Quarterly* 28 (2): 264–84.

Naresh, S. 2017. "Role of Communication in Human Resource Management—an Exploratory Study." *Imperial Journal of Interdisciplinary Research* 3 (5): 385–91.

Oppel, E., D. Mohr, and J. Benzer. 2017. "Let's Be Civil: Elaborating the Link Between Civility Climate and Hospital Performance." *Health Care Management Review* 44 (3): 1–10.

Parsons, P. J. 2001. *Beyond Persuasion: The Healthcare Manager's Guide to Strategic Communication*. Chicago: Health Administration Press.

Prause, D., and B. Mujtaba. 2015. "Conflict Management Practices for Diverse Workplaces." *Journal of Business Studies Quarterly* 6 (3): 13–22.

Raines, S. 2012. *Conflict Management for Managers: Resolving Workplace, Client, and Policy Disputes*. Hoboken, NJ: John Wiley & Sons.

Rubino, L., S. Esparza, and Y. Chassiakos. 2014. *New Leadership for Today's Health Care Professionals*. Burlington, MA: Jones & Bartlett.

Rue, L. W., and L. L. Byars. 2004. *Supervision: Key Link to Productivity*. Boston: McGraw-Hill Irwin.

Shannon, C. E., and W. Weaver. 1949. *The Mathematical Theory of Communication*. Urbana, IL: University of Illinois Press.

Weger, H. Jr., G. Bell, E. Minei, and M. Robinson. 2014. "The Relative Effectiveness of Active Listening in Initial Interactions." *International Journal of Listening* 28 (1): 13–31.

Whitworth, B. 2006. "The Corporate Communicator: A Senior-Level Strategist." In *IABC Handbook of Organizational Communication*, edited by T. L. Gillis, 205–14. San Francisco: Jossey-Bass.

Wombacher, J., and J. Felfe. 2017. "The Interplay of Team and Organizational Commitment in Motivating Employees' Interteam Conflict Handling." *Academy of Management Journal* 60 (4): 1554–81.

CHAPTER 8

TEAMWORK AND COLLABORATION

Important Terms

- Adjourning stage
- Authoritarian leadership style
- Collaboration
- Democratic leadership style
- Forming stage
- Groupthink
- Interprofessional team
- Laissez-faire leadership style
- Norming stage
- Organizational culture
- Performing stage
- Storming stage
- Team
- Teamwork climate

Learning Objectives

After reading this chapter, you will be able to do the following:

- ➤ Explain the role of teams in healthcare organizations
- ➤ Describe the importance of effective teams to patients and staff members
- ➤ Evaluate the impact of organizational culture on team success
- ➤ Identify characteristics of effective teams
- ➤ Understand the concept of groupthink
- ➤ Evaluate how peer review and teamwork help bring about better patient care

Case Study: Butting Heads

Ben Delozier, director of the stroke recovery unit at St. John's Rehabilitation Institute, closed his office door and sighed. Most of the time, he liked his work. Helping someone lead as normal a life as possible after a stroke was gratifying. The patients exerted great effort to recover, and they appreciated his and his staff's help in the rehabilitation process. Most of the time, he also liked the professional staff members with whom he worked. They were smart and worked independently, which allowed him to adopt a laissez-faire leadership approach, and the culture of the recovery unit reflected this laissez-faire style. Most team members did their jobs without involving Ben directly. And, most of the time, this organizational culture that stressed independence and a team orientation worked well.

Interprofessional team A team that forms when two or more professionals from different disciplines collaborate to enable better patient outcomes.

St. John's staff members were divided into **interprofessional teams** that focused on each individual's therapy. A nurse, a speech pathologist, an audiologist, a physical therapist (PT), and an occupational therapist (OT) would come together to plan, implement, and evaluate the specific rehabilitation treatment for a patient. The team members, who came from about the same hierarchical level, worked together to help the patient recover. "Restore the body, empower the spirit" is a philosophy to which the team members subscribed. That is, they subscribed to it most of the time.

Ben sighed again and said to himself, "Today is not one of those times." Nurse Julie Turner, audiologist Amelia Torres, and speech pathologist Martin Smith had all come to him to discuss the behavior of two of their interdisciplinary team members: Joseph Sarducci from PT and Vince Antoni from OT. Amelia had explained that Joseph and Vince never get along with each other, although each one is great to work with individually.

Joseph is friendly and helpful. He was one of the first PTs St. John's hired 30 years ago. He knows the rehab unit's procedures better than anyone, and is a well-respected PT. He conscientiously keeps up-to-date with treatments and protocol, and many of the other PTs come to Joseph for consultation. Joseph says he likes helping staff help patients "restore the body and empower the spirit."

Vince Antoni is 26 years old and graduated from the local university's OT program last year. This is his first full-time employment, and he is full of energy, full of ideas, and always ready to take on the next task. In fact, Vince sometimes gets so excited about an idea it is difficult to get him to stop talking so others can express their opinions.

Martin told Ben that when Joseph and Vince work on the same team, they never get along. They argue about anything and everything. If Vince recommends a particular course of action, Joseph opposes it. And it is difficult for Joseph to get a word in, so when he does have the opportunity to talk, he ends up shouting at Vince. Their interaction does not help them help the patient.

Amelia added, "When we tell them to stop fighting and get back to discussing the patient, they pout and refuse to participate."

Julie concluded by saying, "We just end up frustrated with the time wasted. They are both so busy trying to lead the team and telling everyone else what to do that we don't accomplish as much as we could."

Introduction

We see in the case study the failure of **collaboration** among professionals who are supposed to work effectively on a **team**. Their failure is the opposite of what you read in chapter 4's opening case about Maryland's Local Overdose Fatality Review Teams (LOFRTs). The interprofessional team members of the LOFRTs exhibited mutual respect and trust, and they collaborated to share pertinent information. There does not seem to be any trust or respect between Joseph and Vince, and they are not able to collaborate because they are busy disagreeing with each other. Their failure to collaborate is also affecting the performance of other team members who cannot focus on providing patient-centered care because they are busy trying to cope in a dysfunctional team environment. Until Vince and Joseph come to a resolution so they may work together better, their fellow team members will find it more difficult to focus on their shared purpose of delivering patient-centered care and to perform their tasks timely and well, because time is wasted.

Collaboration
Working together to achieve designated goals.

Team
A group of people who work toward a shared task and hold themselves mutually accountable for effective performance.

The organizational culture that favors a team orientation with laissez-faire leadership may be contributing to the problem. Perhaps Ben should reflect on two outcomes of his leadership style. First, he has not provided direction to his teams regarding his support for innovative patient care. Second, his hands-off approach has contributed to the growth of a competitive environment between two team members. Competition is not necessarily a negative variable among team members; however, if the competition affects their ability to collaborate on behalf of the patient, it is a problem that warrants attention.

In the last chapter, we saw that managers' clear communication skills are vital for a healthcare organization to serve patients effectively, efficiently, and safely. This chapter will address the healthcare management practice of employing teams and discuss the importance of team development and management to providing quality patient care. You will learn how to create teams comprising professionals who work toward the common goal of providing patient-centered care, as well as how to overcome barriers for effective collaboration. On a more personal level, you will read about the importance of your responsibility to create and sustain an organizational culture that lets teams operate well.

Healthcare Teams and Organizational Culture

It is standard practice for healthcare organizations to use teams. Dedicated clinical teams administer patient care, and management teams develop and implement a healthcare organization's strategy, rules, and protocol—all with the goal of improving the healthcare system and the delivery of healthcare services.

Discussing the history of team development in the US healthcare system, Heinemann (2002) noted that in the 1900s physicians initiated the use of teams as a strategy for communicating about the patient. By the 1930s, nurses—via their state associations—officially supported the team approach to coordinating patient care (Washington State Nurses Association 2018). Interdisciplinary healthcare professionals continued to endorse the use of teams in clinical practice. By the end of the twentieth century, The Joint Commission had mandated that patient care plans document interdisciplinary input and included teamwork as one of its corporate values (Joint Commission 2009):

> We believe that a productive work environment requires teamwork, active collaboration, and clear and open communication within and across organization units.

Collaboration and cooperation among professionals on a healthcare team have resulted in improvements in patient care. In a review of the literature, Lemieux-Charles and McGuire (2006) found a positive relationship between the presence of teams and patients' clinical outcomes (Caplan et al. 2004; Cohen et al. 2002).

Members of healthcare teams adhere to the principle that quality improvement is achievable by the way healthcare is delivered. To illustrate, let us examine the practice of providers who wash their hands before and after seeing a patient, as they know this reduces infection risk (Polacco et al. 2015). The World Health Organization (WHO) offers recommendations for providers to wash their hands through their "Save Lives—Clean Your Hands" promotion (WHO 2017). Healthcare team members who exhibit appropriate handwashing, as recommended by WHO, and encourage team members to do so as well exemplify improved quality of patient care, which, in turn, positively affects patient satisfaction and patient outcomes.

This focus on teams adopting quality improvements to improve patient care is supported by healthcare organizations such as the American Society for Quality (ASQ), an international organization focused on continuous quality improvement in various organizations. Its mission is to "increase the use and impact of quality in response to the diverse needs of the world" (ASQ 2018). Applied to the healthcare environment, this quality philosophy focuses on the fact that patients' satisfaction depends on outstanding performance and requires input from all the healthcare professionals involved in their care. In fact, ASQ (2018) notes that the overall goal of quality improvement is to

> engage all members of an organization to participate in improving processes, products, services, and the culture in which they work.

Quality improvement will be more fully discussed in chapter 14. For now, let us look at an example of quality improvement and teams. Virtua, a four-hospital system serving southern New Jersey and Philadelphia, reduced length of stay for congestive heart failure (CHF) patients by adopting a model of quality improvement known as Six Sigma (Ettinger 2001).

Six Sigma encourages team members to watch for variances in performance, with the goal to reduce or eliminate inefficiencies in patient-care processes (Spath 2018). To accomplish this goal, the team determines the problem that needs improvement, analyzes the way the services are currently being delivered, identifies ways to improve, implements those improvements, and assesses the outcomes. By following these steps, the team at Virtua identified a problem with length of stay for CHF patients.

CHF patients tend to be elderly, and exposure to unfamiliar surroundings and germs in a healthcare facility increase their risk for negative health outcomes. By working together and identifying potential causes of extended inpatient stays, the Virtua team could discuss, and then implement, best-practice solutions that reduced hospitalizations.

When they analyzed current processes, the team identified four factors that affected length of stay: family expectations and education regarding CHF, nursing protocol for patient care, specific care procedures, and post-hospital care instruction. Implementing changes in communication to educate families and in nursing protocol reduced the average length of a patient's stay from 6.2 days to 4.6 days, which improved outcomes for the older patients. These changes and effective teamwork also benefited the Virtua organization, thanks to the use of more efficient processes.

For another example of the importance of effective clinical teams on patient outcomes, let us consider the impact of the **teamwork climate**. Researchers or interested human resource administrators may measure teamwork climate by surveying health professionals' responses to questions about the quality of their collaboration with one another. The Agency for Healthcare Research and Quality supported research regarding the creation and use of the Safety Attitudes Questionnaire that has become widely accepted to assess the culture of safety among healthcare teams (Pronovost et al. 2003; Sexton et al. 2006; Smits et al. 2017). The survey includes a section on teamwork climate and asks respondents to rate their agreement with the following statements in the intensive care unit (ICU) setting (Sexton et al. 2006, 7):

Teamwork climate
How well healthcare team members perceive they work together to provide patient care.

- It is easy for personnel in this ICU to ask questions when there is something they do not understand.
- I have the support I need from other personnel to care for patients.
- Nurse input is well received in this ICU.
- In this ICU, it is difficult to speak up if I perceive a problem with patient care.
- Disagreements in this ICU are resolved appropriately (i.e., not who is right, but what is best for the patient).
- The physicians and the nurses work here together as a well-coordinated team.

Other research has found that a strong teamwork climate is associated with better patient care. For instance, teamwork climate is associated with lower rates of healthcare-associated infections in very low birth weight infants (Profit et al. 2017), and with outcomes for adult patients in the ICU (Huang et al. 2010; Pronovost et al. 2008).

In particular, a study by Pronovost and colleagues (2008) examined whether the Comprehensive Unit-Based Safety Program (CUSP) improved the teamwork climate in ICUs and led, in turn, to improved safety culture and better patient care. First, clinical professionals working on ICU teams answered the Safety Attitudes Questionnaire to determine a baseline teamwork climate. Then, evidence-based research on ways to improve patient safety was introduced to the teams, and members identified potential problems in their respective ICUs that might have a negative effect on patient care. Senior leadership was asked to prioritize and provide support for actions that might be taken to improve safety. Clinical staff monitored and assessed any actions taken to improve safety conditions and they, along with senior leaders, conducted a "culture checkup" that examined and reflected on ways to improve teamwork (Pronovost et al. 2008). In the end, the study found that exposure to CUSP improved teamwork climate scores in the ICU setting. And, this improved teamwork climate positively affected patient care.

Given these findings, research has also examined how healthcare managers can help create and sustain the culture of an effective teamwork climate. This research is based on the premise that **organizational culture** affects healthcare professionals' perception of their workplace climate, which in turn affects patient care quality.

Organizational culture
The shared values, beliefs, and taken-for-granted assumptions of an organization's employees.

It is the healthcare managers' responsibility to help shape an organizational culture that allows for effective teamwork. Edgar H. Schein, social psychologist and noted scholar on organizational culture, proposed that organizational culture may be analyzed at three levels (Schein 2010, 53):

1. Visible artifacts;
2. Espoused beliefs, values, roles, and behavioral norms; and
3. Tacit, taken-for-granted, basic underlying assumptions.

The term *visible artifacts* refers to what you can see, such as the uniforms worn by various staff members in a healthcare setting, the layout of the nurses' station on hospital floors, and the appearance of patient waiting rooms in a clinic. Espoused beliefs, values, roles, and behavioral norms all refer to what employees learn about the organization and adopt as organizationally sanctioned. This does not mean all employees will accept these as their own beliefs, values, or norms, but those who do not may risk "excommunication" (Schein 2010, 26) from the group. For instance, if managers at a teaching hospital support the inclusion of students as interns but do not encourage departmental employees to serve as preceptors, then the behavior contradicts what the espoused beliefs state. Also, if an employee refuses to serve as preceptor when management has endorsed student interns, then that employee risks management and peers perceiving she is not a good team member.

The last level identified by Schein (2010) regarding organizational culture refers to the taken-for-granted, or the unspoken expectations. As you learn about an organization's culture, you may see that these taken-for-granted, underlying assumptions about the way employees conduct themselves, what senior management considers important regarding employee behavior, and how work is actually done can help you predict how the organization may respond in future circumstances. You can, thus, determine your actions accordingly.

For example, the firm Medical Management (MedMan) illustrates the importance of culture and effectiveness in the workplace. Jim Trounson (2018a) founded MedMan in 1977 with the thought that managing medical clinics was best conducted by a team, not an individual. If the MedMan team managed the physician practice, then the physicians could devote their time to their patients. Today, 11 MedMan managers and seven corporate-based officers are responsible for ten medical groups located in Idaho, Oregon, Washington, Montana, Wyoming, and Utah.

The MedMan culture rests on the principles of respect, integrity, loyalty, and sharing (MedMan Medical Management 2018):

> Respect—We constantly strive to earn and express respect for ourselves, our clients and our employees;
>
> Integrity—We do the right thing;
>
> Loyalty—We build the trust required of a high-performance team; and
>
> Sharing—We improve each other's performance through aggressive information transfer.

Given that these culture statements are published on MedMan's website, you know the firm is built on the *principles* of effective teams and active individual participation. But are they an accurate indicator of the *true* culture? The sharing habits among MedMan's managers and employees tell us more.

Since the firm's managers are located in six states, it is not possible for them to gather at a conference table frequently to share. To ensure they do meet face-to-face on a scheduled basis, MedMan holds annual retreats. Trounson (2018a) explained:

> We are a virtual company spread all over the Northwest. The retreat is one way to create a sense of company, to encourage a team spirit without people having a collective "water cooler" to gather around.

MedMan also holds "think tanks" through video conferencing. Better than mere conference calls, these let managers share documents and see one another—in real time—which improves communication. Staff members often participate in think tanks three times a day regarding committee meetings, problem-solving sessions, or task force updates.

Each week, MedMan also holds 30-minute meetings through video conferencing, during which each manager talks about what is going on in her clinic and describes something she is proud of or something she is worried about. For example, recruiting was the topic of a March 2018 weekly meeting. One manager was having difficulty recruiting an appropriate nurse practitioner (NP) or physician assistant (PA) for her practice. A fellow manager provided the contact information for a reputable recruiting company she had used successfully to recruit an NP. Another manager reported he knew a PA that was looking for a position in that area and thought they would work well together. Thus, the 30 minutes spent by MedMan team managers talking with each other offered solutions to a pressing problem.

Monthly one-hour educational colloquiums also are held to share knowledge that may be of interest to managers. During the March 2018 session, the focus was on generational challenges and how to effectively manage employees from different cohorts (e.g., baby boomers, Generation Xers, millennials), who all have different expectations and work behaviors. The colloquium described each group and identified what managers might face at different times, such as during recruiting. For example, millennials, born between 1982 and 2004, often want to work at a company that has purpose and will help make the world a better place. Thus, a manager can address how MedMan may fit that profile when discussing corporate culture.

Lastly, each quarter Trounson leads a town hall meeting over video conferencing. In March 2018, the topic was the business of MedMan—its stock price, the opportunity for employees to buy into the firm, and succession planning, as Trounson was preparing to retire after 41 years of leadership. In addition, all practice financial information is posted so each manager knows how well his or her clinic is performing compared to all the other MedMan clinics. Managers also may discuss who needs support or training.

Given all these opportunities for managers to share information, you might surmise that sharing is indeed a taken-for-granted, underlying core of the MedMan culture. However, what happens when the sharing helps clinics do well also is an important indicator of the firm's culture. At MedMan, salary increases are tied to client satisfaction scores. The clients, usually a physician group, are the owners of the clinics. And, the salary increases of MedMan managers are partially based on client scores from *all* the firm's clients. The rationale for this compensation practice rests on the assumption that clinic performance improves with good teamwork, advice, and solutions offered. Thus, sharing is not only tied to the face-to-face or online opportunities to talk with each other; the salary policy underscores the importance to MedMan of communicating and sharing well.

A strong culture like this is characterized by employees' devout commitment to the organization's values, beliefs, and taken-for-granted assumptions regarding the way things are done. Organizational culture affects healthcare professionals' perception of their workplace climate, which in turn affects patient care quality. And, as we turn our attention to characteristics of effective teams, it is important to note that a strong culture also promotes better outcomes for staff working on effective teams.

Research regarding the team approach supports beneficial outcomes not only for patients, but also for staff members. Collaboration and cooperation among healthcare team members are positively associated with job satisfaction; in addition, recruitment and retention are influenced by the organizational environment. If upper management supports team efforts, if team leaders are positive regarding the team, if communication is clear regarding the team's goals, and if communication among members supports the charge's importance to organizational success, positive outcomes are more likely (Amos, Hu, and Herrick 2005; Anderson 1993; Barczak 1996; Borrill et al. 2000; Korner et al. 2015; Weisman et al. 1993).

Characteristics of Effective Teams

Given the positive outcomes associated with teamwork, researchers have investigated the characteristics of effective teams. For example, Hellriegel and Slocum (2003) developed a self-assessment tool to determine team effectiveness. Team members are asked if they

- know why the team exists,
- have a procedure for making decisions,
- communicate freely among themselves,
- help each other,
- deal with conflict among themselves, and
- identify and address ways to improve the team's functioning.

Looking back to this chapter's opening case study, if Julie, Martin, Amelia, Joseph, and Vince completed this self-assessment, their team probably would score poorly. While the team members understand why the team exists, the evidence indicates they do not communicate freely among themselves. Vince and Joseph do not help one another, Joseph dismisses Vince's ideas, and Vince resists allowing others to speak. In addition, the team members do not deal with conflict among themselves; Julie, Amelia, and Martin all turned to Ben, their supervisor, for help.

The Academic Health Center Task Force on Interdisciplinary Health Team Development (1996) lists ten competencies team members should strive to achieve. These competencies form the basis for team self-assessment:

1. Do team members focus on the patient as their first priority?
2. Have the members established common goals regarding patient outcomes?
3. Do the members understand the roles of other team members from different professions?

4. Do the members have confidence in each other's abilities?
5. Are members flexible in their roles to accommodate team goals?
6. Do the members share group norms and expectations?
7. Do they deal with conflict among themselves?
8. Do members communicate freely among themselves?
9. Do team members share responsibility for actions made by the team?
10. Do the members evaluate themselves and their team performance?

If we apply the assessments of Hellriegel and Slocum (2003) and the Academic Health Center Task Force on Interdisciplinary Health Team Development (1996) to the interdisciplinary team of Julie, Martin, Amelia, Joseph, and Vince, we would conclude that this team is not as effective as it could be. Their uncooperative behavior has resulted in the team's accomplishing less than it could. Their team lacks the needed communication and conflict-management skills to address the problems that have occurred. Hence, members have turned to Ben for help.

The problem confronting Ben Delozier from the opening case study is that he has a team that lacks collaboration and cooperation. Ben has three concerns to address: the conflict between Joseph and Vince; the potential effect of this conflict on other team members' commitment; and, most important, the conflict's potential interference with patient care. In addition, Ben should be aware that these team dynamics have developed in part because he has not created and established a culture that supports mutual respect and sharing. Ben knows the conflict is a barrier to effective team performance, and he has several options for addressing this problem.

First, he can reassign responsibilities so Joseph and Vince are not on the same interdisciplinary team. Second, he can talk with them separately to ascertain why the conflict exists and to develop a plan to address their concerns effectively. Third, he may choose not to get involved and let team members address the conflict themselves. Ben rejects the first option, because St. John's Rehabilitation Institute is about patient care. The staff members need to learn how to behave in a professional manner to help patients. At the same time, however, Ben knows the context in which the team operates needs to be addressed to prevent this problem from happening again. He needs to rally the team and help establish a department-wide culture that encourages effective team construction and maintenance. Ignoring the problem is not a viable option. Ben needs to work on the immediate issue regarding Joseph and Vince, who, in turn, need to work on a plan of corrective action. But Ben also needs to devote time to communicating his vision of how the department teams should work, and he should create opportunities for employees to communicate more effectively. Ben could take some lessons from the MedMan culture.

Strategies for Developing Team Effectiveness

Team effectiveness depends on how well team members work together. Tuckman (1965) and Tuckman and Jensen (1977) propose that individuals move through stages of team development and behavior. These stages are forming, storming, norming, performing, and adjourning. The **forming stage** is an orientation phase in which members are given their charge or purpose for the team. During this stage, team members learn about one another's personalities. The **storming stage** is characterized by conflict and emotional issues that may inhibit a team's progress toward performing the task with which it was charged. How effectively (or not) team members learn to work with one another depends on their personalities.

The St. John's Rehab team is stuck in this storming stage. Joseph and Vince have allowed their conflict to overshadow work efforts, and the other team members are frustrated by the time that has been wasted. The ultimate concern is that Joseph and Vince are more focused on their conflict than they are on developing, implementing, and evaluating the patient's rehabilitation care plan.

If this team is able to move forward, it will experience the **norming stage** that Tuckman (1965) proposed. In this stage, team members agree upon working styles and make compromises. Conflict is reduced as the team unifies. The energy that had been directed toward the conflict is now devoted to the charge of patient care. The team then enters the fourth stage, **performing**, and they work productively together. The final stage is **adjourning**, during which the team goes over its successes and individuals disengage from the team. As the patient is discharged from the rehabilitation unit, the team regroups to focus on a new task, or a new team is created, and the process begins again.

Managers can establish an organizational context that is conducive to team success. They communicate the team's charge clearly; set the stage for a positive and supportive environment; and focus on the team's goal. Staff members expect managers to take the lead to establish a positive work environment (Harmon, Brallier, and Brown 2002). During the forming stage of the rehab team, Ben could have met with the members and reviewed the team's purpose, discussed the patient load for the team, and endorsed a positive work environment in which team members treat one another with respect, listen to one another's ideas, and allow one another to contribute.

Moreover, at this stage of team formation, a shared mental model may be identified. Shared mental models give team members a common understanding of the work at hand (Weller, Boyd, and Cumin 2014). The team gains a sense of the treatment plan and each member's individual role and responsibilities. Without a shared mental model, team members are less likely to contribute to decision-making about a patient or to solve problems (Stout et al. 1999).

To move the St. John's team out of the storming stage, Ben needs to decide how to deal with the problem before it escalates or leads to poor patient care. As mentioned earlier, he could ignore the problem, but this action would only encourage the team members

Forming stage
The first stage of teamwork, during which members are given their charge or the purpose of the team.

Storming stage
The second stage of teamwork, during which team members learn about one another. This stage is characterized by conflict and emotional issues that may inhibit a team's progress.

Norming stage
The third stage of teamwork, during which team members agree upon working styles, conflict is reduced, and group cohesiveness emerges.

Performing stage
The fourth stage of teamwork, during which team members are engaged in the work and purpose of the team.

Adjourning stage
The final stage of teamwork, during which team members review outcomes and successes and individuals disengage from the team.

who approached him to conclude he does not support them or the team's goals. He might encourage the three team members to talk with Joseph and Vince and let the team solve the problem. However, Amelia tried that without success. So Ben opted to meet with Joseph and Vince separately, and they developed a plan of correction. He also met with the team as a whole, the first step in creating a cultural climate of support and encouragement—a characteristic of effective teams. Ben's intervention was critical, as this conflict was on track to cause errors and poor patient care (Salas et al. 2015).

Authoritarian
A leadership style in which power is concentrated in the leader.

As the team resolved its storming experiences and regrouped, leadership style was also addressed. Leadership in teams may be authoritarian in style, laissez-faire, or democratic. Joseph and Vince had each been vying for **authoritarian** rule, but the resulting conflict suggested this leadership style might not be the best for this team. **Laissez-faire**, or hands-off, leadership might not have been the best approach either, as team members needed to bring in their expertise from their different disciplines and discuss patient care specifics.

Laissez-faire
A "hands-off" leadership approach.

At various times, different team members may need to take the lead in a conflict or process—what is known as **democratic**, or shared, leadership. This may be the best approach for the five team members in the case study, as they each come from approximately the same hierarchical level and can pool their expertise to help the patient "restore the body and empower the spirit." Research also favors democratic leadership, as studies have indicated teams who share leadership tend to perform better than those with one authoritarian leader (Solansky 2008).

Democratic
A leadership approach in which team members share governance.

Going forward, Ben's challenge is to figure out the best way to ensure Joseph and Vince fulfill their roles as team members. Fisher, Ury, and Patton (1991) offer advice on principled negotiation among people who are in conflict with one another. The first step is to define the problem and outline the options. Ben already accomplished this. Second, the authors recommend separating the people from the issues and encouraging each person to understand the other's position. When Ben met with Joseph and Vince, he asked Joseph why he ignores Vince's ideas. Joseph replied that Vince is very new to the profession and could learn more if he took time to listen. Vince then offered his opinion that Joseph had been there more than 30 years and was a "know-it-all." As the supervisor, Ben directed Joseph and Vince to propose what they thought might work for both parties so the team would function better. Fisher, Ury, and Patton (1991) suggest that the more the conflicting parties are involved in the negotiation process, the more likely they are to support any initiative that addresses the problem. Ben's involvement of Joseph and Vince in the process was more likely to result in a successful outcome. As they brainstormed possible solutions, they were focusing on the ultimate goal of any healthcare team: working together to help patients.

Fisher, Ury, and Patton (1991) also stress that each team member should allow other team members to express their emotions and should listen actively to improve communication. Active listening is discussed in detail in chapter 7; its basic principles are that the receiver of the message should pay attention to the sender (i.e., the speaker) and focus on the contents of the message. The receiver may summarize the message to ensure it was delivered clearly and correctly. Last, the speaker and receiver should respect one another throughout the process. If one party is unwilling to engage in this principled negotiation process, the other parties should keep guiding the conversation back to the problem at hand. This helps keep the attention focused on solving the problem, which lets the team move on to the performing stage, the ultimate goal of Ben's meeting with Joseph and Vince.

A Word About Groupthink

While research indicates that cohesive team efforts benefit patients and staff, evidence also suggests that mistakes may occur precisely because a team is especially cohesive. Janus (1972, 1982) proposed the term **groupthink** to illustrate this phenomenon. Groups whose members are well informed and intelligent but who also define themselves and their work as morally superior, are isolated from outside ideas and practices, have a stressful work environment, possess illusions of invulnerability, and experience strong in-group cohesiveness may make decisions that are not in the best interests of patient care (Janus 1972, 1982).

Groupthink
Conformity to group values and ethics that can lead to negative outcomes.

Healthcare teams in the performing stage are generally cohesive, and of course all healthcare team members are extremely busy and work under time constraints. Healthcare professionals often spend less time outside the healthcare arena because of the profession's demands and, as a result, they may become isolated and form an even more cohesive group with other team members. In addition, healthcare is a stressful occupation, and team members may be pressured to contain costs. Combined, these factors may lead to groupthink and cause a good team to make poor decisions.

Heinemann, Farrell, and Schmitt (1994) applied Janus's groupthink theory to the geriatric healthcare environment. They presented the case of an older couple in which the husband was paralyzed from the neck down and the wife had served as his primary caretaker for more than 18 months. Not surprisingly, the wife became exhausted from the physical toll of caring for her husband, and she regularly let the provider team members know she was overwhelmed. The team members did not hear her concerns; rather, they were strictly focused on the needs of their patient, her husband. Two members of the man's healthcare team were extremely domineering; the rest were busy, under stress, and focused on containing costs.

Communication among team members was left to the two most vocal; other member input was nil. One option for the husband was nursing home care, but some team members exhibiting a morally superior stance looked down on this care, an opinion they felt was justified by the husband's preference not to go to a nursing home. Again, they ignored the wife's communications regarding the toll the care was taking on her mental and physical well-being.

However, after a year and a half of providing care at home, the wife knew she could not continue to deliver the care her husband needed. When she again expressed concern regarding her abilities, the team members did not listen to her, and options such as respite care or nursing home care were never suggested as viable options. The result was that the wife threatened to abandon her caregiving role completely. Thus, while the team members felt the wife's caring for the husband was best for the patient, their inability to listen to her and examine other options resulted in the team's failure. The wife's leaving would certainly not have been in the patient's best interest.

Healthcare delivery team members need to be conscious of the potential for groupthink. They should avoid assuming a morally superior stance, because other healthcare options may fit a patient's needs well. They should also avoid isolation from other healthcare practices and protocols. A commitment to sponsor outside speakers may help a healthcare organization decrease the isolation factor. To provide an effective treatment plan, team members should commit to listening to others who care for a patient, such as a spouse, and to the patient's desires. Determined to follow the patient's wishes and fortified by their disdain for nursing home care, the team members in this example almost caused a disaster because the groupthink had created an environment in which the primary caregiver was ignored. The result was that the wife thought she had no other option than to abandon her supportive, caregiving role for her husband.

To avoid future groupthink, this team needs to reform to discourage disdain for one type of caregiving over another and to adopt a willingness to hear from current caregivers. Furthermore, this team was dominated by two members; it is important to allow each team member's input. Open communication, respect for team member participation, and regularly scheduled evaluation of team behavior and performance will help prevent groupthink.

Best Practices for Team Formation

Healthcare managers who rely on team output need professional staff members who understand why the team was formed; allow for respectful, open communication among team members; share leadership; deal with conflict effectively; and evaluate team performance on a regular basis (Couzins and Beagrie 2004; Hellriegel and Slocum 2003; Weaver, Dy, and Rosen 2014). Healthcare managers may help by clearly defining the team goals. The team then should adhere to the following best practices:

1. Determine the best way to attain goals (what protocol may help the patient improve).
2. Agree on team norms (how team members will collaborate and communicate with one another).
3. Advocate shared leadership for interprofessional teams.
4. Assign specific team member functions (e.g., one member may schedule meetings, another may make certain that documentation for the patient is complete).

5. Hold regularly scheduled meetings.
6. Handle conflict with team members directly, but seek assistance from the supervisor if internal mechanisms do not work.
7. Evaluate team performance on a regular basis, addressing the team's strengths and weaknesses. Healthcare managers provide a positive environment, intervene as necessary to help solve problems, and evaluate team performance. As a result, the team members are supported so they may work to "restore the body and empower the spirit."

Conclusion

At the beginning of this chapter we met Ben, who had to address a conflict between two team members in his department. We quickly surmised that the problem was larger than just two employees disagreeing. Rather, a culture of mutual respect was missing, as team members made clear through their frustration with the dysfunctional team and the lack of collaboration and cooperation among them. Throughout this chapter, we put forth that Ben's solution to the problem rested with his intervention on two levels—the team level, to confront both Joseph and Vince, and the department level, to confront the need for a culture of team excellence. Ben could learn from our example of MedMan, where a strong culture helps lead to better team performance. Ben's success—as well as yours when you manage teams—will depend on mastering an understanding of team formation and assessment, which are essential for quality patient care and employee satisfaction.

Mini Case Study: MedMan and Its Cultural Climate

As discussed earlier, Jim Trounson (2018a) founded MedMan Medical Management in 1977 with the strategy that placing quality on-site healthcare managers in physician-controlled practices would create clinics that work well. His philosophy was that clinics are best managed by a team, not an individual, and that if a high-functioning team managed a physician practice, the physicians could devote their time to their patients and improve patients' quality of care. The business model worked like this: The physician-led clinic hired MedMan to place a healthcare manager on the clinic site. Through a team approach, MedMan managers, based in Idaho and the five surrounding states, served as experts and resources for each other, providing continual support on- and off-site for its clients.

To create and reinforce a culture based on respect, integrity, loyalty, and sharing, Trounson established a "taken-for-granted assumption" of the MedMan approach to teamwork. Newly hired MedMan managers undergo a two-day orientation in Boise that introduces the MedMan culture and reviews best clinic practices. To maintain the positive teamwork environment, numerous communication channels have been established so knowledge is shared among practice managers, to the benefit of all the clinics. The MedMan managers team up with each other in person twice annually at retreats, and at other times of the year during regular virtual meetings. These virtual conferences include the "think tanks" (held three times per day), the 30-minute weekly meetings, the monthly colloquia that last 60 minutes, and the quarterly town hall meeting, led by Trounson.

Along with the face-to-face and virtual encounters, all managers have a mentor with whom they talk once a week. In addition, they regularly e-mail each other questions such as the following:

> *While we are familiar with dogs as service animals, what do we do about a support parrot, if anything?*
>
> *We have a patient who is a jail inmate, and his wife is authorized to receive health information about him. However, the jail does not want us to give out information about appointment dates outside the jail. Can we release the personal health information, but not include the next appointment date with the wife?*

Along with the managers and Trounson to provide responses, MedMan can forward e-mails to their attorney on retainer or the board of directors, which is made up of physicians and clinic and hospital executives. MedMan also deploys a monthly newsletter and publishes an ongoing corporate blog. All communications, whether in person, virtual, or in writing, are centered on the same theme of providing excellent administrators to client practices to facilitate better patient care. Overall, MedMan's activities reinforce a culture of teamwork, which helps improve physician and patient lives, helps the clinics perform better, and increases access so patients receive quality healthcare.

A recent blog post illustrates the MedMan culture (Trounson 2018b):

> We've gone overboard inconveniencing ourselves and our patients.
>
> "If this in an emergency, hang up and dial 911" is my favorite example of an assault on patients. There are clinics with locked doors needing secret codes to get the patients from the reception to exam areas. I hate sliding glass windows at reception desks allegedly for HIPAA privacy.
>
> When trying to find actual requirements for these kinds of restraints I'm being referred anecdotally to some "recommendation" by an attorney, insurance company or advisor. Unlike consultants who achieve full employment scaring physicians into hyper-compliance, MedMan stays around to manage clinics and, while complying with regulations, rationally balances safety with practicality.
>
> The price is too high in terms of productivity and quality of our and our patients' lives for mindless acceptance of all safety considerations. In a one-physician practice,

patients listening to the 911 admonition takes them a combined thirty hours per year. Was that a consideration, and who made this decision to annoy them anyway?

I prefer a world in which the masses have fewer restrictions and delays, and we deal bravely with the occasional exceptions and offenders.

Mini Case Study Questions

1. Explain how the virtual meetings allow for team development at MedMan.
2. Explain how the blog post, "We're Becoming Too Safe," illustrates the MedMan culture.
3. MedMan was founded in 1977 and remains a successful business to date. Why do you think MedMan enjoys such success with its clients? Refer to the MedMan Medical Management website, www.medman.com, as you consider your answer.

Points to Remember

- Teams have an important role in providing quality patient care. The Joint Commission has mandated interdisciplinary input and included teamwork as one of its corporate values because of the relationship between effective teamwork and patient outcomes.
- Organizational culture affects teamwork climate, which in turn affects patient care.
- Healthcare professionals who experience effective teamwork report better job satisfaction.
- Groupthink may yield negative outcomes, for the team members as well as for the patients. Too much conformity to group values and ethics may lead team members to fail to consider alternative ideas.
- Effective teamwork results from a culture that supports open communication among team members that is respectful yet can deal with conflict effectively.

Challenge Yourself

1. Think of a team you have been a part of (e.g., a sports team or musical group). With reference to Hellriegel and Slocum (2003) and the Academic Health Center Task Force on Interdisciplinary Health Team Development (1996) assessment plan, evaluate your team. Was it successful, according to the assessment criteria? Why or why not?
2. When is an authoritarian leadership style more effective for teams? A democratic style of leadership? A laissez-faire style? Which do you think is more appropriate for teams dedicated to healthcare delivery? Why?
3. The mini case, "MedMan and Its Cultural Climate," quoted from two e-mailed questions. Conduct your own research. How would you respond to these e-mails? Interview local

clinic or hospital administrators. How would they respond to the queries? What insight do their answers give into their corporate culture?

For Your Consideration

1. Explain why effective teams are important for better outcomes. Give an example to illustrate.
2. This chapter's discussion of groupthink presented a case in which the healthcare team did not pay attention to the wife's concerns. Why do you think they did not listen to her?

Exercise 8.1 Groupthink and the Board of Governors

The physicians of Beachside Medical Group had spent more than five years combining seven local practices into a single, multispecialty group practice. The goal of this merger was to bring the best, most respected practices together to create efficiencies in clinic management. It also gave the doctors a more powerful bargaining position in negotiations with insurance companies on policies and payment structures. The group had also introduced a radiology center, which would not have been possible if the practices had remained separate. Beachside Medical Group was now made up of 20 physicians, five physician assistants, ten nurses, three radiology technologists, one clinic manager, and six general staff and office assistants.

The governing board of Beachside Medical Group made decisions about third-party contract negotiations, resource allocations, and strategy for the group's future. The six board members were all physicians. They noted that the board's makeup was skewed toward a physician perspective, but they were satisfied that they would represent all interests and take their commitment to the group seriously. After all, they were the ones who were in charge and had volunteered to serve on the board.

The board met on a monthly basis for the first year to deal with all of the new clinic's business activities. Sometimes they asked Leslie Duncan, the clinic manager, to attend; sometimes they did not include Leslie. They made resolutions and passed them without input from the other physicians in the practice or from the clinic staff. After all, they knew best. They were the doctors who had volunteered. The result was that the board often met without notifying other clinic physicians and staff. Closed-door meetings became the norm.

Some of the new rules being passed frustrated Leslie. "The board is creating a series of problems for the staff. They are creating a mess, and I do not know how much longer I can continue to clean up after them." The previous month, the board had mandated a change in work schedules for the office staff, converting eight-hour days into ten-hour shifts without consulting

Leslie or the staff members affected by the change. This change in working hours meant that those staff members with children needed to change their childcare arrangements to accommodate the board's rules, and all staff members needed to change their day-to-day routines.

Two office assistants quit out of frustration, and Leslie was left to find qualified assistants to fill the positions quickly. She had just succeeded when the board issued two new mandates. The first was that all promised annual pay raises for staff would be postponed until the following quarter because profits had been lower than expected. The second was that all office personnel except for the physicians would punch a time clock so their hours could be documented. The staff members who had not quit after the schedule changes had stayed primarily because they were proud of their contributions to the multispecialty practice. Leslie questioned the decision not to follow through on a promised pay raise because of lower-than-expected profits while at the same time incurring an expense to add a monitoring system (the time clock). Leslie asked the board if she could talk about the new policy with them, and they agreed to meet with her today.

Exercise 8.1 Questions

1. What do you think Leslie should say to the board members when she meets with them?
2. With reference to the concept of groupthink, how do you think the board made the decisions Leslie is questioning?
3. What will the repercussions be if the board members go unchecked? What do you think will happen to staff–physician relations?

Exercise 8.2 New Team Formation and the Reduction of Patient Errors

Grace Hunter, the vice president for strategic management, listened to Oli Bordeux, the CEO. They were discussing a new strategic initiative to eliminate patient errors. In the past five years, the 336-bed hospital where they worked had reported nine adverse patient errors that had resulted in death or a permanent vegetative state. Grace knew these statistics did not compare favorably with numbers for other hospitals in their area. Virginia Hope, 50 miles away and licensed for 1,400 beds, had reported four incidents and no deaths in the past five years. Swan Valley Medical Center, 80 miles away and licensed for 450 beds, had reported five incidents and three deaths over the same time period.

Oli said to Grace, "I need you to form a team to deal with this. And Grace, I need this team to find us some answers. Put together a team that can underscore the need for every staff member to step up. We need to identify potential problems before they become errors that affect our patients and their families."

Grace promised Oli she would do what he had asked. As she left Oli's office, she said to herself, "I just need to get the right people to commit to making a difference, and then to get them to make the difference. Not an easy task."

Exercise 8.2 Questions

1. What advice would you offer Grace regarding who should be on this team? What advice would you offer regarding the team's forming phase?
2. How should the team evaluate its own performance?
3. How should Grace evaluate the team's performance?

References

Academic Health Center Task Force on Interdisciplinary Health Team Development. 1996. *Developing Health Care Teams*. Published September 1. https://conservancy.umn.edu/handle/11299/103777.

American Society for Quality (ASQ). 2018. "Who We Are." Accessed July 19. https://asq.org/about-asq.

Amos, M., J. Hu, and C. Herrick. 2005. "The Impact of Team Building on Communication and Job Satisfaction of Nursing Staff." *Journal for Nurses in Staff Development* 21 (1): 10–16.

Anderson, L. 1993. "Teams: Group Processes, Success, and Barriers." *Journal of Nursing Administration* 23 (9): 15–19.

Barczak, N. 1996. "How to Lead Effective Teams." *Critical Care Nursing Quarterly* 19 (1): 73–82.

Borrill, C., M. West, D. Shapiro, and A. Rees. 2000. "Team Working and Effectiveness in Health Care." *British Journal of Health Care Management* 6 (8): 364–71.

Caplan, G., A. Williams, B. Daly, and K. Abraham. 2004. "A Randomized Controlled Trial of Comprehensive Geriatric Assessment and Multidisciplinary Intervention After Discharge of Elderly from the Emergency Department—The DEED II Study." *Journal of the American Geriatric Society* 52 (9): 1417–23.

Cohen, H., J. Feussner, M. Weinberger, M. Carnes, R. Hamdy, F. Hsieh, C. Phibbs, D. Courtney, K. Lyles, C. May, C. McMurtry, L. Pennypacker, D. Smith, N. Ainslie, T. Hornick, K. Brodkin, and P. Lavori. 2002. "A Controlled Trial of Inpatient and Outpatient Geriatric Evaluation and Management." *New England Journal of Medicine* 346 (12): 905–12.

Couzins, M., and S. Beagrie. 2004. "How To . . . Build Effective Teams." *Personnel Today*, February, 29–30.

Ettinger, W. 2001. "Six Sigma: Adapting GE's Lessons to Healthcare." *Trustee* 54 (8): 10–16.

Fisher, R., W. Ury, and B. Patton. 1991. *Getting to Yes: Negotiating Agreement Without Giving In*. New York: Penguin Books.

Harmon, S., S. Brallier, and G. Brown. 2002. "Organizational and Team Context." In *Team Performance in Health Care*, edited by G. Heinemann and A. Zeiss, 57–70. New York: Kluwer Academic/Plenum Publishers.

Heinemann, G. D. 2002. "Teams in Health Care Settings: Assessment and Development." *Team Performance in Health Care*, edited by G. D. Heinemann and A. M. Zeiss, 3–17. New York: Kluwer Academic/Plenum Publishers.

Heinemann, G. D., M. P. Farrell, and M. H. Schmitt. 1994. "Groupthink Theory and Research: Implications for Decision Making in Geriatric Health Care Teams." *Educational Gerontology* 20 (1): 71–85.

Hellriegel, D., and J. Slocum. 2003. *Organizational Behavior*, 10th ed. Cincinnati, OH: Southwestern College Publishing.

Huang, D. T., G. Clermont, L. Kong, L. Weissfeld, J. Sexton, K. Rowan, and D. Angus. 2010. "Intensive Care Unit Safety Culture and Outcomes: A US Multicenter Study." *International Journal for Quality in Health Care* 22 (3): 151–61.

Janus, I. 1982. *Groupthink: Psychological Studies of Policy Decisions and Fiascoes*, 2nd ed. Boston: Houghton Mifflin.

———. 1972. *Victims of Groupthink: A Psychological Study of Foreign-Policy Decisions and Fiascoes*. Boston: Houghton Mifflin.

Joint Commission. 2009. "The Joint Commission Mission Statement." Published August. www.jointcommission.org/assets/1/18/Mission_Statement_8_09.pdf.

Korner, M., A. M. Wirtz, J. Bengel, and S. A. Goritz. 2015. "Relationship of Organizational Culture, Teamwork and Job Satisfaction in Interprofessional Teams." *BMC Health Services Research* 15 (243): 1–12.

Lemieux-Charles, L., and W. McGuire. 2006. "What Do We Know About Health Care Team Effectiveness? A Review of the Literature." *Medical Care Research and Review* 63 (3): 263–300.

MedMan Medical Management. 2018. "Our Culture: We Do the Right Thing." Accessed April 29. www.medman.com/culture.

Polacco, M., L. Shinkunas, E. Perencevitch, L. Kaldjian, and H. Reisinger. 2015. "See One, Do One, Teach One: Hand Hygiene Attitudes Among Medical Students, Interns, and Faculty." *American Journal of Infection Control* 43 (2): 159–61.

Profit, J., P. Sharek, P. Kan, J. Rigdon, M. Desai, C. Nisbet, D. Tawfik, E. Thomas, H. Lee, and J. Sexton. 2017. "Teamwork in the NICU Setting and Its Association with Healthcare-Associated Infections in Very Low Birth Weight Infants." *American Journal of Perinatology* 34 (10): 1032–40.

Pronovost, P., S. Berenholtz, C. Goeschel, I. Thom, S. Watson, C. Holzmueller, J. Lyon, L. Lubomski, D. Thompson, D. Needham, R. Hyzy, R. Welsh, G. Roth, J. Bander, L. Morlock, and J. Sexton. 2008. "Improving Patient Safety in Intensive Care Units in Michigan." *Journal of Critical Care* 23 (2): 207–21.

Pronovost, P., B. Weast, C. Holzmueller, B. Rosenstein, R. Kidwell, K. Haller, E. Feroli, J. Sexton, and H. Rubin. 2003. "Evaluation of the Culture of Safety: Survey of Clinicians and Managers in an Academic Medical Center." *Quality and Safety in Health Care* 12 (6): 405–10.

Salas, E., M. Shuffler, A. Thayer, W. Bedwell, and E. Lazzara. 2015. "Understanding and Improving Teamwork in Organizations: A Scientifically Based Practical Guide." *Human Resource Management* 54 (4): 599–622.

Schein, E. 2010. *Organizational Culture and Leadership*, 4th ed. San Francisco: John Wiley & Sons.

Sexton, J. B., R. L. Helmreich, T. B. Neilands, K. Rowan, K. Vella, J. Boyden, P. R. Roberts, and E. J. Thomas. 2006. "The Safety Attitudes Questionnaire: Psychometric Properties, Benchmarking Data, and Emerging Research." *BMC Health Services Research* 6: 44.

Smits, M., E. Keizer, P. Giesen, E. Deilkas, D. Hofoss, and G. Bondevik. 2017. "The Psychometric Properties of the 'Safety Attitudes Questionnaire' in Out-of-Hours Primary Care Services in the Netherlands." *PLoS ONE* 12 (2): e0172390.

Solansky, S. 2008. "Leadership Style and Team Processes in Self-Managed Teams." *Journal of Leadership and Organizational Studies* 14 (4): 332–41.

Spath, P. 2018. *Introduction to Healthcare Quality Management*, 3rd ed. Chicago: Health Administration Press.

Stout, J. R., A. J. Cannon-Bowers, E. Salas, and M. D. Milanovich. 1999. "Planning, Shared Mental Models, and Coordinated Performance: An Empirical Link Is Established." *Human Factors* 41 (1): 61–71.

Trounson, J. 2018a. Interview with L. Cellucci, April 16.

———. 2018b. "We're Becoming Too Safe." MedMan Blog. Published April 18. www.medman.com/single-post/2018/04/18/Were-Becoming-Too-Safe.

Tuckman, B. 1965. "Developmental Sequences in Small Groups." *Psychological Bulletin* 63: 384–99.

Tuckman, B., and M. Jensen. 1977. "Stages of Small Group Development Revisited." *Group and Organizational Studies* 2 (4): 419–27.

Washington State Nurses Association. 2018. "The 1930s." Accessed July 23. www.wsna.org/about/centennial/1930s.

Weaver, S., S. Dy, and M. Rosen. 2014. "Team-Training in Healthcare: A Narrative Synthesis of the Literature." *BMJ Quality & Safety* 23 (5): 359–72.

Weisman, D., D. Gordon, S. Cassard, M. Bergner, and R. Wong. 1993. "The Effects of Unit Self-Management on Hospital Nurses' Work Process, Work Satisfaction, and Retention." *Medical Care* 31 (5): 381–93.

Weller, J., M. Boyd, and D. Cumin. 2014. "Teams, Tribes and Patient Safety: Overcoming Barriers to Effective Teamwork in Healthcare." *Postgraduate Medical Journal* 90 (1061): 149–54.

World Health Organization (WHO). 2017. "Save Lives—Clean Your Hands." Accessed August 15. www.who.int/gpsc/5may/en/.

CHAPTER 9

EXECUTION: GETTING THINGS DONE WITH DECISION-MAKING, DELEGATION, AND TIME MANAGEMENT

Important Terms

- Bias
- Delegation
- Dustbin delegation
- Effective
- Efficient
- Ethics
- Four Rights approach
- Internalize
- Level of authority
- Multitasking
- Nonprogrammed decision
- Open door management
- Rational decision-making process
- Risk
- Running a morning dash
- SSLL dilemma
- Socialization process
- Stakeholder
- Time inventory log
- Time management
- Working memory

Learning Objectives

After reading this chapter, you will be able to do the following:

- ➤ Explain the significance of effective decision-making to get things done
- ➤ Discuss and apply the decision-making process
- ➤ Explain the critical role of ethics in decision-making
- ➤ Evaluate your decision-making skills
- ➤ Explain the significance of effective delegation to get things done

- Explain why it is often difficult to delegate
- Define the "Four Rights" approach to delegation
- Explain the significance of time management for getting things done
- Analyze how you use your time
- Plan how to better use your time
- Explain work/life balance

Case Study: Strange Behavior

Robin Pearhill, RN, MHA, has a problem. One of his student interns is acting strangely, and Robin needs to act swiftly. Robin is the director of patient care at Atlantic Hills Treatment Center, a residential rehabilitation facility that treats adults recovering from alcohol and drug dependency. The center helps addicts and their families begin the recovery process. Robin worked at the center as a staff nurse for 12 years before he was promoted to director of patient care, a position he has held for two years. He is proud to be associated with the physicians, psychologists, counselors, and rehabilitation professionals who understand the recovery process and provide highly effective treatment in a caring and compassionate manner. The center also employs clinical psychology interns working toward their PhDs. Robin thoroughly enjoys mentoring these student employees. The residents have consented to the students' presence, and the staff appreciates their excellent work habits and enthusiasm.

However, Robin is concerned about one of the psychology interns, Jay Brennecke. Jay is one of the brightest interns the center has ever employed, but recently he has been coming to work tardy, his notes on the residents have gotten sloppy, and he has been missing appointments. This morning, Robin noticed that Jay came to work with dilated pupils and was exhibiting hyperactive behavior. Robin immediately asked Jay to meet with him in his office, for he is concerned that Jay may have a substance abuse problem. Robin has worked with substance users for years now, and he prides himself on his diagnostic abilities. As a manager, Robin needs to decide what to do about Jay.

Introduction: The Significance of Decision-Making to Get "Things" Done

People make decisions every day. The difference between decisions such as what to wear to work and decisions such as the one Robin Pearhill faces rests in their complexity, their strategic implications, and the **decision-making process** involved. The decision of what to wear reflects the requirements of an organization's dress code and indicates how an individual

Decision-making process
The thought and action that lead one to choose from a set of options.

would like to manage others' impressions (Goffman 1959). Robin's decision-making dilemma is different, as he needs to make a decision in the best interest of the **stakeholders** (i.e., interns, residents, resident families, the staff of the center) and the facility so that work on behalf of the residents may be accomplished. For a manager in a healthcare organization, dilemmas like the one Robin is addressing are part of the job, and he needs to make an effective decision so the interns learn as they work and so they provide quality care to the residents. He needs to decide so he can get "things" done. In this case, the "things" refer to Robin's need to decide how to address the student and his behavior so that the center's work may get done and get done well.

Stakeholder
An individual, group, or entity that has an interest in organizational success.

Herbert Alexander Simon, a Nobel laureate for his research into the decision-making process within organizations, proposes that decision-making is "almost synonymous with managing" (Simon 1977, 1). Peter Drucker, management consultant and the "father of management," notes that the "first managerial skill is . . . the making of effective decisions" (Drucker 1974, 465). Simon's and Drucker's writings provided a framework for subsequent understanding of the importance of effective decision-making for managers. Research confirms their conclusions. Simply put, a manager's value lies in the quality of the decisions she makes (Kopeikina 2006; Peer and Rakich 1999; Sutton 2002).

A manager who makes effective decisions searches for satisfactory solutions to his own problems, taking into consideration how others are solving theirs. To do this, an effective manager follows a **rational decision-making process**. There are typically five steps in the rational decision-making model, as illustrated in exhibit 9.1.

Rational decision-making process
Steps that assist when one is determining what course of action to take.

Identifying the problem correctly is essential to management success. What is the issue at hand? The old adage that a problem well defined is a problem half solved applies to this discussion. Correct identification of the problem may generate ideas for solutions. Drucker

EXHIBIT 9.1
The Rational Decision-Making Process

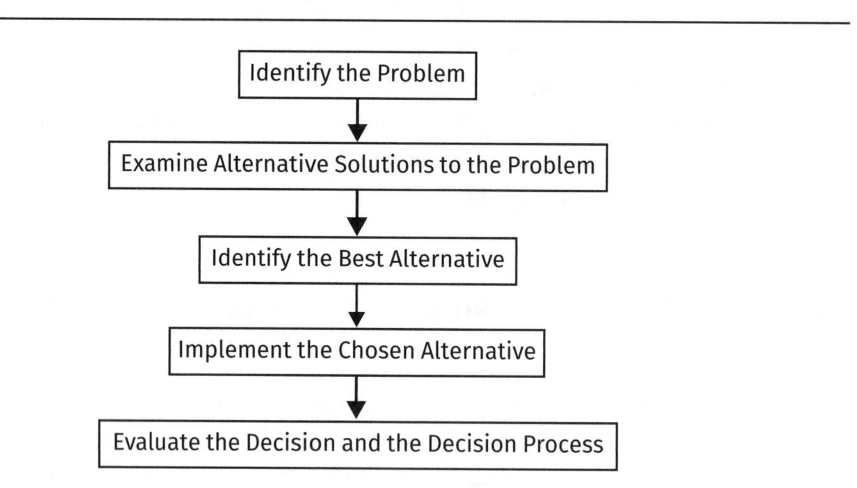

Source: Adapted from Robbins (2000).

proposes that asking the wrong questions is a dangerous misstep, and he illustrates this with reference to the medical profession (Flaherty 1999).

A physician must come to the proper diagnosis before she can approach a patient's problem. She needs to examine the patient, listen to what the patient has to say, refer to research about the symptoms, and rule out various disease alternatives before coming to a diagnosis. An effective physician will get the diagnosis right and can then turn her attention to preventive or curative action. A misdiagnosis may result in an ineffective or even life-threatening outcome. An incorrect identification of the problem leads to inappropriate action, and the problem is not addressed effectively.

Consider Robin's dilemma in the case study. He suspects that Jay is impaired by alcohol and/or drug abuse. Healthcare professionals may abuse substances. For instance, estimates suggest that 15 percent of practicing physicians will become impaired during their careers, and impairment is estimated at 5 to 15 percent of practicing psychologists (American Psychological Association 2006). As a result, policies have been created to address professional impairment in healthcare facilities, and Atlantic Hills Treatment Center has such a policy. How does Robin determine whether this is indeed the problem? To make the proper diagnosis, he should first talk with Jay. If he still suspects substance abuse after the meeting, Robin should review corporate policy regarding potential staff impairment.

When Robin was promoted to director of patient care, he attended a one-day training session conducted by the center's assistant director of human resources (HR). The manual distributed during this training included the policy for impaired employees. Since Jay receives remuneration, he is considered an employee. The policy clearly explains the intervention plan, which was updated by a task force at the center and adopted as policy in 2017. If Robin's suspicions are correct, he already has a recommended course of action to follow. However, proper identification of the problem first requires consultation with Jay.

Robin should listen to Jay's response just as a physician listens to a patient. Communication is such an important managerial skill that this book devotes an entire chapter to it (chapter 7). When they meet, Robin asks Jay about his declining work efforts, his hyperactive behavior, and his dilated pupils. At first, Jay avoids the questioning and will not look Robin directly in the eye. But then he begins to talk about his recent professional and personal stresses. He admits to using a drug, but immediately promises he will not do so again. The outcome is that Robin knows Jay has violated the center's policy by using an illegal substance. Robin has been able to identify the problem correctly, and as the adage says, it is now a problem half solved.

Examining the alternative solutions to the problem is essential to selecting the best course of action once the problem has been identified. A manager should begin by considering what action has been taken in the past and what actions might be appropriate given the particulars of the problem. Consider a professor who catches a student cheating on an exam. The professor reviews the university's code of **ethics** and policies on cheating. Alternative solutions for the professor may include (1) giving the student no credit on the exam,

Ethics
An internalized understanding of how one should behave.

(2) giving the student an F for the course, (3) reporting the student's behavior to the university's honor code committee, or (4) pretending nothing happened. Having examined the alternative solutions to the problem and having researched policies regarding the behavior, the professor can now identify the best option.

After Robin reviewed the policy at Atlantic Hills Treatment Center, and after he talked with Jay, he determined his options were to (1) follow center policies, (2) pretend nothing happened, or (3) provide individual counseling to Jay to help prevent him from doing this again. Robin's effectiveness as a manager lies in the quality of his decisions. He knows the corporate policy and is clearly aware of the center's values. Hence, he has the information he needs to identify the best option for this situation.

Identifying the best alternative is more than simply selecting one option over another. One should evaluate the possible outcomes of each potential decision. **Risk** and uncertainty accompany any decision. Consider the Atlantic Hills Treatment Center again. Robin may consider the effect of reporting Jay's behavior on future residents. There is risk in reporting, because knowledge of an intern's substance abuse problem may discourage potential future residents from seeking care at this facility. However, there is also risk if Robin does not report it. Discovery of this cover-up could generate doubt about the center's integrity. Thus, future potential residents may decide not to come to the center because of its dishonest reputation.

Risk
A possible, usually negative, outcome. Managers must eliminate as much risk as possible, although in healthcare it is impossible to eliminate all risk.

Robin should also consider the critical factor of ethics. As Drucker (1967, 134) asserts, "one has to start out with what is right rather than what is acceptable." *Business ethics* is not an oxymoron. The decision-making process should include an evaluation of professional codes and corporate policy and an examination of the interests of those who hold a stake in the outcome in healthcare as well as other industries (Law et al. 2017; Van den Bulcke et al. 2018). Robin should not only examine corporate policy, he should also consider the interests of the residents, their families, and the staff members.

Robin is an employee of the center, and any decision he makes reflects on the organization and its responsibilities to residents. Sociologist Theodore Caplow (1983) noted that a manager of a stable organization is more a representative than an initiator and that his success is measured by how well the constituents' wishes are followed. Robin knows that the task force who wrote the corporate policy regarding impaired staff had followed a democratic process that included stakeholder input and well-researched action plans. Thus, he determines that the best option is to follow this corporate policy.

Implementing the chosen alternative is essential once the best course of action has been determined. The center policy for impaired staff calls for placing Jay on a leave of absence from his work responsibilities. He may take his accrued sick leave, and the center will pay for evaluation and treatment costs that are not covered by Jay's health insurance. Jay's counseling and drug treatment are to be overseen by one of the center's staff psychologists, and depending upon the psychologist's reports and the staff team members' assessment of Jay's progress, Jay may resume his duties after three to six months. To ensure stability, there is a process to replace any team member who must exit the team.

The result is that Jay has an opportunity to address his addiction issues, recover, and work again in the future. However, his progress toward his PhD is delayed, and his future as a professional clinical psychologist is no longer certain. Nonetheless, Robin's decision to follow the corporate policy and implement the chosen alternative ensures that the stakeholders' wishes are followed, and his decision is in the best interest of the facility and residents so their work may be done well. Robin notifies the HR director, who then takes over as plan implementation leader and chair of the team that will follow Jay's progress.

Caplow (1983) stated that the main factors for managing a stable organization include the following:

1. Adherence to traditional procedures
2. Slow-moving, intensive problem-solving efforts
3. Democratic participation in decision-making
4. Meticulous and accessible records and accounts
5. A system for the designation of successors designed to prevent surprises

Robin followed traditional procedures by selecting the best alternative from among those he identified. The HR director, Robin, and the monitoring psychologist will follow the problem-solving efforts on behalf of Jay (his recovery) and the institution (the stakeholders' wishes were followed, and employee impairment was identified and addressed before any stakeholder was harmed). In this case, the democratic decision-making rests with the task force that wrote the professional impairment policy and the team that will follow Jay's rehabilitation process. This latter team will decide whether or not to reinstate Jay. They will create meticulous records to ensure the center's policies are followed before they assess Jay's ability to return to work. The team will designate successors to follow Jay's progress and prevent any surprises so the work of the center may be done well.

Evaluating the decision and the decision process ensures that the problem was identified correctly and assesses whether the implemented plan addressed the problem appropriately. For Robin, the problem was that an employee was impaired. The implemented plan was to follow the corporate policy and procedures regarding an impaired professional. The team that follows Jay's recovery should assess his progress and the appropriateness of the policies for impaired professionals. Can the policy be improved? Is the time frame indicated (three to six months) appropriate for recovery? How much supervision should Jay have if he returns to work? Should all staff be tested for drugs? Evaluating the decision and the decision process may help ensure that the institution's needs and the stakeholders' wishes are met effectively as problems are identified and addressed within an organization.

Why did Robin follow this rational decision-making process when the center had a policy regarding suspected employee drug use? Fortunately for Robin, the center is stable and prepared to address the presence of an impaired professional. Robin also had support and guidance from the director of the HR department. However, not all managers have the support Robin enjoys at work. The rational decision-making model is particularly valuable where a stable system is not in place. It is valuable because in an unstable system, effective decision-making may not ensure things get done, but the process may help a manager determine if her professional reputation is in jeopardy and guide her as she decides if it is time for her to take her talents, skills, and hard work and go where she can get things done.

Consider the situation of Sherron Watkins, once the vice president of corporate development at Enron, an energy trading company formerly based in Houston, Texas, that has become an example of corporate scandal, fraud, and unethical behavior. The firm collapsed in 2001 when its questionable accounting practices, including the generation of fake revenue streams, were exposed, spurring the downfall of investor confidence (Keller 2002). Enron chief executives Lay and Skilling were found guilty of lying to stakeholders, which included stockholders, investors, employees, and government regulators. Lay died before sentencing; Skilling was to spend 14 years in jail (Barrionuevo 2006; Johnson 2006; Wilbanks 2013). While the Enron incident occurred in 2001, it is still notable today because the term "Enron Effect" has emerged to refer to a workplace that is low in ethical culture, but has high financial yield for corrupt behavior. In Enron's case, an estimated 70 billion dollars were lost—the largest bankruptcy filed in US history up to that time (CNN Library 2018; Tang et al. 2018).

Sherron Watkins became known as the "Enron whistleblower." She was suspicious of wrongdoing when she analyzed certain assets Enron expected to sell and determined that Enron was using its own stock to post a gain or loss on its income statement, which is prohibited by the United States' Generally Accepted Accounting Principles (GAAP). Concerned that she would lose her job if she confronted her direct supervisor, Watkins reported her concerns to Lay, Enron's CEO. In court, Watkins testified that her supervisor did want her "out of Enron" after he learned of her meeting with Lay (United Press International 2002). Given the obstacles Watkins faced and her concern for her livelihood, why did she make the decision to confront Lay? Watkins wrote in her memo to Lay that her personal history and who she was spurred her action. She had worked for Enron for eight years, and her work efforts would mean nothing on her resume, given Enron's actions. Thus, her decision-making followed a rational decision-making model, but without the support that Robin enjoyed. Watkins's professional reputation was not marred by the experience; in fact, she was praised for her honesty and ethical actions resulting from the decisions she had made regarding Enron's accounting fraud (BBC News 2006; Lucas and Koerwer 2004; Wearing 2005).

Improving Decision-Making Skills

As discussed in chapter 7, communicating effectively is essential in the daily work of a healthcare manager. Communicating effectively is also essential in identifying a problem and gathering the facts and relevant information. Consider Robin's dilemma again. What if Jay had explained that his pupils were dilated from an eye exam and had shown Robin proof of his appointment? This explanation would have addressed Robin's concerns. However, it would not have addressed Jay's declining work performance. Robin needs to listen closely to Jay's explanation for why his work efforts have slowed. He needs to avoid distractions, such as answering the phone or reading his mail. Open, positive, nonverbal communication, such as looking at Jay as he speaks and encouraging him to continue, will aid Robin in the process (Lear, Hodge, and Schulz 2015; Ross 2018). Finally, summarizing what Jay has told him will help Robin ensure that he has heard correctly and may help him determine whether there is an impairment problem.

Avoiding ***bias*** is also important. Through the process of socialization, an individual acquires a self-identity and **internalizes** (to a degree) a cognitive frame of reference for interpersonal relations and a moral conscience (Parsons 1951). Parents, other family members, teachers, colleagues, bosses, and others play a role in this lifelong process. Reutter and colleagues (1997) examined student nurses and the role of socialization on their learning. The **socialization process** in nursing school helps ensure the students internalize the nursing profession's values, norms, and behaviors. We not only internalize the values, norms, and behaviors associated with our culture as a consequence of the socialization process, but we also internalize biases, often based on gender, race, religion, socioeconomic status, or other cultural designations. Recognizing our biases enables us to understand that they influence our decisions. This awareness improves our ability to make decisions.

Bias
A tendency to apply a negative or positive bent to a situation because of prejudicial thought.

Internalize
To incorporate values, beliefs, or norms as self-guiding principles.

Socialization process
The process whereby people learn values, beliefs, and norms.

Recognizing a programmed decision and being able to differentiate it from a **nonprogrammed decision** is important for managers approaching a potential problem. Programmed decisions are routine and recurring. For example, Robin regularly makes decisions regarding daily operations activities for the residents. Decisions regarding supplies for the residents' rooms and room assignments for individual and group therapy sessions are examples of programmed decisions because they are frequent, routine decisions needed for operational activities. Nonprogrammed decisions address unusual problems. Robin's decision regarding Jay was nonprogrammed because there is nothing recurring or routine about Jay's behavior. Hence, while the center had a policy regarding impaired professionals, addressing the issue as nonprogrammed was in the best interest of the institution and its stakeholders because it involved a staff member who could have harmed a resident or a staff member, hurt the center's reputation, and hurt himself.

Nonprogrammed decision
A decision for which there is no set procedure in place and that must be resolved via rational thinking and action.

Being timely is significant because even the best decisions are not helpful if they are made too late. Robin immediately removed Jay from working with patients and met with him to discuss his concerns. He did not wait to initiate action until he had gathered more information or talked with others. Had he waited, Jay might have caused harm. Timely response to problems is essential to effective decision-making.

Making assurances one can keep builds trust. A manager may promise pay raises to generate a temporary positive response, even though he does not have the authority to ensure raises will be given. However, promising only what one can deliver develops professional trust based on honesty. Robin did not promise Jay that his work would continue as usual. Rather, he met with Jay and communicated his concern about Jay's behavior. He expressed concern instead of making promises he could not keep.

Creativity in a rational decision-making process should be supported. Brainstorming alternative solutions to a problem allows for expansion on standard, conventional approaches to problem solving. Creative thinking may generate innovative, appropriate solutions.

Including an ethical checklist will ensure better decision-making. Managers' positions make them more visible and give them higher levels of responsibility in the organization. Therefore, viewing ethics as an essential factor in effective management decisions recognizes that managers should consider their role as one of responsibility. Drucker (2001) proposes that managers should observe the ethics of responsibility. It is the manager's responsibility to consider the needs of the stakeholders and of the institution and to decide what is right. Ross, Wenzel, and Mitlyng (2002) discuss ethics and values as personal healthcare leadership competencies. They refer to Nash's (1989) list of questions designed for ethical guidance. Answering the following questions may reaffirm the manager's decision regarding the problem, if he is content with the answers (Ross, Wenzel, and Mitlyng 2002, 133–34) :

1. Have you accurately defined the problem?
2. How would you define the problem if you stood on the other side of the fence?
3. How did this situation occur in the first place?
4. To whom and to what do you give your loyalty as a person and as a member of the corporation?
5. What is your intention in making this decision?
6. How does this intention compare with the probable results?
7. Whom could your decision or action injure?
8. Can you discuss the decision with the affected parties before making the decision?
9. Are you confident that your decision will be as valid over a long period of time as it seems now?
10. Could you discuss without qualm your decision or action to your boss, your CEO, the board of directors, your family, and society as a whole?
11. What is the symbolic potential of your action, if understood? If misunderstood?
12. Under what conditions would you allow exceptions to your stance?

How do you think Robin at the Atlantic Hills Treatment Center would answer these questions? Do you think he would be at ease with his answers?

The Significance of Delegation to Get "Things" Done

For a healthcare manager to get things done well, it is essential to develop both her decision-making and delegating skills. **Delegation** can be difficult: As managers assign tasks to others, they potentially lose control over how the task is performed. However, there is a plus side to delegation, as it lets managers demonstrate trust and encourage employees to handle a work assignment. Delegation affects team performance positively, as well (Lorinkova, Pearsall, and Sim 2013). And, if delegation is handled properly, the manager will now have time to work on another task while the employee to whom the task was delegated can demonstrate her skills. In chapter 4, we discussed the places where healthcare professionals work and described the teams needed to do the work so healthcare may be delivered in a manner that is mindful of cost, quality, and patient access. One person cannot do all the work required to meet healthcare's Triple (or Quadruple) Aim. Hence, delegation is a necessity rather than a luxury (Marquis and Huston 2000). Those to whom tasks are delegated have the opportunity to demonstrate their abilities, master new tasks, enhance their leadership and decision-making skills, gain a greater understanding of the work of the department and organization, network, and experience greater ownership over their work and the work of their colleagues.

Delegation
Assigning tasks to others; the ability to get work done through others.

Understanding the criticality of developing delegation skills is different than managers being able to let go of tasks. This is a sentiment that many leaders share. As South African family physician and professor Ian Douglas Couper (2007, 261) described it,

> If I feel important, I start to do everything myself instead of delegating responsibilities. I fear passing tasks on to others because they will not do it the way I would or as well as I would (so I believe), but I become unable to do everything myself. I become an obstacle for myself and for others because I am doing too much. Delegation is an important aspect of leadership and, distinct from offloading work, it requires that I have a balanced view of myself. I sometimes believe that "my" hospital would collapse without me, yet it has continued to function at times when I was not there.

We can all relate to feeling that it is easier to do something yourself than to teach someone else how to do it (Culp and Smith 1997, 30):

> It may seem that you can do the task better or faster than anyone else, but then you might be overestimating the uniqueness of your skills and underestimating those of others. Clearly, if you don't break out of this trap there is a very real limit on what you can accomplish.

People who climb the career ladder have been rewarded for their technical skills, knowledge, and task performance. As a result, managers may be concerned that delegating will diminish the importance of their own contributions in the eyes of their superiors or will be seen as a way to get out of doing the work themselves (Portny 2002). No one likes to look inadequate, and managers who feel powerless tend to be less willing to delegate (Haselhuhn, Wong, and Ormiston 2017).

According to an old joke, even God delegates. He asked Noah to build the ark, and He had Moses led the Israelites out of Egypt. Then Moses delegated some of his tasks to his brother Aaron, who was a better public speaker. One way of thinking about delegation, then, is that it is the ability to get work done through others (Curtis and Nicholl 2004; Kourdi 1999; Marquis and Huston 2000; Rocchiccioli and Tilbury 1998). Delegation extends results beyond what one person can do (Culp and Smith 1997). It enhances efficiency, time management, and productivity by distributing the workload (Ales 1995).

President Woodrow Wilson (1914) supposedly said, "I not only use all the brains I have, but all I can borrow." This provides another way to think about delegation. Done right, it can ensure that the most capable people available are working on the most appropriate tasks (Portny 2002). Delegation can allow employees to demonstrate their abilities, stretch, and learn new skills.

Delegation is not about finding a way to make employees work harder so managers have to do less. Delegation benefits the delegator and the delegatee. Delegators have more time for other managerial activities. They can focus on doing a few things well rather than too many things poorly. By delegating, they mentor and prepare employees for their own career advancement, resulting in higher-level performance. If work is done and decisions are made at the lowest appropriate level, everyone benefits from faster and more effective decision-making.

The Craft of Delegation

How does a manager know when he needs to delegate tasks? The signs may include the following (Culp and Smith 1997, 30):

- You work longer hours than your staff.
- You take work home regularly.
- You constantly rush to meet deadlines.
- You miss deadlines.
- You do or redo work that has been assigned to your staff.
- You regularly help with tasks you have delegated to others.
- Your own top-priority items remain undone.

- You are the only person you can identify as being able to handle the next big project.
- Your staff has low initiative.
- You have high turnover among your "rising stars."

To determine if you have an issue with delegation, read through the following statements. If you agree with more than three of them, you may want to reread this section on delegation (Daft 1991, 253):

- I tend to be a perfectionist.
- My boss expects me to know all the details of my job.
- I don't have the time to explain clearly and concisely how a task should be accomplished.
- I often end up doing tasks myself.
- My subordinates typically are not as committed as I am.
- I get upset when other people don't do the task right.
- I really enjoy doing the details of my job to the best of my ability.
- I like to be in control of task outcomes.

To further determine if you have an issue with delegation, consider the following question: If you had to take an unexpected week off work, would your initiatives and priorities advance in your absence (Sostrin 2017)? If your answer is no or you are not certain, you also may want to reread this section on delegation.

Delegation should not necessitate surrendering control of the process or of the outcome. Smart delegation is about giving employees the appropriate **level of authority** to carry out their assigned tasks (Kahn 2004). At the lowest level, an employee might be asked to look into a problem and to report back to the boss, who will then make the decision or take the action. A higher level of authority would involve the employee developing a recommendation, informing the boss about alternatives or pros and cons, and recommending a course of action. Even more authority would allow the employee to develop an action plan for the boss's approval. At the highest level, the boss might pass the authority to take action on to the employee and ask to be kept informed (Culp and Smith 1997).

Effective delegation takes thought, insight, and commitment. One way to simplify delegation is to use the **Four Rights approach**: the right task, the right person, the right communication, and the right feedback (Hantsen and Washburn 1992).

Level of authority
An employee's empowerment to carry out delegated tasks. Levels include the authority to search for information, the authority to provide recommendations, and the authority to fully implement a task.

Four Rights approach
Delegating by identifying the right task, the right person, the right communication, and the right feedback.

Dustbin delegation Delegating only unpleasant, boring tasks that the manager does not want to do.

Before delegating, the manager must accurately assess the work situation and environment. She must know the skills, abilities, interests, and limits of her employees. This does not mean she can only delegate a task to someone who already has the skill. Sometimes, a delegated task is an excellent opportunity for an employee to stretch and learn something new. The manager must have a grasp of her own skills and abilities and must know what responsibilities she should pass on to others and what tasks she should complete herself. She should beware of **dustbin delegation**—only delegating unpleasant, boring tasks that she simply does not want to do herself. Delegated tasks should include enjoyable, appealing, and challenging tasks that are assigned according to skill and ability (Kourdi 1999).

Managers need to recognize the talents and personalities of their employees (Lewis 2000). As Culp and Smith (1997, 30) recommend, "Choose a capable person, someone with intelligence, aptitude, and willingness to learn." Matching the right person to the right task can be a challenge. Sometimes, the best way to pursue this is to look at each employee's "toolbox" and see whose background, previous work, and skills best fit the task at hand. Another option is to think about not only "who can do this," but also "who would enjoy this," or "who needs to acquire this particular skill," or "who is eager to stretch."

Delegated assignments also need to be clear and well defined, as several leading authors suggest:

> Successful delegation includes information on what, when, who, and, perhaps, how. The employee must clearly understand the task and the expected results. (Daft 1991, 253)

> It is best to stress desired outcomes, not details or methods of production. (Lewis 2000)

Moreover, the manager should

> point out the potential failure paths and what not to do, but don't specify every detail of how to do the task. Identify the human, financial, technical, and organizational resources the person can draw on to accomplish the desired results. (Covey 1990, 174)

Agree upon the standards for performance that will be used to evaluate the results, a timeline, and the deliverables. Last, make certain the resources needed to do the task right are available.

Throughout the project, keep the lines of communication open. Establish checkpoints and provide objective feedback. If the delegated task is not moving ahead as it should, address your concerns promptly; do not allow the task to go completely awry. It can be difficult to provide negative feedback, but letting the employee continue down a path of inappropriate or unsatisfactory progress helps no one. Provide negative feedback in private, and try to address the ineffective behavior or poor outcomes. Discuss specific, objective details, and ask the employee to provide alternatives for improvement.

If the task is on target, provide praise as appropriate. Be certain to deliver any agreed-upon rewards. Give credit where credit is due; a manager who takes the credit for his employees' good work will not be respected and will have difficulty delegating in the future. And, it is the right thing to do.

The Significance of Time Management to Get "Things" Done

Along with a healthcare manager's improving her decision-making skills and practicing delegation appropriately, her **time management** skills are key for her to get things done well. We have all heard a myriad of platitudes about time: A stitch in time saves nine; time waits for no one; time is of the essence; timing is everything; do not waste time, for that is the stuff from which life is made; time is money. Why do some people seem so much better able to manage time than others? It almost seems as though they simply have *more* time, yet everyone has the exact same amount of time: 60 seconds in every minute, 60 minutes in every hour, 24 hours in every day. One way to approach time is to think of it as a limited resource, a tool to use and control. No one is completely **efficient**; everyone wastes some time. The key to time management, however, is to minimize time wasting and maximize productive time use. Books, tools, websites, and technologies are available to help managers do just that, both at work and in their personal lives.

Time management
The practice of using time effectively to achieve professional and personal goals.

Efficient
Productive, with minimum waste or effort.

This section focuses on helping you develop your time management skills by showing you ways to analyze how you actually spend your working hours and plan how to better spend your time. Last, this section offers tips to help you waste less time and use time more productively so that you can do things well.

One way to analyze your time at work is to prepare a **time inventory log** (Rue and Byars 2004). The log should briefly note how you are spending your time at regular intervals, perhaps each hour or half hour, during your work day. Choose a week that is typical of your working life, not a week when special tasks or events are planned for you or for your department. For example, part of one day of your log might read something like this:

Time inventory log
A tool that illustrates how time is used by briefly noting activities at regular intervals, such as each hour or half hour, during the workday.

Monday
9:30 phone call with Mary
10:00 e-mail
10:30 meeting with department heads
11:00 meeting
11:30 meeting
12:00 lunch break at desk reading reports
12:30 reading reports
1:00 preparing budget
1:30 talking with Bob

While this exercise may feel a bit tedious, it is well worth your while. Once you have a record of your time and tasks for the week, sort each entry into specific categories, such as scheduled meetings, telephone, e-mail, report writing, walk-ins, break times, and planning and analysis. Pay attention to trends and to which times of day you seem to be most productive or most unproductive. You might be surprised at how much time you are spending in some categories, and how little in others. After keeping a running tally of your time, how you spend your working hours should become clearer. The next question is, "Am I spending my time in the most productive ways?" Last, ask yourself about the time spent: "Does it match my key priorities?" (Kaplan 2010, 154).

Once you have conducted a self-assessment, seriously reflect on planning to organize your day. First, set your goals and priorities. Working without daily goals and priorities is like driving without a map—you get nowhere fast. Identify what you need to accomplish, and plan your time accordingly. It is far too easy to lose hours of time tidying up your desk, sorting through mail, answering phone or e-mail messages, and dealing with unexpected visitors.

Open door management
Always working with your office door open to show you are available to everyone all the time.

SSLL dilemma
The basic conflict between "smaller-sooner" (short-term, more immediate costs and benefits) and "larger-longer" (long-term, and perhaps riskier, future payoffs).

Effective
Having a definite or desired effect.

Clearly, part of being a manager is taking the time to talk with colleagues, coworkers, and employees about their work, tasks, issues, and concerns. Work would be a cold and boring place with no friendly talk or interactions. In our culture, we have a myth of "**open door management**." The idea of being available to everyone all the time is appealing, but not very practical. To become a skilled time manager, you must protect your time so you can address the tasks you have prioritized. And if you have an office door, it is okay to close it and work uninterrupted for part of the day.

But just what is it you should do when you close your door? Management tasks vary, not only in their immediate importance, but also in their long-term usefulness. This is called the "smaller-sooner" versus "larger-longer" **(SSLL) dilemma** (Bixter, Trimber, and Luhmann 2017; Dickson and Fongoni 2015; Konig and Kleinmann 2007). This is a basic conflict between short-term costs and benefits and long-term, perhaps riskier, future payoffs. Research indicates that people often prefer an SS outcome to an LL outcome (Bixter, Trimber, and Luhmann 2017; Dickson and Fongoni 2015). **Effective** time managers need to find the right balance between both, while ignoring neither.

The first tool you need to spend your time productively is a calendar. Before leaving work each night, check your calendar for the next day's meetings and appointments to make certain you are prepared for them, or have allocated time to prepare for them in your next day's schedule. At the very least, your calendar (whether it is on paper or kept electronically on your phone or laptop) helps you know when meetings are and when you have a project deadline forthcoming.

Next, create a running to-do list. Your work life is busy and your tasks will become increasingly complex and time-consuming. So, start now to keep a list of things to be done and their deadlines. A working to-do list includes daily, weekly, and perhaps monthly tasks. It includes tasks that may not be priorities now but will become priorities at a later date.

Some people simply keep a running list on a pad of paper at their desks; some people use a calendar with enough room to write in tasks; some people use electronic calendar systems. None of these is inherently better than the others; the key is to find a system that keeps things from falling through the cracks and keeps you from having to call your colleagues for vital information.

Your to-do list should be reorganized and reprioritized regularly—perhaps daily, if necessary (Trunk 2008). Some people prioritize by noting if the tasks are "must do now," "important," "desirable to do," and "can wait." Some people simply number tasks or arrange them by deadline. There is no one perfect system; the best system is the one that works for you as you get things done. "**Running a morning dash**" (Trapani 2006) is an example of prioritization in action. It involves spending an hour on the most important thing on your to-do list first thing each morning, even before checking your messages or e-mail. Running the dash ensures your most important tasks get started and get at least one hour of undivided attention each day.

Running a morning dash
Spending an hour on the most important thing on your to-do list first thing each morning, even before checking your messages or e-mail.

You may have heard the joke about the structured person who has to schedule "time to be spontaneous" in her or his weekly calendar. This might sound amusing, but work becomes tedious and stressful with no breaks or social interactions. While there may be days when you close your door, work on creating a balance in your own life. Rituals may help with creating and sustaining this balance. Consider taking breaks at set times and spending daily time doing activities you like (Schwartz and McCarthy 2010). For example, spend a few minutes before the workday begins and a few minutes after the workday ends practicing yoga (if you like yoga). Walk a few minutes each hour and stand to read your e-mails. Turn your e-mail off at set times during the day. Write an appreciative note to a colleague who did a job well. During your commute to and from work, play an audiobook that you have been wanting to read, but have not had the time to. All of these actions may help create balance among your physical, emotional, mental, and spiritual energies so you may add value to your work and personal life and get things done well (Schwartz and McCarthy 2010).

Finally, with the work stacked up on your desk, creating and working on your to-do list might feel like a waste of precious time, particularly at first. This is a good example of the SSLL dilemma. The long-term advantages of taking time with your to-do list will almost always pay off in long-run productivity and efficiency, so take the time. It will help you get things done—both the "smaller-sooner" and "larger-longer" tasks.

A Note on Wasting Time

The list of ways to waste time at work is endless. However, there are tips that seem to help most people manage their time more effectively and efficiently.

Handle each piece of paper or e-mail only once (St. James 2001). Give each piece of paper or e-mail enough time and attention to absorb its message and then either (1) handle it right now, (2) file it in the appropriate folder so you can handle or use it later, (3) pass it on to someone else, or (4) simply throw it away or delete it. With the advent of standing desks, try going through e-mail while standing up; it is too easy to waste time reading unimportant materials while sitting down. Standing up gives the task a feeling of urgency and gets a manager through a stack of papers or a backlog of e-mails more quickly than sitting down to do the tasks.

Also, become aware of your own internal clock. Are you particularly alert early in the day? Do you encounter a mid-afternoon slump, or do you finally hit your stride after 2:00 p.m.? Try to schedule your most important and most difficult tasks for your best, most productive times. These might also be the best times to close your door if you can and run a morning (or "afternoon," as the case may be) dash.

Manage your technology; do not let it manage you. Not every phone call, e-mail, tweet, or Facebook post must be accessed immediately or dealt with that very minute. If technology interruptions are your downfall, try looking at your e-mail or answering your phone messages only at one or two specific times each day. As previously suggested, try to handle each message only once, and fight the urge to click on every link that looks interesting.

What are your most tempting distractions? Is it answering your cell phone, surfing the Internet, getting a snack, or chatting with coworkers? These are part of work life, and you cannot avoid them all the time. However, as you become aware of which of them is most likely to lure you away from your work, plan in advance for ways to handle them. Strategies such as only chatting with colleagues at certain times of the day or bringing a snack from home can sometimes help you bypass your most tempting distractions.

Nearly every time management book, website, or technology has a list of the most common time wasters (see, for example, Allen 2015; Blair 2008; Credit Suisse Learning 2008; Harvard Business School 2005; Rue and Byars 2004). Our own list of time wasters includes the following:

- Telephone interruptions
- Visitors dropping in
- Reading and sending nonessential e-mail
- Lack of objectives or priorities
- Cluttered desk and disorganization
- Indecision and procrastination
- Perfectionism
- Inability to say no
- Social media, such as Facebook, Twitter, Instagram, and Snapchat

In brief, time management is about controlling two "eff" words (Blair 1992):

- Effective: having a definite or desired effect
- Efficient: productive with minimum waste or effort

We sometimes think we can become more effective and more efficient by **multitasking**, or doing more than one thing at a time. Multitasking has been the time management tip for the past few decades. However attractive it might seem to be able to do many things at once, it may be better to focus on one task or one person at a time. Neurological research has shown that one unit of focused time is equal to four units of broken focus (Vaccaro 2003). Multitasking as a method to improve at getting things done is a myth. Multitasking tends to have negative consequences on learning (Carrier et al. 2015); it is less efficient than single-task performance (Courage et al. 2015); and heavy media multitaskers exhibit lower **working memory** performance, which, in turn, negatively affects long-term memory (Uncapher, Thieu, and Wagner 2015).

Multitasking
Doing more than one thing at a time.

Working memory
Part of short-term memory associated with storing and managing information for learning, reasoning, and comprehension.

As Blair (2008) writes, "The absence of time management is characterized by last minute rushes and hours and days that seem to slip unproductively by." Time management is not a genetic characteristic. We all know people who say they just cannot seem to get organized or cannot stop procrastinating or being late. With all due respect, they are wrong. It is hard to break old time-wasting habits and to learn new time-productive skills, but it is, again, an SSLL issue. Invest the effort now to learn how to use time to your advantage so you can get things done.

Conclusion

At the beginning of this chapter we met Robin, who was deciding what he should do about a student intern at a rehab facility. Working through a rational decision-making model, we learned how managers such as Robin make decisions that will add benefit to the organization while being mindful of employees. We then discussed the need for appropriate delegation that will not only allow a manager to get work done, but also help employees develop professionally. Last, we discussed the importance of time management to allow managers to get things done in a timely manner, with the caveat that they can and should create a work/life balance. Throughout this chapter, we put forth that these are skills to be developed—we can make good decisions, based on rational thinking; we can develop our delegation skills so our colleagues participate and know they contributed; and we can manage our time more effectively so we get "things" done well while we create and sustain a balance between our professional and working lives.

Mini Case Study: What Do We Do About Joe?

Joe, a surgery nurse, was outgoing, energetic, and athletic. He enjoyed telling stories about his cross-country ski races. However, his talkative nature bothered Sue, the nursing manager of the operating room. Sue noticed that the whole surgical nursing team often stopped and encouraged Joe to continue telling his racing stories. It did not seem to interfere with surgery or daily work tasks, but Sue was concerned because it did not seem to bother Joe that he was doing it during working hours or that someone other than his coworkers might be listening. Joe seemed to just enjoy being in the spotlight, and the other nurses enjoyed his stories. Joe's nursing team performed extremely well. The surgeries went smoothly, and the surgeons often requested that Joe's nursing team assist with their scheduled surgeries. From the surgeons' perspective, this nursing team made certain that all was ready and that few, if any, errors were made. But the frequent storytelling breaks bothered the OR supervisor. Sue believed that Joe's team was setting a bad example for the other nursing teams and the rest of the nursing staff.

Sue had just recently taken charge of the surgical ward. She was determined to do her job well, and she wanted her staff to do things well, too. She thought she could point out to Joe that his behavior was inappropriate, and he would change. In addition, she knew she could tell the other nurses that they should not be listening to Joe's nonsense. Sue called Joe in to discuss the situation. She told Joe that he and his colleagues could make better use of their time. Joe promised he would try.

Things did improve, but after a few weeks, the old pattern reemerged. Sue then met with the other members of the nursing team individually. However, the nursing team maintained their habits, and Sue was left to ponder what to do about Joe.

Mini Case Study Questions

1. With reference to the rational decision-making model, identify the problem in this mini case.
2. What options would you recommend to address the problem identified? Based on these options, make a recommendation to Sue. Explain why you recommended what you did.
3. How could the chapter discussion about time management and life balance have influenced your thoughts about your answers to questions 1 and 2 for this mini case?

Points to Remember

- Rational decision-making is important, as a manager makes decisions that are in the best interest of the stakeholders and the workplace.

- Rational decision-making is important, as the process may help a manager determine if her professional reputation is in jeopardy and guide her to decide it is time for her to take her talents, skill, and hard work and go where she can get things done.
- Delegation allows for better productivity for managers, as well as opportunities for employees' professional development.
- Effective delegation has four rights: right task, right person, right communication, and right feedback.
- Accurate self-assessment of your time management skills, and corresponding changes in behavior, can improve job performance.
- Multitasking does not bring about increased efficiencies or effectiveness.

Challenge Yourself

1. Evaluate this statement: The value of a manager lies in the quality of the decisions he makes. Consider an example from your own work experience that illustrates the importance of quality decisions.
2. Keep a time inventory log for a week. Analyze how you spent your time. What are some ideas specific to you for making better use of your time?
3. In the section on time management, we discussed the notion that balancing our physical, emotional, mental, and spiritual energies offers positive outcomes (Schwartz and McCarthy 2010). Tony Schwartz is part of an organization entitled "The Energy Project." Go to the firm's website, https://theenergyproject.com, and click on the blog link. Select a recent post and discuss how its subject relates to the theme of managing our energy.

For Your Consideration

1. This chapter's opening case study lists several options Robin could have considered regarding what to do about Jay. Would you have chosen the same option Robin did? Why or why not?
2. Explain why time management is an important skill to master. Offer an example to illustrate its importance.

Exercise 9.1 Effective Time Management and Alicia's Day—Oxymoron?

Alicia Benson entered the Cardio Planning Committee meeting late—as usual. It seemed Alicia was always arriving late to meetings. This one was focused on a presentation from the Utah Consultant Group (UCG). The hospital where Alicia worked as a health educator was in the process of expanding its cardiovascular services. UCG had been hired to present its architectural design for the new cardiovascular unit.

Alicia was asked to join the Cardio Planning Committee because she could represent the health educators' perspective on the expansion project and help keep communications open between the administration and the health education staff members. However, Alicia rarely spent enough time in a meeting to know what information to communicate back, and she was so busy apologizing for being late that she rarely contributed a health education perspective to the discussion.

Alicia settled in and examined the floor plan that UCG had presented. She did not see any space designated for community education regarding the influences of healthy lifestyle behavior on cardiovascular health. Why, she wondered, had UCG forgotten to include such an important aspect of cardiovascular care?

After the meeting concluded, Cal Hermans, the director of strategic planning, asked Alicia to come with him to his office. When they entered his office, he emptied a glass vase full of fresh flowers and water into the sink. He handed the empty vase to Alicia. Then he removed two pouches—one small and one large—from a desk drawer. The small pouch contained sand; the larger was filled with rocks.

Cal said, "Alicia, I want you to pour the sand into this vase."

Alicia felt this was a silly exercise and thought of the long list of things she still had to do today. However, since Cal was the director of strategic planning, she knew she needed to go along with his game, even if it was a waste of her time. Alicia poured the pouch of sand into the vase.

Then Cal said, "Okay, add the rocks." Alicia placed a few of the rocks in the vase, but could not add many because the sand was taking up too much of the space.

Cal took the vase from Alicia, removed the rocks, and emptied the sand back into its pouch. "Now," he said, "put the rocks in the vase first."

Now Alicia was curious. What was Cal up to? She put the rocks into the vase.

"Okay, Alicia," Cal continued. "Now put in the sand." Alicia turned the pouch upside down and all of the sand flowed into the vase. Both the rocks and the sand fit inside.

Alicia looked at Cal and said, "I get it, Cal. Thanks."

Exercise 9.1 Questions

1. What did Alicia "get"? What was Cal's purpose for the sand and rocks demonstration?
2. Why is it important to plan for the bigger projects first and then the smaller ones?

Exercise 9.2 Joy's Complaint

Carla Kasiska has been the clinic manager for the Medgroup Management Practice in Nashville, Tennessee, for 12 years. She is responsible for all staff and business operations in the practice. The practice is made up of three dermatologists, two plastic surgeons, and three nurses. Minor surgeries are conducted on the premises. It is Carla's responsibility to ensure the office runs smoothly, patients' calls are received promptly, medical records are in order, billing is conducted on a timely and regular basis, and materials and equipment are ordered and stored properly.

Carla is also responsible for all personnel issues. She hires, motivates, evaluates, and sometimes fires employees. Carla finds she is constantly hiring office assistants, as turnover is higher than at comparable practices. She finds herself working late to review the billing system for which Joy, the billing officer, is responsible. Joy has worked at the practice for two years and is very comfortable with her ability to bill appropriately. She knows the coding procedures and has a good record regarding billing collections. She has asked why Carla stays late to review her billing work all the time, or to do work that other assistants could do during the day.

Joy says, "Carla, my work is excellent. Do you really think you need to review my efforts on such a regular basis? You are busy. If you want to review, why don't you ask Linda to help? She has been working in the practice for almost nine months now, and she has been asking for more responsibility in the office. All she does is answer the phones, and she would like to have more variety."

Carla responds, "Joy, I am ultimately responsible for all operations in the practice. I need to conduct the review."

Joy tries again. "Carla, I don't want to lose Linda. She has a lot of talent, and she is getting bored doing the same task over and over. You are overworked. Can't you allow us to take on some of the jobs you do?"

Carla waves away Joy with a shake of her head. "Oh, Joy. I need to do it."

The next week, Linda resigns from the Medgroup Management Practice. Carla sighs to herself, "Now I have to go out and hire somebody else. I don't understand why Linda is leaving us. She was very competent and Joy was right—she had a lot of talent. Oh well, I need to move forward with writing the advertisement and posting it on the website. Then I'll need to interview. Nobody else can handle this."

Exercise 9.2 Questions

1. Do you think Carla is a good practice manager? Why or why not?
2. Consider the signs that Daft (1991) lists regarding difficulty delegating. Does Carla seem to have difficulty with delegating?
3. With the information provided, how can Carla become a better practice manager? What would you recommend she do to retain good staff members at the practice?

References

Ales, B. 1995. "Mastering the Art of Delegation." *Nursing Management* 26 (8): 32A–33A.

Allen, D. 2015. *Getting Things Done: The Art of Stress-Free Productivity*. New York: Penguin Books.

American Psychological Association. 2006. *Advancing Colleague Assistance in Professional Psychology*. Published February 10. www.apa.org/practice/resources/assistance/monograph.pdf.

Barrionuevo, A. 2006. "Enron Chiefs Guilty of Fraud and Conspiracy." *New York Times*. Published May 25. www.nytimes.com/2006/05/25/business/25cnd-enron.html.

BBC News. 2006. "Whistleblower Recalls Enron Crisis." Published September 12. http://news.bbc.co.uk/2/hi/business/5335214.stm.

Bixter, M., E. Trimber, and C. Luhmann. 2017. "Are Intertemporal Preferences Contagious? Evidence from Collaborative Decision Making." *Memory & Cognition* 45 (5): 837–51.

Blair, G. M. 2008. "Personal Time Management for Busy Managers: The 'Eff' Words." Accessed May 11, 2018. www.see.ed.ac.uk/~gerard/Management/art2.html.

———. 1992. "Personal Time Management for Busy Managers." *Engineering Management Journal* 2 (1): 33–38.

Caplow, T. 1983. *Managing an Organization*. New York: Holt, Rinehart, and Winston.

Carrier, L., L. Rosen, N. Cheever, and A. Lim. 2015. "Causes, Effects, and Practicalities of Everyday Multitasking." *Developmental Review* 35: 64–78.

CNN Library. 2018. "Enron Fast Facts." Updated April 23. www.cnn.com/2013/07/02/us/enron-fast-facts/index.html.

Couper, I. D. 2007. "The Impotence of Being Important—Reflections on Leadership." *Annals of Family Medicine* 5 (3): 261–62.

Courage, M., A. Bakhtiar, C. Fitzpatrick, S. Kenny, and K. Brandeau. 2015. "Growing Up Multitasking: The Cost and Benefits for Cognitive Development." *Developmental Review* 35: 5–41.

Covey, S. R. 1990. *The Seven Habits of Highly Effective People*. New York: Simon & Schuster.

Credit Suisse Learning. 2008. *Time Management: Fight Your Time Bandits*. Accessed May 11, 2018. http://emagazine-creditsuisse.com/app/article/index.cfm?aoid=27815&fuseaction=OpenArticle&lang=en.

Culp, G., and A. Smith. 1997. "Six Steps to Effective Delegation." *Journal of Management in Engineering* 13 (1): 30–31.

Curtis, E., and H. Nicholl. 2004. "Delegation: A Key Function of Nursing." *Nursing Management* 11 (4): 26–31.

Daft, R. L. 1991. *Management*. Chicago: Dryden Press.

Dickson, A., and M. Fongoni. 2015. "People and Policy: Behavioral Economics and Its Policy Implications." *Fraser of Allander Economic Commentary* 38 (3): 93–106.

Drucker, P. 2001. *The Essential Drucker*. New York: HarperCollins.

———. 1974. *Management: Tasks, Responsibilities, Practices*. New York: Harper & Row.

———. 1967. *The Effective Executive*. New York: HarperCollins.

Flaherty, J. 1999. *Peter Drucker: Shaping the Managerial Mind*. San Francisco: Jossey-Bass.

Goffman, E. 1959. *The Presentation of Self in Everyday Life*. Garden City, NJ: Doubleday.

Hantsen, R., and M. Washburn. 1992. "How to Plan What to Delegate." *American Journal of Nursing* 92 (4): 71–72.

Harvard Business School. 2005. *Time Management: Increase Your Personal Productivity and Effectiveness*. Boston: Harvard Business School Press.

Haselhuhn, M., E. Wong, and M. Ormiston. 2017. "With Great Power Comes Shared Responsibility: Psychological Power and the Delegation of Authority." *Personality and Individual Differences* 108: 1–4.

Johnson, C. 2006. "Enron's Lay Dies of Heart Attack." *Washington Post.* Published July 6. www.washingtonpost.com/wp-dyn/content/article/2006/07/05/AR2006070500523.html.

Kahn, R. A. 2004. "Records Management and Compliance: Making the Connection." *Information Management Journal* 38 (3): 28–36.

Kaplan, R. 2010. "What to Ask the Person in the Mirror." In *On Managing Yourself*, 147–68. Boston: Harvard Review Press.

Keller, B. 2002. "Enron for Dummies." *New York Times.* Published January 26. www.nytimes.com/2002/01/26/opinion/enron-for-dummies.html.

Konig, C. J., and M. Kleinmann. 2007. "Time Management Problems and Discounted Utility." *Journal of Psychology* 141 (3): 321–34.

Kopeikina, L. 2006. "The Elements of a Clear Decision." *MIT Sloan Management Review* 47 (2): 19–20.

Kourdi, J. 1999. *Successful Delegation*. London: Hodder and Stoughton.

Law, E., N. Bennett, C. Ives, R. Friedman, K. Davis, C. Archibald, and K. Wilson. 2017. "Equity Trade-Offs in Conservation Decision Making." *Conservation Biology* 32 (2): 294–303.

Lear, J., K. Hodge, and S. Schulz. 2015. "Talk to Me!! Effective, Efficient Communication." *Journal of Research in Business Education* 57 (1): 64–77.

Lewis, B. J. 2000. "Management by Delegation." *Journal of Management in Engineering* 16 (2): 21.

Lorinkova, N. M., M. J. Pearsall, and H. P. Sim. 2013. "Examining the Differential Longitudinal Performance of Directive Versus Empowering Leadership in Teams." *Academy of Management Journal* 56 (2): 573–96.

Lucas, N., and V. Koerwer. 2004. "Featured Interview: Sherron Watkins, Former Vice President for Corporate Development of Enron." *Journal of Leadership and Organizational Studies* 11 (1): 38–47.

Marquis, B. L., and C. J. Huston. 2000. *Leadership Roles and Management Fuctions in Nursing*. New York: Lippincott, Williams & Wilkins.

Nash, L. 1989. "Ethics Without the Sermon." *Ethics in Practice: Managing the Moral Corporation*, edited by K. R. Andrews, 243–56. Boston: Harvard Business Review.

Parsons, T. 1951. *The Social System*. Glencoe, IL: Free Press.

Peer, K. S., and J. S. Rakich. 1999. "Ethical Decision Making in Healthcare Management." *Hospital Topics* 77 (4): 7–13.

Portny, S. E. 2002. "The Delegation Dilemma: When Do You Let Go?" *Information Management Journal* 36 (2): 60–64.

Reutter, L., P. A. Field, I. E. Campbell, and R. R. Day. 1997. "Socialization into Nursing: Nursing Students as Learners." *Journal of Nursing Education* 36 (4): 149–55.

Robbins, S. P. 2000. *Managing Today!* 2nd ed. Upper Saddle River, NJ: Prentice Hall.

Rocchiccioli, J. T., and M. S. Tilbury. 1998. *Clinical Leadership in Nursing*. Philadelphia, PA: WB Saunders.

Ross, A., F. J. Wenzel, and J. W. Mitlyng. 2002. *Leadership for the Future: Core Competencies in Healthcare*. Chicago: Health Administration Press.

Ross, J. 2018. "Effective Communication Improves Patient Safety." *Journal of PeriAnesthesia Nursing* 33 (2): 223–25.

Rue, L. W., and L. L. Byars. 2004. *Supervision: Key Link to Productivity*. Boston: McGraw-Hill Irwin.

Schwartz, T., and C. McCarthy. 2010. "Manage Your Energy, Not Your Time." In *On Managing Yourself*, 61–78. Boston: Harvard Business Review Press.

Simon, H. A. 1977. *The New Science of Management Decision*. Englewood Cliffs, NJ: Prentice-Hall.

Sostrin, J. 2017. "To Be a Great Leader, You Have to Learn How to Delegate Well." *Harvard Business Review*. Published October 10. https://hbr.org/topic/leadership-transitions.

St. James, E. 2001. *Simplify Your Work Life*. New York: Hyperion.

Sutton, R. I. 2002. *Weird Ideas That Work*. New York: Free Press.

Tang, T. P.-L., T. Sutarso, M. A. Ansari, V. K. G. Lim, T. S. H. Teo, F. Arias-Galicia, I. E. Garber, R. K.-K. Chiu, B. Charles-Pauvers, R. Luna-Arocas, P. Vlerick, A. Akande, M. W. Allen, A. S. Al-Zubaidi, M. G. Borg, B.-S. Cheng, R. Correia, L. Du, C. Garcia de la Torre, A. H. S. Ibrahim, C.-K. Jen, A. M. Kazem, K. Kim, J. Liang, E. Malovics, A. S. Moreira, R. T. Mpoyi, A. U. O. Nnedum, J. E. Osagie, A. M. Osman-Gani, M. F. Ozbek, F. J. C. Pereira, R. Pholsward, H. D. Pitariu, M. Polic, E. G. Sardzoska, P. Skobic, A. F. Stembridge, T. L.-N. Tang, C. Urbain, M. Trontelj, L. Canova, A. M. Manganelli, J. Chen, N. Tang, B. E. Adetoun, and M. F. Adewuyi. 2018. "Monetary Intelligence and Behavioral Economics: The Enron Effect—Love of Money, Corporate Ethical Values, Corruption Perceptions Index (CPI), and Dishonesty Across 31 Geopolitical Entities." *Journal of Business Ethics* 148 (4): 919–37.

Trapani, G. 2006. *Lifehacker: 88 Tech Tricks to Turbocharge Your Day*. New York: John Wiley & Sons.

Trunk, P. 2008. *10 Tips for Time Management in a Multitasking World*. Published December 10. http://blog.penelopetrunk.com/2006/12/10/10-tips-for-time-management-in-a-multitasking-world/.

Uncapher, M., M. Thieu, and A. Wagner. 2015. "Media Multitasking and Memory: Differences in Working Memory and Long-Term Memory." *Pyschonomic Bulletin & Review* 23 (2): 483–90.

United Press International. 2002. "Enron Whistle-Blower Testifies to Congress." Published February 14. www.newsmax.com/archives/articles/2002/2/14/165328.shtml.

Vaccaro, P. J. 2003. "Forget About Time Management." *Family Practice Management* 10 (5): 82.

Van den Bulcke, B., R. Piers, H. I. Jensen, J. Malmgren, V. Metaxa, A. K. Reyners, M. Darmon, K. Rusinova, D. Talmor, A.-P. Meert, L. Cancelliere, L. Zubek, P. Maia, A. Michalsen, J. Decruyenaere, E. Kompanje, E. Azoulay, R. Meganck, A. Van de Sompel, S. Vansteelandt, P. Vlerick, S. Vanheule, and D. Benoit. 2018. "Ethical Decision-Making Climate in the ICU: Theoretical Framework and Validation of a Self-Assessment Tool." *BMJ Quality & Safety* 27 (10): 781–89.

Wearing, R. 2005. *Corporate Governance*. London: Sage Publications.

Wilbanks, C. 2013. "Ex-Enron CEO Jeff Skilling to Leave Prison Early." CBS News. Published June 21. www.cbsnews.com/news/ex-enron-ceo-jeff-skilling-to-leave-prison-early/.

Wilson, W. 1914. "Speech to the National Press Club." *Independent Weekly* 77: 439.

PART III

BUSINESS SKILLS

CASE STUDY

THE DECISION TO ADMIT OR NOT TO ADMIT*

INTRODUCTION

This book addresses many of the conceptual, interpersonal, and business skills associated with healthcare management. Among the material covered in part III are business skills related to healthcare law and ethics; strategic planning; healthcare operations and quality; financial management; human resources management; and healthcare information technology. Much of the knowledge and skill set needed to solve the complexities presented in this case require a practical application of the ideas presented in part III, as well as in parts I and II. Discussion questions at the end of the case will facilitate insight and learning.

BACKGROUND

Over the past five years, Bob Allred, administrator at Mountain State Hospital, had noticed that magistrate and district judges across his rural state were increasingly directing that dangerous and severely mentally ill patients be placed under the charge of the state's Department of Health & Human Services (DHHS). Although Allred was deeply conflicted and troubled about this trend, as administrator of a hospital under the auspices of DHHS, he was not entirely surprised when he was directed to admit a mentally ill patient who had a history of violent crime, including aggravated assault and murder.

Allred's rural state was one of only a few US states that did not own, operate, or contract with a secure forensic mental hospital—mainly because of poor funding and other institutions' unwillingness to receive transferred patients because of limited capacity or overcrowded conditions of their own. As a result, severely mentally ill criminals who required significant mental health care often languished without needed psychiatric care and medications in secure, lockdown units in county jails or the state penitentiary. Alternatively, many were admitted to minimally secure civil units in hospitals contracted with, owned, or operated by the state, where they received much-needed care, despite the risk they posed to others.

The Hippocratic imperative to physicians—"Bring benefit and do no harm"—expresses both the principles of nonmaleficence ("do no harm") and beneficence ("bring benefit"). By its very declaration, the Hippocratic Oath invites trust. Doctors, and those who work with and for them, voluntarily promise they can be trusted to "bring benefit" while, above all, "[doing] no harm" (Paola, Walker, and Nixon 2010). However, as Allred and his colleagues would learn, balancing these imperatives is, at times, extraordinarily difficult.

State Law, Social and Political Realities, and Incompatibility

Consistent with other states, Allred's local state legislature had enacted statutes that required DHHS, notably the state's network of clinics and state hospitals, to evaluate and treat all citizens with severe and persistent mental illness who were not otherwise treated by private mental hospitals and clinics. Allred's state statutes also required that dangerously mentally ill patients or criminals be treated in properly designated forensic hospitals—that is, secure hospitals able to keep patients on lockdown—or related facilities. In 2015, Allred's state did not have separate and distinct facilities for civil and nondangerous mentally ill citizens and patients deemed dangerous, criminal, or forensic. Thus, two great conflicts routinely, and increasingly, came into play:

1. Dangerous patients were frequently placed and cared for alongside vulnerable patients and staff in nonsecure settings, thus violating state law.
2. Dangerous or forensic patients who, for reasons beyond their control—often mental illness—were denied access to the desperately needed care and medication available in state hospitals and instead left to languish in county jails and state prisons for unreasonable lengths of time.

While most states had long since resolved these difficulties, Allred's state—with its limited funds and highly conservative views on welfare and state-provided mental health care—continued to operate without the needed facilities and ranked near the bottom nationally in mental health care spending per capita.

Allred's state law provided that severe and persistent mentally ill citizens were to be cared for in a safe, secure environment. But without a separate forensic health facility to serve violent patients, the nonviolent mentally ill were not afforded a safe, secure environment. Notwithstanding this dilemma, the violent mentally ill needed healthcare, too.

The Risk

As at other state mental institutions, personnel at Mountain State Hospital were regularly trained and oriented in matters of personal safety as they relate to the risks inherent in caring for mentally disturbed patients. Although these risks are commonly understood and protective measures are routinely employed, employees and vulnerable patients still, on occasion, get injured. These injured staff and patients have even been known to file battery charges against their psychotic aggressors.

Given these conditions, admitting and caring for extremely aggressive or dangerously violent mentally ill patients at Mountain State Hospital created a heightened risk for several constituencies. First and foremost were the other patients. If a violent, mentally ill patient were admitted, how could the other patients be protected from potential harm?

Second were the hospital staff members providing healthcare. How could their safety be ensured, given that their work environment had not been set up to deal with violent patients? And how could they guarantee safe care for the nonviolent mentally ill when violent mentally ill patients were nearby?

The third group at increased risk were members of the public. What dangers would they face when visiting the hospital? And, what if a violent patient escaped the building, into their community? Although potentially dangerous patients are guarded more carefully, the facility was not designed nor staffed to be a high-security hospital. If the public knew it was now accepting dangerous, mentally ill patients, they likely would object, making public opinion a concern.

The Tipping Point

Allred sighed as he read the documents sent over from DHHS. A district judge had directed Mountain State Hospital to admit Mr. Harold Bentley, a middle-aged man who, several years earlier, had violently murdered his supervisor. In his delusional state, Bentley believed his boss was out to kill him, and he had determined to strike first. After being tried and convicted of first-degree murder (Allred's state did not have a "guilty but mentally ill" law), Bentley was sentenced to life in prison at the state penitentiary. For four years, he had sat in near isolation, in a four-by-eight-foot cell, 23 hours per day. He had been given limited psychotropic medications and little other mental health evaluation or treatment. Thus, while the public was safely protected from this man whom most regarded as a truly violent criminal, mental health advocates pleaded Bentley's case, insisting he was not receiving needed mental health care services.

The media had followed Bentley's case for more than three years, resulting in various feature stories from television and newspaper outlets. During this time, repeated appeals on Bentley's behalf were entered into court. Advocacy groups that proposed Bentley's removal from prison and placement into an acute mental health care facility had garnered favorable mental health evaluations. Coupled with the state statute that required DHHS to arrange for or directly treat all severe and persistent mentally ill citizens, the media were able to keep the Bentley story alive. In the most recent appeal, the judge, citing the favorable mental health professions, evaluations, directed that Bentley be released from prison and admitted to Allred's hospital.

Allred and the Decision

Upon learning of the judge's ruling, various members of the Mountain State Hospital medical staff responded quickly. They told Allred they viewed the judge's order negatively and demanded he ignore the ruling and refuse admittance to Bentley. They argued that Mountain State Hospital did not have the ability to care for a violent, mentally ill patient and that the medical staff leaders were within their rights to argue this point. Moreover, state law provided that the state hospital administrator consult with the hospital's medical director on matters related to hospital admissions, and because of this consultation, the medical staff had the legal right to accept or reject patients based on the hospital's ability to care for such patients in a safe and effective manner. To further protest Bentley's admittance, two of the seven staff psychiatrists threatened to resign if Bentley were admitted.

Other hospital caregivers, including many psychologists, nurses, and social workers, had mixed opinions regarding Bentley's admittance. Some sympathized with Bentley and argued his need for care, even noting "we should be the obvious providers of that care." Others supported the medical staff's view. One nurse said, "We should care for our patients—the nonviolent mentally ill; the violent should not be allowed in the facility. I can't keep my vulnerable patients safe with dangerous and violent patients around!"

Beyond the medical staff, Allred had another constituency with a markedly different demand. Because of its state hospital status, Mountain State Hospital operated under the direction of DHHS. Any decisions made by Allred or the medical director were subject to influence by DHHS officials. Thus, despite the medical staff leaders' position, DHHS officials strongly encouraged Allred to accept Bentley. In fact, Allred's supervisor at DHHS essentially demanded that Allred follow the judge's directive and admit Bentley to Mountain State Hospital.

Allred reread the documents. What should he do? Should he follow the judge's order and DHHS's directive to admit Bentley? Should he follow the demand by his medical staff leadership not to admit? To facilitate his decision-making process, Allred made a list of the hospital's key stakeholders and their positions regarding Bentley's potential admission. He also considered various decision-making models he had studied in college and read more recently in management books. A number of questions coursed through his mind (Nash 1989):

- Have you defined the problem correctly?
- How did we get to this point in the first place?
- What are the short- and long-term implications of your potential decision(s)?
- What are the legal and ethical frameworks for your position?
- What strategic, operational, human resources, or quality/safety considerations affect your potential decisions/positions?
- Under what conditions would you allow exceptions to your positions?

Allred hoped that by clearly identifying key stakeholder positions, and by following a thoughtful, rational decision-making model, he would make a wise decision in the Bentley case.

Discussion Questions

1. What was the gist of the conflict surrounding Bentley's admission to Mountain State Hospital? Identify the stakeholders involved and their positions regarding whether or not Bentley should be removed from prison and placed at Mountain State Hospital. Consider how their positions might have been influenced by the state statutes and what they want regarding hospital action.
2. In his effort to balance the competing interests of public safety with Bentley's rights as a citizen and potential patient, do you think the judge acted wisely in relocating Bentley from the state prison to the state hospital? Consider both the legal and ethical conflicts involved. Explain why you made the decision you did.
3. Although they could provide the psychiatric care Bentley desperately needed, why did the medical staff object to his admission to Mountain State Hospital? In view of their commitment to the Hippocratic Oath—namely, to bring their patients benefit and to do no harm—was the medical staff's objection professional or otherwise appropriate? Why or why not?
4. Do you recommend Allred admit Bentley? Why or why not?
5. What is the role of ethics for Allred as he makes his decision?

Note

* A version of this case was originally published by the Society for Case Research as Farnsworth, T., and L. W. Cellucci. 2011. "Admit or Not Admit." *Journal of Critical Incidents* 4: 34–37.

References

Nash, L. 1989. "Ethics Without the Sermon." In *Ethics in Practice: Managing the Moral Corporation*, edited by K. R. Andrews, 243–56. Boston: Harvard Business Review Press.

Paola, F. A., R. Walker, and L. A. Nixon. 2010. *Medical Ethics and Humanities*. Sudbury, MA: Jones & Bartlett Publishers.

CHAPTER 10

ETHICS AND LAW

Important Terms

- Autonomy
- Beneficence
- Bribe
- Clinical ethics
- Competencies
- Confidentiality
- Corporate citizenship
- Emergency Medical Treatment and Labor Law Act of 1986 (EMTALA)
- Fidelity
- Good stewardship of resources
- Health Insurance Portability and Accountability Act (HIPAA) Privacy Rule
- Informed consent
- Justice
- Kickback
- Liability
- Litigious
- Malpractice
- Managerial ethics
- Nonmaleficence
- Organizational ethics
- Organizational politics
- Positive duty
- Protected health information (PHI)
- Quality improvement
- Tort
- Trust
- Truth telling
- Worker's compensation

Learning Objectives

After reading this chapter, you will be able to do the following:

- Understand and explain four foundational tenets of Western philosophy that influence ethical decision-making and legal requirements:
  - Autonomy
  - Nonmaleficence
  - Beneficence
  - Justice
- Understand and explain the four major points of managerial ethics and address the healthcare manager's role in relation to each:
  - Excellence in patient care
  - Respect for employees
  - Corporate citizenship
  - The appropriate use of resources
- Outline the broad and overarching federal legislation
- Discuss the legal duties and responsibilities shared among healthcare organizations, patients, physicians, and employees

Case Study: The Ethics Committee

This discussion can be witnessed in the boardrooms of healthcare organizations across the country:

"Can you believe this? As if we don't have enough to do, now we have to be on this silly ethics committee?"

"Does anyone know how long this is going to take? I've got a desk full of stuff to do and I don't have time to sit here talking about stuff that has nothing to do with me."

"Well, I don't know about you, but I'm not going to rat on any of my coworkers."

"Whose idea was this, anyway?"

"I bet it is just a kneejerk reaction to that crazy woman who complained that other people had seen the results of her lab work."

"No, I don't think that's it. . . . I think they know The Joint Commission is coming soon and they need to make it look like we actually pay attention to this kind of stuff. Mark my words—once The Joint Commission comes and goes, this so-called ethics committee will just fade into the background."

"What time was this meeting supposed to start, anyway? Who's running this meeting?"

"Well, actually, I am. Sorry I'm a few minutes late. Some of you might not know me yet; I just started a few months ago. I'm the new director of operations. The CEO asked me to chair this committee, and she gave me a few agenda items for us to start with."

"Wait a minute, before we get into that stuff, why are we here? Why us? What do we know about ethics? We aren't experts. I mean, we all do the best we can every day, but the job changes every day, and there are no hard and fast rules that are ever going to cover everything."

"Hey, I don't even do patient care. I never touch patients, and I don't think I need to be here."

"So are we going to be talking about professional codes of conduct or philosophy, or how everyone is supposed to be a good person all the time?"

"I think the people who should start thinking about this kind of stuff are the VPs, not us. I mean, whose brilliant idea was it to remodel the radiology department before fixing the entrance to the ER? And how do they think they are going to be able to find a new head nurse for intensive care when they won't pay us what we are worth and they work us to death with ridiculous hours? Most of us could earn more working at the mall."

"Yeah, let the folks earning the big bucks and making the big decisions start talking about ethical conduct. Did you hear how much the CEO is earning this year?"

"I don't think that's the kind of thing we're supposed to be talking about. If we're supposed to be fixing ethical problems, we should be talking about those poor people in the long-term care center who are just lying around waiting to die. Doesn't anyone care that they don't ever get out of their rooms? My best friend's husband works there, and he says that often the patients don't get their meds on time, and sometimes they don't get them at all! Remember that old lady who died last week and left her life insurance to us? He says she died because she wasn't getting the right meds."

"If you want to talk about things that shouldn't be happening, how about all the lead paint and asbestos in the old hospital wing? And you know that the shielding in the X-ray room isn't actually up to code, don't you?"

"I heard the janitors just empty all the recycling bins right into the regular garbage dumpsters, so why should we worry about the environment and recycling when they just dump sharps and dirty dressings and the recycling stuff right into the garbage? Doesn't that stuff just end up in the landfill?"

"Sounds like we do have lots to talk about, doesn't it? I understand your concerns, and I know that everyone here is very busy. The CEO asked me to chair this committee because I was on the ethics committee at my last job, and even though it wasn't always easy or fun, we felt that we made a difference. We all face challenges and hard decisions every day. I think having a few basic principles to fall back on really helps. How should we start?"

Introduction

Although in-depth study of Western philosophy is beyond the scope of this book, understanding some of its core principles that guide our ethical reasoning in general is not. In particular,

Autonomy
The state of being self-governing. The liberty to rule one's self, free of the controlling influence of others.

Truth telling
A positive duty to provide accurate, complete, and honest information at all times as part of the respect for other persons.

Fidelity
The quality of being faithful, accurate, and steadfast to an ideal, obligation, trust, or duty.

Nonmaleficence
The quality of causing no injury or harm and committing no misconduct or wrongdoing.

Beneficence
An obligation to help and provide benefits to others.

Positive duty
The duty of commission. The requirement to engage in an action actively and intentionally.

Justice
Fairness. Ensuring that everyone is treated equitably.

four tenets derived from Western philosophical thinking are at the root of virtually every ethical consideration in healthcare: autonomy, nonmaleficence, beneficence, and justice. Virtually every ethical consideration in healthcare emanates from one or more of these tenets. To a noteworthy degree, these tenets also serve as the foundation for many of the legal requirements that apply to healthcare providers and organizations. The tenets *should* be the guideposts that lead decision makers to make ethically sound decisions. What follows is a brief look at these four central tenets.

Autonomy. Having respect for another is a critical ethical touchstone. Autonomy means to respect the person and his or her capacity to make informed decisions. It also means a commitment to **truth telling**. Patients (or a colleague, whether clinical or administrative) can only be autonomous effectively if they know the truth. Autonomy also means treating communications with them, and information about them, confidentially. Finally, it means the relationship should be treated with **fidelity**, meaning that you will be faithful to the other person. This means keeping your commitments and being accurate with your facts as they relate to others.

Nonmaleficence. There is an adage in healthcare, particularly for physicians but it relates to administrators as well: "First, do no harm." Clearly if the patient is seeking care, the notion to avoid doing harm to them is instinctive. It also means taking a reasonable risk, if the patient has provided informed consent, in advancing care. In a broad sense, this dictate means that one should avoid doing those things that might damage a relationship. As we shall see in later sections, this has applications in managerial ethics as well.

Beneficence. This duty extends beyond nonmaleficence to create a **positive duty** to do all one can to aid patients. In addition, it means being charitable and kind to others. The manager has a duty to treat all patients with beneficence. Likewise, the alert administrator always approaches other stakeholders with this standard. This concept also weighs the benefit of an action against the harm caused by not taking it, which means one should do what is in the best interest of those involved.

Justice. The concept of justice speaks to the allocation of resources. How are scarce resources distributed? Are patients treated equally? Equitably? What is the difference? Are more funds dedicated to those who are sicker than those who have slightly better health? Does the organization make resources available to treat patients without means in the same fashion as patients who are insured or can pay directly for the care they receive? The answers to these questions help illustrate the concept of justice.

Together, these four tenets of Western philosophy are not only foundations for ethical thinking in healthcare, but also provide an underpinning for a number of legal standards presented later in this chapter.

Professional Ethics: Clinicians and Managers

The people in the "dreaded" ethics committee meeting transcribed at the beginning of the chapter are right about one thing: Everyone in healthcare is busy. Sometimes, in our fast-paced work world, we forget that it helps to sit back and look at the big picture. While each patient has individual needs, problems, and concerns, overarching moral and ethical issues underscore our work and affect our organizations.

One fallacy about ethics is that it is only for caregivers; another is that ethical discourse is solely the business of philosophers and ethicists. The person in the case study who said the committee members are not experts and that everyone just does the best they can is missing the point. Each of us must live with the consequences of our actions and decisions. Whether we acknowledge it or not, we each have a framework that we use for making hard decisions about the right thing to do. Legal requirements may serve as a "bright line" for what is out of bounds, but sometimes that which is ethical is also illegal; likewise, sometimes something legally permissible may be unethical. A professional's framework for ethical decision-making often has its foundation within his or her field, as each profession has its own code of ethics and professional standards.

Professional Ethical Standards for Clinicians

We often classify the ethical principles applied to clinical practice in terms of rights and duties—the rights every person holds and the duties we have toward others. The four tenets certainly do not encompass the entire field of **clinical ethics**, nor are they a conclusive list of ethical principles for healthcare professionals. However, these foundational principles are considered the most pertinent to clinical practice, and we can see how they guide many key aspects of a healthcare provider's job:

Clinical ethics
The overarching framework of morals and principles underscoring the provision of medical care to patients.

- Autonomy ➔ Provide informed consent and privacy
- Nonmaleficence ➔ Ensure a safe environment for care
- Beneficence ➔ Provide competent care
- Justice ➔ Treat all patients equitably

The Agency for Healthcare Research and Quality (AHRQ) has espoused six domains of care, establishing the standard that care should be safe, effective, patient-centered, timely, efficient, and equitable (AHRQ 2016). Think about those domains carefully against the backdrop of the four principles discussed earlier. Can you see where some elements of those domains have roots in autonomy, for example? In justice? To put it simply, good clinical care is also good ethical care. That is not to say that if clinicians make mistakes they have violated ethical guidelines, but it is very likely that if a clinician behaves unethically he or she is most likely providing substandard care.

Professional Ethical Standards for Managers

Clinical care providers are not the only ones who need to think about ethics. Even managers and other professionals who do not directly provide patient care still have ethical

Organizational ethics
The ethics of an organization; how an organization responds to an internal or external stimulus.

Managerial ethics
A set of principles and rules that define what is right and what is wrong in an organization. It is the guideline that helps direct a lower manager's decisions in the scope of his or her job when presented with a conflict of values.

responsibilities to patients, colleagues, organizations, and society. Winkler and Gruen (2005) propose four ethical principles of **organizational ethics** for healthcare organizations and managers: provide care with compassion, treat employees with respect, act in a public spirit, and spend resources reasonably. Slightly reworded, these principles provide the framework for our discussion of **managerial ethics** in healthcare: excellence in patient care, respect for employees, corporate citizenship, and the good stewardship of resources. As exhibit 10.1 shows, these are drawn from, and overlap with, the ethical tenets previously discussed.

Excellence in Patient Care

This first principle mirrors the biomedical ethics principles for clinical practice listed above, yet it goes beyond hands-on patient care to the patient-centered organizational values of "competence, compassion, and trust," which are at the heart of excellence in patient care (Winkler and Gruen 2005, 112). The committee member who argues that she does not touch patients and thus does not need to be on the committee has a very narrow view of ethics. Patient care is not the sole domain of caregivers. Managers are responsible for creating an environment of excellent care. One way to do so is to make certain all hospital employees are qualified and able to meet the criteria and demands of their positions. This is a two-sided coin: Healthcare organizations must be diligent in performing criminal background checks and confirming licensure and education; in addition, they must provide all employees with the opportunity to continue their education. The other side of the coin is the organization's duty to have policies and procedures in place to identify, intervene with, and assist impaired or inadequately prepared workers (ACHE 2017b).

Confidentiality
Holding information as secret and private.

Ensuring the **confidentiality** of health information is another essential component of excellence in patient care. Confidentiality goes beyond simply following "the laws

Exhibit 10.1 Healthcare Organizational Ethics and Selected Tenets of Western Philosophy

		Selected Tenets of Western Philosophy			
		Autonomy	Nonmaleficence	Beneficence	Justice
Healthcare Organizational Ethics	Excellence in patient care	X	X	X	
	Respect for employees	X			X
	Corporate citizenship		X		X
	Appropriate use of resources			X	X

governing the use and release of information, limiting access to patient information to authorized individuals only" (ACHE 2016), and extends to providing the organizational resources—including personnel, hardware, software, policies, and procedures—needed to safeguard confidential information. As the American College of Healthcare Executives (ACHE 2016) says, "Society's need for information rarely outweighs the right of patients to confidentiality."

The person on the ethics committee whose best friend's husband talks about poor care in the long-term care (LTC) unit and refers to a specific patient's medication has violated a number of ethical principles. Any discussion of a specific patient's care outside the direct care setting can be, and in this case is, a serious breach of confidentiality. In addition, while we do not know the context of the husband's comments, such an unguarded and potentially harmful disclosure about the organization is disloyal and ethically inappropriate. If the husband truly believes the care in the LTC unit is negligent, he has an ethical obligation to report his concerns to the appropriate person.

Technology also has a significant place in patient care, though it, too, is a double-edged sword. While it has led to the miracles of organ transplantation, remarkable pharmaceutical therapies, and science fiction–like procedures that formerly were mere figments of the imagination, these and other advances prompt difficult decisions regarding length and quality of life. Providing excellent care with compassion, **competency**, and **trust** depends on an environment in which patients have the knowledge, ability, and right to govern their lives; it is care that respects their decisions. Comments about patients lying around waiting to die are callous, insensitive, and uninformed. This committee member is reacting to gossip and perhaps projecting her own feelings onto these patients. She could not possibly know the life decisions of the patients being talked about.

Competencies
A set of professional and personal skills, knowledge, values, and traits that guide a leader's performance, behavior, interactions, and decisions.

Trust
Assured reliance on character, ability, strength, or truth. Putting confidence in a person, place, or thing.

Since the release of the Institute of Medicine (2001) report *To Err Is Human*, healthcare organizations and individual providers have acknowledged an ethical responsibility to participate in **quality improvement** (QI). QI is defined as "systematic, data-guided activities designed to bring about immediate improvements in healthcare delivery in particular settings" (Lynn et al. 2007, 666–67). However justified and important, QI endeavors may inadvertently cause harm, waste scarce resources, or affect some individuals unfairly. Healthcare managers must ensure that patient and employee participation in QI is subject to standards of reasonableness and guarantee the confidentiality of those involved. Furthermore, individuals, both patients and employees, must be able to opt out if the QI endeavor presents unacceptable risk to themselves.

Quality improvement
A systematic, formal approach to analyzing performance and efforts to improve service.

Last, the healthcare industry is fraught with personnel shortages and budget constraints. Attracting and retaining qualified staff is increasingly a challenge, and severe understaffing can endanger patients. If staff shortages become severe, healthcare leaders need to have plans for "closing units or diverting patients . . . to ensure that patient care is not compromised and high quality care is maintained" (ACHE 2017a).

Respect for Employees

Businesses should involve their employees by giving them an opportunity to influence decisions (Bayraktar et al. 2017). Employers' duties to employees include, but are not limited to, offering fair salaries, safe working conditions, equitable rewards and disciplinary actions, a voice in policy and procedure decisions, and protection from discrimination in the workplace (Robinson et al. 2005; Wynia, Latham, and Kao 1999). Organizations and managers can ensure fair and just treatment of all employees in these areas by having clear, legal, and up-to-date policies and procedures on hiring and firing, salaries and raises, grievances, and inappropriate behavior. Creating an ethical culture is a prerequisite for allowing employees to take responsibility for their own actions rather than hiding behind rules and structures (Margolis 2001).

Treating employees with respect and justice means that those of equal organizational rank or stature are treated as equals, while those at different employment levels are treated differently but still equitably. This makes sense when you think about it in reference to age, for example. Children of different ages might have different bedtimes, different allowances, different chores, and different curfews. In healthcare, practitioners in different professions are allowed to perform different treatments, those with different levels of education within a profession are allowed to provide different levels of care, and people in different jobs get paid differently. One committee member commented on the CEO's salary, implying that the "folks making the big bucks" might not be acting ethically. The adage about "walking a mile in someone else's shoes" before judging their actions should be taken seriously before making accusations and judgments about another person's ethical actions.

Healthcare organizations are stressful workplaces. Perhaps it is the life-and-death nature of the work. Perhaps it is the tight budgets. Or perhaps it is the fast pace and the difficulty of meeting all patients' needs and being all things to all people. Staffs are composed of a hierarchy of professions and egos, accompanied by knowledge and power differentials. Rumor mills flourish. Combined, these factors create a highly political stew of coworkers, bosses, decisions, and situations, sometimes devolving into a game of **organizational politics**.

Organizational politics
Informal, unofficial, and sometimes behind-the-scenes efforts to sell ideas, influence an organization, increase power, or achieve other targeted objectives.

Mintzberg (1983) defined organizational politics as actions that are inconsistent with accepted organizational norms, designed to promote self-interest, and taken without regard for—and even at the expense of—organizational goals. Higher levels of absenteeism, turnover intentions, anxiety, and stress are likely to occur when employees have this perception of organizational politics. Furthermore, those views correspond to lower levels of job satisfaction, job performance, and organizational citizenship (Kacmar and Baron 1999).

Later research has indicated, however, that organizational politics can be both "good" and "bad" in terms of their impact on the organization. "The phenomenon of organizational politics subsumes all forms of influence in organizations; therefore, organizational politics can take on both negative and positive connotations. Many are aware of astute managers or individuals who use political influence to successfully conduct the organization's work"

(Valle and Witt 2001, 388). This thought directly contravenes Mintzberg's definition. Thus, there can be "good" organizational politics when an organization is fair (Byrne 2005) and values teamwork (Valle and Witt 2001), and when employees understand why events at work take place (Sutton and Kahn 1986) and perceive they can influence decisions and work outcomes in a constructive fashion (Witt, Andrews, and Kacmar 2000).

One clear demonstration of respect and care for employees is a safe workplace. Employees want to know they will be safe with patients and visitors, other employees, unwanted intruders, and technologies, and physically safe from injuries, as evidenced by the committee member's comment about asbestos and radiation shielding. Healthcare organizations have a responsibility to teach employees proper techniques and afford them proper equipment to safeguard themselves. Wiggins and Bowman (2000) found that feelings of safety while working affect not only work satisfaction, but also the life satisfaction of healthcare managers. Healthcare has a predominantly female workforce, and women healthcare managers report significantly more actual experience with danger—such as harassment and being accosted by strangers—in the workplace than men (Wiggins 2000).

Another clear demonstration of respect for employees is to create a climate of empowerment—that is, one in which employees see meaning in their work, feel competent to do the work assigned, believe their work will make a difference, and enjoy some degree of self-determination in how to approach their tasks (Houghton et al. 2015).

Corporate Citizenship

Organizations are expected to be good corporate and community citizens. As participants in a democratic society, organizations have a duty to obey the laws concerning issues such as employment, pollution, taxes, and building codes. Healthcare is one of the most complex, transaction-intense, highly regulated industries in our nation (Wiggins et al. 2006). As such, healthcare organizations must comply with federal, state, and local laws regarding licensure, privilege to practice, staffing, continuing education, physical plant safety, the safeguarding of information, and disposal of medical waste, to name just a few. (Several of these will be discussed at greater length later in the chapter.) Corporate citizenship also goes beyond adherence to mere legal requirements and speaks to the level of charity care and engagement in the community at large.

Corporate citizenship
The social responsibility of both not-for-profit organizations and for-profit businesses, and the extent to which they meet legal, ethical, and economic responsibilities, as expected by stakeholders.

The old idea that businesses exist to narrow-mindedly pursue profit to the exclusion of all other considerations has been widely challenged. Society is entitled to expect from business a significant net positive contribution to the general good (Hutton and Mayer 2010). Obviously, this is particularly true for healthcare organizations. Today's broader corporate culture includes responsibility and respect toward staff and customers, help for the wider community, and a responsible approach to the environment (Andriof and McIntosh 2001; Birch 2001; Waddock and Smith 2000). This expands the corporate focus from strictly increasing the wealth of *stock*holders to also serving the needs of organizational *stake*holders, "such as employees, suppliers, customers, and neighbors in the wider community" (Warburton et al. 2004, 118). Healthcare organizations should be sponsors of, and participants in, a variety of activities that raise awareness of disease as well as promote good health. Hinckley (2002, 19) suggests the following words be added to the description of duties for board members and directors regarding increasing profits: "but not at the expense of the environment, human rights, public health or safety, the community, or the dignity of employees."

Research indicates most employees want "meaningfulness" in their work, which is defined as work that provides a venue for human authenticity, affirmative moral commitment, and dignity. It is, in short, work that serves an "ultimate concern" (Lips-Wiersma and Morris 2009). The comment from the committee member about recycling and the landfill illustrates the employee's desire to do the right thing and the frustration that results when he perceives the organization is not supporting his efforts.

This idea of good corporate citizenship seems like a natural for healthcare. Most healthcare organizations—for-profit and not-for-profit alike—mention caring for others in their mission statements (Wiggins, Hatzenbuehler, and Peterson 2008). Many traditionally fulfill their duty of corporate citizenship via community-strengthening activities, such as care for the uninsured, reinvestment of profit into hospital improvements and employees, community health education, staff education, involvement with research, and other community benefits.

Good Stewardship of Resources

Good stewardship of resources
The careful and responsible management of something entrusted to one's care.

Today's healthcare organizations have multiple and complex responsibilities; tensions between these responsibilities often result. For example, while caregivers have responsibilities to their patients, healthcare organizations have the responsibility to care for entire patient populations, employees, payers, and stakeholders (Winkler and Gruen 2005). Indeed, new payment models urge healthcare organizations to focus on the community at large and take steps to improve the health status of entire communities. The values, wants, and needs of these groups are often in conflict, though each has a meritorious claim on precious resources.

As healthcare becomes more competitive, economic incentives blur. Healthcare organizations must walk the tightrope between financial success and living their mission and values. Some might naively say there isn't a choice: Healthcare organizations must serve patients and stakeholders. However, a more sophisticated understanding of the business of healthcare shows a delicate balance often stated as "no margin, no mission." Take, for example, the committee member's complaint that the radiology department was remodeled before the emergency room (ER). Radiology is often one of the most profitable services a hospital offers, whereas the ER frequently loses money. At first glance, it may seem that choosing radiology over the ER is mercenary—preferring expensive new technology for the doctors over serving people with an immediate and dire need for care. However, the money made by the improved radiology department might be reallocated to other departments, enabling them to provide care that might not have otherwise been possible.

It is also important to remember that money is not an organization's only resource. Healthcare organizations' other resources include employees, time, physical plant, talent, knowledge, skill, and community goodwill. Not only must a healthcare organization use its financial resources wisely, but it also must leverage all its resources for the greatest benefit to the organization and stakeholders.

Discussion

Ethical conduct in healthcare organizations flourishes if moral principles are routinely applied in issues of workplace fairness by rewarding ethical conduct, disciplining unethical conduct, and emphasizing the fair treatment of employees (Cropanzano, Goldman, and Folger 2003). The formation of the ethics committee, dreaded or not, is one way for the organization in the case study to institutionalize agreed-upon ethical values, policies, and procedures (Giganti 2004). Ethical problems and concerns, such as those voiced in the committee meeting, need to be examined and discussed from a broad ethical perspective before solutions can become institutionalized (Winkler and Gruen 2005). The first step, and seemingly a challenge for the leader of the meeting, is to separate the tendency to gossip and complain from the true ethical issues and develop a shared approach to those concerns.

The four principles of managerial ethics—excellence in patient care, respect for employees, corporate citizenship, and the appropriate use of resources—raise awareness of the depth and breadth of ethical responsibilities facing healthcare organizations and managers. While agreeing on these principles will not necessarily provide instant conflict resolution among organization members or members of the ethics committee, one would hope it at least provides consensus on overarching realms of obligation, and perhaps a framework to guide discussion.

The four tenets forming the bedrock of ethical considerations in healthcare—autonomy, nonmaleficence, beneficence, and justice—also can be seen in legal considerations of healthcare organizations. Because much of US law relies broadly on Western philosophical ideas, laws governing the conduct of healthcare organizations and providers also stem from these four tenets.

Ethical Foundations of Legal Requirements and Restraints

The failure to behave ethically and legally, regrettably, occurs much too frequently. Consider the following recent cases:

- Owners and managers of a Massachusetts pharmacy allegedly failed to sterilize a pain drug shipped to hospitals and other healthcare providers, triggering a meningitis outbreak. Two company executives face murder charges (Johnson 2018).
- In June 2015, 243 people were arrested and charged with stealing $712 million from Medicare. This included 43 physicians, nurses, and pharmacy owners (Graham 2015).
- In 2012, GlaxoSmithKline was fined in Argentina when two of its researchers were found to have falsified parental consents during a clinical trial of a vaccine. Subjects were babies recruited from poor families who used public hospitals and whose parents were often illiterate and could not understand the 28-page consent form (Tejan 2012).
- In 2016, New York–Presbyterian Hospital paid $2.2 million for federal regulators to settle an alleged HIPAA violation when it allowed TV crews to film two patients being treated for injuries (Ornstein 2016).

Sadly, the record is replete with innumerable examples of ethical lapses as well as legal wrongdoings in areas of clinical research, administration, and patient care. What happened to make these failures of judgment so prevalent in our culture?

It is imperative that healthcare managers understand their industry's complex legal environment. Healthcare managers face legal issues every day. Of course, all healthcare professionals and organizations must obey the same laws as other businesses and citizens, such as tax law, contract law, and business law. However, the special circumstances of the medical field have resulted in additional, healthcare-specific laws and regulations. These are far too numerous to be discussed in depth in this chapter. Instead, we will present a general overview of important elements of healthcare law, first looking at broad and overarching legislation and then examining the legal duties and responsibilities of healthcare organizations, patients, physicians, and employees. Unless otherwise noted, the term *healthcare organization* applies to any organization or facility that delivers healthcare services, including, but not limited to, hospitals, LTC facilities, behavioral and mental health facilities, physician group practices, and all types of clinics. The term *provider* applies to any and all caregivers.

This chapter also will not go into detail on state law, despite its importance in healthcare. Because of the many variations in state law, it is impossible, within the scope of this book, to give the topic comprehensive attention. However, understand that the Tenth Amendment to the US Constitution, through the "police power" clause, delegates to the states the authority to protect the health and safety of their citizens. This means that actions intended to directly protect the health and safety of citizens residing in any given state are the sole province of that state. Thus, healthcare professions are licensed and regulated by the states. Because states' laws are intended to protect the public's health within the boundaries of a state, the state may agree to whatever licensure and regulatory schemes it decides are reasonable. Those requirements may be quite different across the state line. Likewise, the state's authority to impose things like certificate-of-need (CON) laws also is derived from the Constitution's police power clause. Some states have CON laws, while others do not. Of those that do, the requirements for a CON vary from state to state. So while treatment of state law is limited in this book, in some circumstances, when very broad generalizations are possible, you will notice a brief reference to state legal requirements. In addition, students are advised to become acquainted with the laws pertaining to healthcare organizations within their state.

Federal Law

For the most part, federal laws that affect healthcare organizations and providers are intended to prevent fraud, abuse, corruption, and the waste of government funds. They present the nexus of the ethical tenets justice and nonmaleficence. While government funding for healthcare organizations and providers comes from various sources, the federal laws discussed here have been primarily designed to protect the government's investments in the Medicare and Medicaid programs.

Antitrust legislation exists to ensure competition. The Sherman Antitrust Act of 1890 prevents restraint of trade and formation of monopolies, and the Federal Trade Commission Act of 1914 outlaws unfair competition and deceptive acts or practices. The Clayton Act of 1914 addresses contracting and exclusive dealing arrangements, and the Robinson-Patman Act of 1936 stops price discrimination. These antitrust acts have been in place for many years and were not specifically directed at healthcare. However, they have become increasingly pertinent to the healthcare industry. Mergers, acquisitions, joint ventures, and novel contractual relationships among healthcare organizations, providers, insurers, physician groups, and vendors are occurring across the United States at a record pace. Because these laws are aimed at keeping the marketplace "fair," it is easy to see how they find their source in the tenets of justice and respect for the person.

Emergency Medical Treatment and Labor Act of 1986 (EMTALA)
Legislation created to address the perceived problem of "patient dumping"—the refusal to treat uninsured patients, who are instead transferred to charitable hospitals without being seen by a clinician or receiving care. EMTALA requires hospitals and their affiliated physicians to screen and to continue to treat emergency patients until they are stabilized or transferred.

Federal Law Governing Healthcare Organizations and Patients

While the direct regulation of hospitals is primarily the province of the states, as discussed earlier, there are several federal laws that bear directly on the relationship between the hospital and the patient.

The **Emergency Medical Treatment and Labor Act of 1986 (EMTALA)** applies to hospitals. EMTALA was created to address the concern of "patient dumping"—the refusal to treat uninsured patients and instead transferring them to charitable hospitals without their having been seen or receiving care (Centers for Medicare & Medicaid Services 2012). Previously, common law in many states held physicians and healthcare organizations under no obligation to treat any person seeking care. To prevent patient dumping, EMTALA requires hospitals and their affiliated physicians to screen and continue to treat emergency patients until they are stabilized or transferred (Fosmire 2009).

While EMTALA clarifies the hospital's duties to patients in need of emergency care, the hospital's obligation to provide care in nonemergency situations is less clear. For example, a hospital may decline to provide care if it does not have adequate facilities or providers. In addition, a hospital may require that patients be admitted by an attending physician who is a member of the hospital's medical staff. On the other hand, Title VI of the Civil Rights Act of 1964, Section 504 of the Rehabilitation Act of 1973, and Title III of the Older Americans Amendments of 1975 protect hospital patients from discrimination. Finally, once a patient has been accepted and treated, a contract is implied—a hospital or provider may not simply stop treating that patient without risking **liability** for abandonment (Pozgar 2016).

Liability
Being in a position to likely incur an undesirable responsibility or obligation, usually monetary.

Whether or not under the dictates of EMTALA, healthcare organizations and providers have the duty to maintain complete, accurate, and timely medical records for all treated patients. The medical record is more than just documentation of the care and treatment provided. Medical records are used to review the appropriateness of care, to provide information for billing, and as a data source for medical research. The medical record is often seen as a legal document, and it may be used as evidence in **malpractice** cases or other legal proceedings. Medical records must be confidential, secure, current, authenticated, legible, and complete (Joint Commission 2013).

Malpractice
Injury or harm to a patient or customer directly caused by negligence, intentional tort, or breach of contract by a professional.

In addition to the obligation to maintain medical records, hospitals are responsible for keeping all patient-specific information safe and confidential. The **Health Insurance Portability and Accountability Act (HIPAA) Privacy Rule** took effect in 2003. It establishes a baseline of acceptable protection for patient privacy and confidentiality and was the first federal law to identify specifically **protected health information (PHI)**. PHI is information that (Wager, Lee, and Glaser 2013)

Health Insurance Portability and Accountability Act (HIPAA) Privacy Rule
The part of HIPAA that establishes safeguards to protect confidentiality and privacy and specifically identifies protected health information.

- relates to a person's physical or mental health, the provision of healthcare, or the payment for healthcare;
- identifies the person who is the subject of the information;
- is created or received by an entity subject to HIPAA; and
- is transmitted or maintained in any form (paper, electronic, oral).

Protected health information (PHI)
Information from which a specific person or patient can be identified and that relates to physical or mental health, the provision of healthcare, or the payment for healthcare.

Conversely, despite the need to protect PHI, healthcare organizations and providers may be required to release information in certain circumstances. For example, federal law requires the reporting of certain incidents relating to the failure or malfunction of medical devices. In addition, most states require providers to report suspected cases of child abuse, elder abuse or neglect, births, deaths, gunshot wounds, and some contagious, infectious, and occupational diseases (Hastings, Luce, and Wynstra 1995). Healthcare providers may also release PHI for QI purposes, such as utilization, and peer review. PHI may also be used to facilitate third-party payment, program evaluation, and medical research.

The legal protection accorded to patients' privacy is easily traceable to the ethical concept of respect for the person, or autonomy. Indeed, in many ways HIPAA's Privacy Rule is a codification of this part of the Hippocratic Oath that doctors take when they finish their training (National Library of Medicine 2012):

> Whatever I see or hear in the lives of my patients, whether in connection with my professional practice or not, which ought not to be spoken of outside, I will keep secret, as considering all such things to be private.

Federal Law Governing Healthcare Organizations and Physicians

The Medicare Fraud and Abuse Amendments of 1977 and the Medicare and Medicaid Patient and Program Protection Act of 1987 are commonly known as *Stark I* and *Stark II*, and they include what is known as the Anti-Kickback Statute. A **kickback**, which is a form of bribery, is providing something of value to induce certain behavior on the part of the recipient. It is a form of "I'll scratch your back if you scratch mine." In general terms, a **bribe** is (Law Dictionary 2018)

> any valuable thing given or promised, or any preferment, advantage, privilege, or emolument, given or promised corruptly and against the law, as an inducement to any person acting in an official or public capacity to violate or forbear from his duty, or to improperly influence his behavior in the performance of such duty.

A kickback is slightly different because it does not necessarily involve a "person acting in an official or public capacity." Instead, it can be, and often is, a private citizen or corporate entity providing something of value in an effort to change the behavior of the recipient to do something in favor of the one providing the thing of value. In this case, the valuable thing is an offer of payment in exchange for referrals. The Stark rules also forbid organizations and providers from referring patients to themselves or to businesses in which they hold an ownership position (Hastings, Luce, and Wynstra 1995). Anti-kickback laws were created to ensure free trade and the patient's free choice of provider. In addition, the regulation of referrals is meant to prevent the creation of closed feedback loops of referrals and services that benefit the organization or providers but may not be in the best interests of the patient. Again, the sense of justice and respect for the person permeate from the core of what Stark represents: a prohibition on self-dealing to profit at the patient's expense.

Kickback
A form of bribery; the offering, giving, receiving, or soliciting of any item of value to influence the actions of another as a result of the recipient's activity to provide illicit value to the giver.

Bribe
Money or favor given or promised in order to influence the judgment or conduct of a person in a position of trust.

Hospitals, however, are required to have an organized medical staff of physicians and other licensed providers who have privileges at that hospital and who are authorized to treat patients at that facility. As we know from Stark, the hospital cannot offer certain inducements to recruit a medical staff. Conversely, hospitals cannot arbitrarily bar physicians from their hospital. Because members of the medical staff are often not employees, the hospital needs a mechanism to ensure the quality of services and care within the organization. Healthcare organizations need clear and enforceable criteria for medical staff membership that, in part, speaks to the quality of care. Usually there is a process by which a provider becomes credentialed as a member of the medical staff. Once credentialed, the physician must comply with established rules and procedures to maintain that medical staff membership.

Because lawsuits are often directed at the provider and the organization, healthcare organizations and their boards of directors need to demonstrate due diligence in allowing the privilege of practicing at their facilities. They, too, can be liable if they should have reasonably known a medical staff member was not meeting the quality standards of care required. These quality standards, however, can also be used as a bar to keep selected providers from becoming part of the medical staff. This becomes a question of antitrust law.

Even when a hospital has clear criteria for appointing and maintaining its medical staff, physicians have challenged staff membership under antitrust laws—primarily the Sherman Act, which prohibits restraint of trade. Physicians in practice groups also must be aware of antitrust activities and are prohibited from acting together to (Wenzel and Wenzel 2005)

- refuse to accept a proposed fee schedule from a payer,
- merge so all physicians within a specialty in a service area belong to one group, or
- vote to refuse hospital privileges for a new physician if that means that physician will not be able to practice in the service area.

Exhibit 10.2 provides a short-hand review of selected federal laws and their ethical roots.

Law Governing Providers and Patients

Physicians and other clinical care providers are generally under no legal obligation to accept or treat any individual. The key exception is if they have entered into a contract for care with a managed care organization, a hospital, or another such entity. In that case, the provider is obligated to provide care under the terms of the contract. However, once a provider has accepted an individual as a patient, a contract for care is implied. Once that provider–patient relationship has been established, the provider must continue to provide care and fulfill her responsibilities to the patient until the relationship is legally terminated, or she may be held liable for abandonment.

Even if the provider–patient relationship exists, the provider must obtain the patient's consent before providing medical treatment, as patients have the right to refuse treatment.

Exhibit 10.2 Selected Federal Laws and Their Ethical Roots

Selected Federal Legislation	Autonomy	Nonmaleficence	Beneficence	Justice
	Selected Tenets of Western Philosophy			
Sherman Antitrust Act of 1890 Clayton Antitrust Act of 1914 Robinson-Patman Act of 1936	X			X
EMTALA		X	X	
HIPAA	X			
Stark I and II		X		X
Americans with Disabilities Act of 1990	X			X
Civil Rights Act of 1964 Rehabilitation Act of 1973 Americans with Disabilities Act	X			X
Family Medical Leave Act of 1993	X		X	
Occupational Safety and Health Act of 1970	X	X		

Note: EMTALA = Emergency Medical Treatment and Labor Act; HIPAA = Health Insurance Portability and Accountability Act.

Informed consent
A legal document in all 50 states that constitutes an agreement for a proposed medical treatment, nontreatment, or invasive procedure. It requires physicians to disclose the benefits, risks, and alternatives to the proposed treatment, nontreatment, or procedure. It is the method by which fully informed, rational persons may be involved in choices about their healthcare.

Obtaining **informed consent** from the patient is the duty of the provider. Informed consent, as a legal matter, is an outgrowth of the ethical concept of recognizing the autonomy of each patient. At its core, it is a reflection of autonomy—respect for the person. The informed consent form is a legal document in all 50 states. It is an agreement for a proposed medical treatment or non-treatment, or for a proposed invasive procedure. It requires physicians to disclose the benefits, risks, and alternatives to the proposed treatment, non-treatment, or procedure. Put another way, "It is the method by which fully informed, rational persons may be involved in choices about their health care" (Encyclopedia of Surgery 2018).

There are two criteria for informed consent. First, the information provided to the patient must meet the standard of the "reasonable provider"—that is, the information any reasonable provider in the same specialty would disclose under the same circumstances. The second criterion is the standard of the "reasonable patient": the information any reasonable patient in the same circumstances would want and need to know to make an informed decision regarding the proposed treatment (Encyclopedia of Surgery 2018). The concept of a "reasonable patient" also includes the fact that the patient has the legal and mental capacity to give consent. A minor, or a person who is incapacitated by reason of injury or mental defect, cannot give an "informed" consent. Failure of a provider to meet both criteria may constitute grounds for liability and perhaps illegal touching in the form of battery (American Medical Association 2016).

A final topic in the area of providers and patients is one with which most people are familiar: the issue of professional liability, or malpractice. While tort and negligence are derived from the common law and not by legislative act, the entire concept of malpractice, which is but a species of negligence, finds its roots in the ethical precept of nonmaleficience: First, do no harm. Malpractice cases can arise because of alleged negligence, intentional **tort**, or breach of contract (Showalter 2017). The most common malpractice cases stem from negligence—seldom do physicians commit an intentional tort to injure a patient! Negligence has four elements that must be proven: (1) that the provider had duty of due care, (2) that the provider breached that duty, (3) that the provider's breach of duty was the direct cause of the injury, and (4) that the injury resulted in damages to the patient (Showalter 2017).

Tort
An intentional wrong that results in injury or harm. Breach of contract is a category of tort.

We live in a **litigious** society, and healthcare managers must understand professional liability and the need to be proactive in the creation and implementation of workable and effective incident-reporting systems. Any unusual or potentially problematic event, medical or interpersonal, between a provider or staff member and a patient should be reported and reviewed by the medical director, the staff member's manager, the human resource office and, as needed, by legal counsel.

Litigious
Contentious and prone to become involved in lawsuits.

Law of Healthcare Organizations and Employees

The precept of "respect for the person" is not limited to the healthcare organization's relationship to the patient. We most commonly think of it in those terms because of the potential for abuse of patients who are, by definition, vulnerable because of their physical condition. But healthcare organizations also must be respectful of the person in other categories of relationships.

Healthcare organizations are labor-intensive and often one of the largest employers in a geographic area. They also employ a range of healthcare professionals and other workers and are subject to the Fair Labor Standards Act of 1938, which ensures all employees access to a minimum wage, overtime pay, and equal pay for equal work, and places restrictions on child labor. The federal government has passed antidiscrimination laws to ensure equal employment opportunities to all qualified workers. The five primary statutes in this area are the following:

- Civil Rights Act of 1964: Bars discrimination based on race, color, religion, sex, national origin, or pregnancy
- Rehabilitation Act of 1973: Bars discrimination against persons with physical disabilities
- Age Discrimination in Employment Act of 1967: Bars discrimination against persons older than age 40
- Americans with Disabilities Act of 1990: Protects individuals with disabilities and requires employers to provide reasonable accommodations
- Family and Medical Leave Act of 1993: Requires employers with 50 or more employees to provide eligible employees up to 12 weeks per year of unpaid leave and continued health insurance coverage

In addition, healthcare facilities also fall within the purview of regulations promulgated by the US Department of Health and Human Services and may face termination, suspension, or the refusal of federal funds should they fail to comply with them (Pozgar 2016).

All employers are required to provide a safe working environment for their employees. The Occupational Safety and Health Act of 1970 was enacted to ensure safe working conditions for all Americans (Pozgar 2016). Potential exposure to blood, bodily fluids, wounds, waste matter, and the diseases that these substances can transmit make healthcare environments a safety challenge. Many healthcare professionals are involved in patient ambulation, lifting, and transport, which present possible injuries. Finally, healthcare is rife with technologies, such as radiation, magnetic fields, and gases, which may endanger employees, particularly with repeated exposure.

An employee who is injured while performing work-related activities is generally eligible for financial payment through **worker's compensation**. Employers are required to provide worker's compensation insurance as a benefit, and the law does not require proof that the injury was caused by the employer's negligence. Because worker's compensation is administered by each state, the scope of coverage varies from state to state. Healthcare managers should acquaint themselves with their state's specific worker's compensation laws and processes.

Worker's compensation
Insurance overseen by the state for employees who are injured while performing work or work-related activities.

A manager's best protection from legal action is to prevent legal problems before they occur. Well-drafted and well-implemented policies and procedures are the first step. Understanding the state and federal requirements for relationships with employees, patients, and other organizations is important. Managers should be familiar with the legal elements discussed in this chapter so they can avoid legal pitfalls.

Conclusion

This chapter has presented the foundational tenets of Western ethical thinking that inform our ethical decisions as managers as well as the core of the legal requirements applicable to healthcare providers and organizations. Respect for the person, nonmaleficence, beneficence, and justice serve as the roots of the tree from which both the limbs of ethics and law have grown. While critically important to their work, ethics are not the sole province of clinicians. Managers, too, must rigorously adhere to ethical guidelines and applicable legal requirements. It is all too easy to turn a blind eye to what appear to be insignificant matters that may not readily present themselves as ethical questions. Good managers should be constantly vigilant of actions that may present ethical dilemmas and take appropriate preventive action.

It is also important for managers to be conversant in laws applicable to healthcare organizations and providers. Understanding the key principles of the legal requirements applicable to the relationships of healthcare organizations to patients and providers; of providers to patients; and to employees and other stakeholders will enable the manager to avoid most legal pitfalls. Understanding these principles will also inform the manager of when to consult with the human resources department or the organization's attorney.

Focusing on "patient first" as a guiding rule will help keep these ethical tenets and legal requirements in mind. By following that path, we can improve healthcare for patients and enhance the treatment of all stakeholders.

Mini Case Study: HIPAA—Where Are the Boundaries?

Ruby Larusso called for an appointment with the Minnesota University Research Institute's legal counsel. She wanted to meet as soon as possible. The secretary informed her that she could come over right away, as the attorney did not have an appointment for the next hour. Ruby hurried from her office to the administration building where the attorney worked.

Ruby sat down in the attorney's office and quickly explained: "This morning, I received an angry phone call from Jake Lawson, a subject in the nutrition research project. It seems that Jake told his boss at a fast-food restaurant that he was coming to the Institute for doctors' appointments. When Jake's boss asked him directly whether he was participating in a research project or coming for medical appointments, Jake lied and answered that he was seeking medical attention. Jake called me because his boss fired him yesterday afternoon for lying to his supervisor. Jake said he was going to sue me and the hospital because I had violated HIPAA regulations regarding his privacy rights."

Ruby further explained, "Yesterday, I received a phone call from someone inquiring whether patients were ever seen at the Institute for medical appointments. I told the caller that the Institute's sole purpose was research, and that any subject who might require medical attention would be referred to the appropriate clinic department at the university. I also said we do not offer medical services to patients in the research institute. I did not disclose any information about Jake, nor did I discuss any of the current research studies with the caller. I think that caller might have been Jake's boss."

Ruby asked, "Am I in trouble? Did I violate HIPAA rules?"

Mini Case Study Questions

1. Do you think Ruby violated HIPAA rules? Why or why not?
2. What action, if any, should Ruby and the attorney take at this time?

Points to Remember

- Managerial ethics are critically important to the life of an organization. They define what is right and wrong in that organization.
- The four central tenets of ethical patient care are autonomy, nonmaleficence, beneficence, and justice.
- Care should be safe, effective, patient-centered, timely, efficient, and equitable (AHRQ 2016).
- Western philosophy is at the root of many rights and responsibilities established by law.
- The concept of patient privacy, codified in HIPAA, has its origins in the Hippocratic Oath.
- State law is an important concept for all healthcare providers; federal law is also important because of its pervasiveness and relationship to providers' funding.

Challenge Yourself

ACHE offers an ethics self-assessment designed to help you identify your ethical strengths and note areas you may want to improve. It is an exercise to help you think about where you stand on the issues. It is not designed to be shared with others or in class.

Go to the ACHE website (www.ache.org/our-story/our-commitments/ethics/ethics-self-assessment) and take the Ethics Self-Assessment you find there. Read carefully how the instrument should be used. Do the best you can, understanding that some of the questions are for people who are further along in their career. Answer those questions hypothetically—what *would* you do? What did you learn about yourself?

For Your Consideration

1. Why do you think the people in the chapter's opening case study dread being on the ethics committee? How would you feel if you were appointed to your organization's ethics committee?
2. If you were the new director of operations, what would your goal be for this first committee meeting? How would you deal with the committee members' comments?
3. Think about the list of four clinical ethical principles and then about the list of four principles for healthcare managers. Is there any overlap between the two lists? What do the two lists have in common? In what ways are they different?

References

Agency for Healthcare Research and Quality (AHRQ). 2016. "The Six Domains of Health Care Quality." Last reviewed March. www.ahrq.gov/professionals/quality-patient-safety/talkingquality/create/sixdomains.html.

American College of Healthcare Executives (ACHE). 2017a. "Ethical Issues Related to Staff Shortages." Ethical policy statement. Revised November. www.ache.org/about-ache/our-story/our-commitments/ethics/ache-code-of-ethics/ethical-issues-related-to-staff-shortages.

———. 2017b. "Impaired Healthcare Executives." Ethical policy statement. Revised November. www.ache.org/about-ache/our-story/our-commitments/ethics/ache-code-of-ethics/impaired-healthcare-executives.

———. 2016. "Health Information Confidentiality." Ethical policy statement. Revised November. www.ache.org/about-ache/our-story/our-commitments/ethics/ache-code-of-ethics/health-information-confidentiality.

American Medical Association. 2016. "AMA Code of Medical Ethics." Accessed August 8, 2018. www.ama-assn.org/delivering-care/ama-code-medical-ethics.

Andriof, J., and M. McIntosh (eds.). 2001. *Perspectives on Corporate Citizenship*. Sheffield, UK: Greenleaf Publishing.

Bayraktar, C., O. Araci, G. Karacay, and F. Calisir. 2017. "The Mediating Effect of Rewarding on the Relationship Between Employee Involvement and Job Satisfaction." *Human Factors and Ergonomics in Manufacturing & Service Industries* 27 (1): 45–52.

Birch, D. 2001. "Corporate Citizenship: Rethinking Business Beyond Corporate Social Responsibility." In *Perspectives on Corporate Citizenship*, edited by J. Andriof and M. McIntosh, 53–65. Sheffield, UK: Greenleaf Publishing.

Byrne, Z. 2005. "Fairness Reduces the Negative Effects of Organizational Politics on Turnover Intentions, Citizenship Behavior and Job Performance." *Journal of Business and Psychology* 20 (2): 175–200.

Centers for Medicare & Medicaid Services. 2012. "Emergency Medical Treatment & Labor Act (EMTALA)." Modified March 26. www.cms.hhs.gov/EMTALA.

Cropanzano, R., B. Goldman, and R. Folger 2003. "Deontic Justice: The Role of Moral Principles in Workplace Fairness." *Journal of Organizational Behavior* 24 (8): 1019–24.

Encyclopedia of Surgery. 2018. "Informed Consent." Accessed June 16. www.surgeryencyclopedia.com/Fi-La/Informed-Consent.html.

Fosmire, S. 2009. "Frequently Asked Questions About the Emergency Medical Treatment and Active Labor Act (EMTALA)." EMTALA.com. Published October 10. www.emtala.com/faq.htm.

Giganti, E. 2004. "Organization Ethics Is 'Systems Thinking.'" *Health Progress* 85 (3): 10–11.

Graham, D. 2015. "The True Face of Medicare Fraud." *The Atlantic*. Published June 19. www.theatlantic.com/national/archive/2015/06/this-is-what-government-fraud-looks-like/396317/.

Hastings, D. A., G. M. Luce, and N. A. Wynstra. 1995. *Fundamentals of Health Law*. Washington, DC: National Health Lawyers Association.

Hinckley, R. C. 2002. "28 Words to Redefine Corporate Duties: The Proposal for Corporate Citizenship." *Multinational Monitor* 23 (7): 18–20.

Houghton, J., C. Pearce, C. Manz, S. Courtright, and G. Steward. 2015. "Sharing Is Caring: Toward a Model of Proactive Caring Through Shared Leadership." *Human Resource Management Review* 25 (3): 313–27.

Hutton, B., and D. Mayer. 2010. "Corporate Social Responsibility and Corporate Excellence." In *Good Business: Exercising Effective and Ethical Leadership*, edited by J. O'Toole and D. Mayer, 94–106. New York: Routledge.

Institute of Medicine. 2001. *To Err Is Human: Building a Safer Health System*. Washington, DC: National Academies Press.

Johnson, C. E. 2018. *Meeting the Ethical Challenges of Leadership*. Thousand Oaks, CA: Sage Publications.

Joint Commission. 2013. *Comprehensive Accreditation Manual for Hospitals*. Oakbrook Terrace, IL: Joint Commission.

Kacmar, K. M., and R. A. Baron. 1999. "Organizational Politics: The State of the Field, Links to Related Processes, and an Agenda for Future Research." In *Research in Personnel and Human Resources Management*, edited by G. R. Ferris, 1–39. Greenwich, CT: JAI Press.

Law Dictionary. 2018. "What Is BRIBE?" Accessed August 3. https://thelawdictionary.org/bribe/.

Lips-Wiersma, M., and L. Morris. 2009. "Discriminating Between 'Meaningful Work' and the 'Management of Meaning.'" *Journal of Business Ethics* 88 (3): 491–511.

Lynn, J., M. A. Baily, M. Bottrell, B. Jennings, R. J. Levine, F. Davidoff, D. Casarett, J. Corrigan, E. Fox, M. K. Wynia, G. J. Agich, M. O'Kane, T. Speroff, P. Schyve, P. Batalden, S. Tunis, N. Berlinger, L. Cronenwett, J. M. Fitzmaurice, N. N. Dubler, and B. James. 2007. "The Ethics of Using Quality Improvement Methods in Health Care." *Annals of Internal Medicine* 146 (9): 666–73.

Margolis, J. D. 2001. "Responsibility in Organizational Context." *Business Ethics Quarterly* 11 (3): 431–54.

Mintzberg, H. 1983. *Power in and Around Organizations*. Englewood Cliffs, NJ: Prentice-Hall.

National Library of Medicine. 2012. "Greek Medicine: The Hippocratic Oath." Updated February 7. www.nlm.nih.gov/hmd/greek/greek_oath.html.

Ornstein, C. 2016. "New York Hospital to Pay $2.2 Million over Unauthorized Filming of 2 Patients." *New York Times*. Published April 21. www.nytimes.com/2016/04/22/nyregion/new-york-hospital-to-pay-fine-over-unauthorized-filming-of-2-patients.html.

Pozgar, G. D. 2016. *Legal Aspects of Health Care Administration*, 12th ed. San Francisco: Jossey-Bass.

Robinson, R., G. Franklin, C. Tinney, S. Crow, and S. Hartman. 2005. "Sexual Harassment in the Workplace: Guidelines for Educating Healthcare Managers." *Journal of Health and Human Services Administration* 27 (3): 501–30.

Showalter, J. S. 2017. *The Law of Healthcare Administration*, 8th ed. Chicago: Health Administration Press.

Sutton, R. I., and R. L. Kahn. 1986. "Prediction, Understanding, and Control as Antidotes to Organizational Stress." In *Handbook of Organizational Behavior*, edited by J. W. Lorsch, 272–85. Englewood Cliffs, NJ: Prentice-Hall.

Tejan, J. C. 2012. "GSK Fined over Vaccine Trials; 14 Babies Reported Dead." *Buenos Aires Herald*. Published January 3. www.buenosairesherald.com/article/88922/gsk-fined-over-vaccine-trials-14--babies-reported-dead.

Valle, M., and L. A. Witt. 2001. "The Moderating Effect of Teamwork Perceptions on the Organizational Politics–Job Satisfaction Relationship." *Journal of Social Psychology* 141 (3): 379–88.

Waddock, S., and N. Smith. 2000. "Corporate Responsibility Audits: Doing Well by Doing Good." *MIT Sloan Management Review* 41 (2): 75–83.

Wager, K. A., F. W. Lee, and J. P. Glaser. 2013. *Managing Health Care Information Systems*, 3rd ed. San Francisco: Jossey-Bass.

Warburton, J., M. Shapiro, A. Buckley, and Y. van Gellecum. 2004. "A Nice Thing to Do but Is It Critical for Business?" *Australian Journal of Social Issues* 39 (2): 117–27.

Wenzel, F. J., and J. M. Wenzel. 2005. *Fundamentals of Physician Practice Management*. Chicago: Health Administration Press.

Wiggins, C. 2000. "Healthcare Managers at Work: Be Careful Out There!" *Hospital Topics* 78 (4): 21–25.

Wiggins, C., J. Beachboard, K. Trimmer, and L. Pumphrey. 2006. "Entrepreneurial IT Governance: Electronic Medical Records in Rural Healthcare." *International Journal of Healthcare Information Systems and Informatics* 1 (4): 40–53.

Wiggins, C., and S. Y. Bowman. 2000. "Career Success and Life Satisfaction for Female and Male Healthcare Managers." *Hospital Topics* 78 (3): 5–10.

Wiggins, C., L. Hatzenbuehler, and T. Peterson 2008. "Hospital Missions and the Education of Our Future Health Care Workforce." *Journal of Allied Health* 37 (3): 132–36.

Winkler, E. C., and R. L. Gruen. 2005. "First Principles: Substantive Ethics for Healthcare Organizations." *Journal of Healthcare Management* 50 (2): 109–19.

Witt, L. A., M. C. Andrews, and K. M. Kacmar. 2000. "The Role of Participative Decision Making in the Organizational Politics–Job Satisfaction Relationship." *Human Relations* 53 (3): 341–57.

Wynia, M. K., S. R. Latham, and A. C. Kao. 1999. "Medical Professionalism in Society." *New England Journal of Medicine* 341 (21): 1612–16.

CHAPTER 11

HEALTHCARE FINANCE AND BUDGETING

Important Terms

- Activity-based budgeting
- Budget
- Charity write-off
- Contractual allowance
- Copay
- Deductible
- Direct costs
- Excess of revenue over expenses
- Expense
- Fixed costs
- Incremental budgeting
- Indirect costs
- Profit
- Revenue
- Rolling budgeting
- Statement of operations
- Variable costs
- Zero-based budgeting

Learning Objectives

After reading this chapter, you will be able to do the following:

- ➤ Discuss sources of healthcare funding
- ➤ Discuss how insurance works
- ➤ Understand the importance of public insurance programs
- ➤ Identify specific types of budgets
- ➤ Illustrate managers' use of budgets in the planning process
- ➤ Explain the use of budgets as a control mechanism

Case Study: Brian's Budget

Brian Sage is the manager of the wellness department at Hope Community Hospital, a nonprofit hospital located on the South Carolina coast. Brian likes working at Hope and is interested in introducing new wellness programs. He has just met with Tony Benton, the chief financial officer (CFO), and he agrees that Tony's directives are right on target. However, the department's programs, while beneficial to patients and the community, were over budget last year, so while Tony is looking to Brian to develop wellness programs, he should do so within the budget. Tony has asked Brian to design a bottom-up budget that includes growth for new programs, and also considers profit-making activities.

Brian hopes he is up to the job. Tony is right—his department's expenses have been exceeding revenues. As a result, Brian knows he will have to ask for additional funds to start up any new programs. Furthermore, he knows that he and his department staff need to brainstorm about programs that might generate a profit to cover the educational programs that cost the hospital money.

Brian received his undergraduate degree in health education and joined the staff of Hope five years ago. His primary activities have been to offer exercise and diet classes to patients and community members. His excellent rapport with patients and his easygoing, friendly manner fit well with Hope. People like him.

While working at the center, Brian earned his MBA online with an emphasis in health services administration. When he received the degree six months ago, he was promoted to department supervisor. The administration had full confidence in Brian's ability as supervisor and his ability to grow the wellness department as a community benefit. The population was growing along the coast, and Hope wanted to be the hospital of choice for new residents. The wellness department was designed to work with patients and members of the community. The wellness services would teach people about healthy lifestyles and market the hospital to the community.

In recent years, the cost of housing along the coast has increased dramatically. Local retirement communities (housing that caters to people older than age 55) offer financially well-off older people a beautiful, albeit expensive, place to live. As a result, the people moving into the area are those who have accumulated personal wealth and are ready to enjoy their retirement years. They also are physically active and in relatively good health, and they lead healthy lifestyles. They are careful about their diet, do not smoke cigarettes, and do not abuse alcohol or drugs. Nonetheless, as they grow older, they acquire health conditions that reflect their age.

The Hope Community Hospital has responded to this population by focusing on the development of its cardiovascular unit. Hope recently became one of the first echocardiography laboratories in the United States to be accredited by the Intersocietal Accreditation Commission for the accreditation of echocardiography. This recognition illustrates the high standards set by Hope in the detection and management of heart disease. Now, the hospital administration has established the goal of developing its wellness program to focus on their cardiovascular patients, and Brian has been given the task of proposing a budget that reflects this goal and, at the very least, generates enough revenue to cover its expenses.

Introduction

As you have seen from previous chapters, managers need to have a variety of teamwork and interpersonal skills to be effective in their work. In addition, they need to possess a variety of technical skills, one of which is budgeting. This chapter will provide a foundation for budgeting in a healthcare organization. You will learn about the various sources of revenue for healthcare organizations. In particular, you will gain an understanding of the differences between public and private insurance, and, more generally, how insurance works. You have already seen that insurance is important to the prospective patient, providing a foundation for access to healthcare. In this chapter, you will see why insurance is important to providers. In addition, you will learn to identify sources of expense and understand how revenue and expenses relate to each other.

Insurance

Before building a budget, a manager should understand the sources of revenue: what they are, how they are derived, and generally how they work. Both public and commercial health insurance are critically important sources of revenue for a healthcare organization. "Private pay" is a very small percentage of revenue, and the phrase frequently is used as a euphemism for "no pay" or "bad debt" or "charity write-off."

Insurance plans, of course, do not send providers money because they want to deliver financial support. Insurance plans pay for services rendered by the healthcare provider that are covered by the insured's policy. That provider can be a physician, a hospital, or some other kind of recognized provider. Understanding the basics of how insurance works and what some of the associated vocabulary is will help the manager in crafting a budget.

There are several kinds of insurance:

Public insurance: The most significant programs for this discussion are Medicare and Medicaid. While there are other much smaller programs, the focus here will be on these two major healthcare funding programs.

Commercial insurance: These are programs typically sponsored by employers and sometimes referred to as "employer-sponsored insurance," or ESI. Employers provide this benefit for employees and their families. Most typically, the employees share in the cost of the coverage, especially for their families. The kinds of plans vary widely.

"Exchange" insurance: These are individual policies purchased through one of the public exchanges created under the Affordable Care Act. Depending on the state, exchanges

can be federally administered, state administered, or fall under a hybrid of federal and state administration. Essentially, insurance issued through the exchanges works the same way as commercial insurance. While the federal government does not subsidize this form of health insurance, it does limit the availability of this insurance on the basis of income. Further, some individuals receive a tax credit to support their purchase of a plan through the exchange.

Private insurance: These individual policies frequently only provide coverage for catastrophic injury only, with very high deductibles and copays.

There are some nuances within each of these categories, but for the purposes of this chapter, this taxonomy is sufficient.

The Fundamentals of How Commercial Insurance Works

Health insurance is essentially a mechanism to spread the risk of illness or injury occurring from any one person to a group of people. When a person has a serious injury or illness, the costs can be so high that a single person cannot afford them. If that individual has insurance, however, the premiums paid by all members of the group, managed by the insurance company, will defray a significant percentage of the costs. Thus, employers, employees, and individuals pay a **premium** that is a contribution to a **risk pool** from which the costs associated with the insured's illness or injury will be paid. Exhibit 11.1 provides a schematic for how this works.

Exhibit 11.1 Schematic of Insurance Payments and Distributions

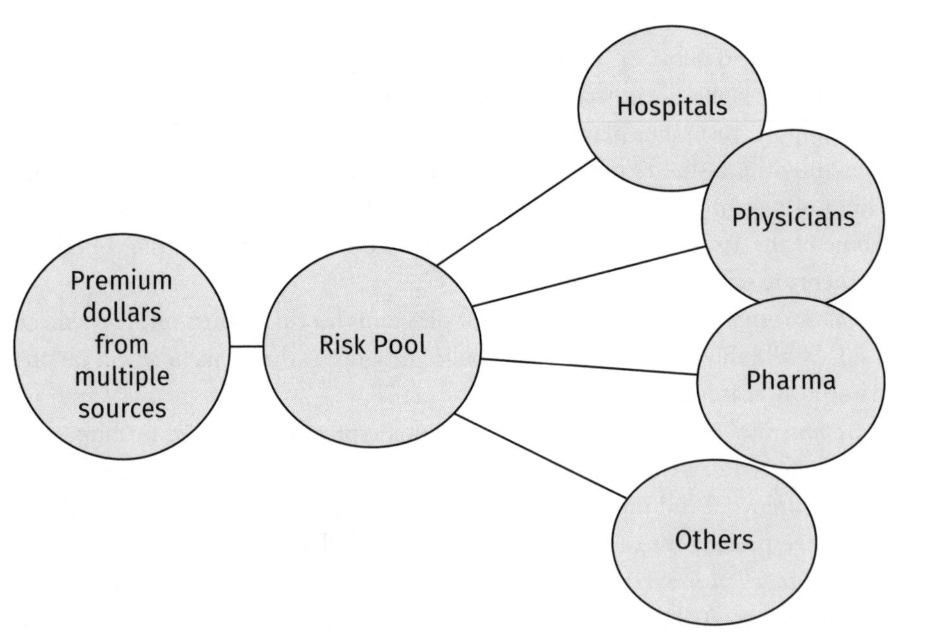

Employers, employees, and individuals pay premiums. The amount of the premium will vary by level of risk. For example, health insurance premiums for coal miners will be higher than health insurance for office workers at a university because the risk of illness befalling coal miners is much higher, compared to office workers who are not exposed to the elements associated with a coal mine.

The function of the insurance company is to assess the risk each person brings to the pool. The basic concept is that the insured expects their costs to be paid in total or in part by the funds deposited in the risk pool by others in the form of premium payments. Indeed, everyone paying premiums into the pool expects that when needed, their insurance will pay the costs associated with their healthcare. The insurance company not only collects premiums and administers payments to providers, but also sets rules about what is or is not a covered expense. In addition, the company invests premium dollars to provide an additional source of funds.

Covered services are usually the subject of a negotiation between the employer and the insurance company, and often an employee union. Because the employer is contributing to the premium payment on behalf of the employee, it has a significant influence on the final structure of the insurance coverage. In most cases, the employees are responsible for paying a portion of the cost for themselves and for their families in the form of a copayment, or **copay**, and through meeting a **deductible** limit. Increasingly, employers are shifting the costs of insurance to employees because of the upward cost spiral in recent years. This shift takes the form of higher copays, higher deductibles, and perhaps still higher deductibles for family members of the employee. Large employers sometimes offer several plans; sometimes they "self-insure" and contract with the insurance company to also administer the plan.

Copay
A fixed amount paid by the patient out of pocket, usually at the time a healthcare service is provided. The copayment is required by the insurance company as a condition of the insured receiving service.

Deductible
The aggregate amount an insured must pay before the insurance begins to pay for the insured's care. For example, a $2,000 deductible means the patient must pay $2,000 before full coverage will begin.

The insurance policy is a form of a contract between the insurance company and the insured, created by the employer for the benefit of the employee. The employer and employee both make payments—premiums—as their obligation under the contract in exchange for the assurance that, when needed, the insurance company will pay providers on behalf of the insured. Insurance plans vary as to what is covered, or how much will be provided, but that is the structure of the contract negotiated by the employer.

The Fundamentals of How Public Insurance Works

Many of the same private insurance principles apply to public insurance. There are, however, several differences. And among the public insurance programs there are also differences. In chapter 2, you read about Medicare and Medicaid. While these each have different sources of funding, the concept of risk pools for the programs is approximately the same.

Medicare

There are several parts of Medicare. For the sake of brevity, and to stay within the scope of this book, the focus here will be on Parts A and B. Part A Medicare covers hospitalization only. Payroll taxes levied on both employees and employers by the federal government provide the funding for Part A. It is for everyone older than age 65. Whether retired or not, and whether an individual wants coverage or not, enrollment in Medicare Part A is mandatory for everyone 65 and older. The tax revenues paid by employers and employees go into the Medicare Trust Fund, which then pays providers for services covered by Part A.

Part B of Medicare is for ambulatory services such as physician office visits. This is funded much like traditional insurance in which the beneficiary pays a premium. Part B is *not* mandatory, but most people enroll in Part B when they retire. The premiums paid by the retiree are subsidized by appropriations from the federal government. Those funds go into a separate part of the Medicare Trust Fund to pay providers for services covered by Part B.

So, for Medicare Parts A and B, special tax revenues (the payroll tax for Medicare Part A), general fund revenues (the federal subsidy for Part B), and premiums paid by enrollees (for Part B) all fund a risk pool from which providers are paid for covered services, just like private insurance.

Medicare has two other parts, Part C and Part D, which deserve mention but are less important here. Part C is a managed care benefit that combines Parts A and B for those who opt for this plan. Part D is a prescription drug benefit, funded by a mix of premiums and general fund allocations, that covers a portion of the prescription drug costs a beneficiary may incur.

Medicaid

Medicaid is somewhat different because it is an entitlement program intended for people whose income falls below certain levels. The program is also different because it is jointly funded by the federal government and the states; the individual states administer the program subject to broad policy parameters set out by the federal government. There is no "trust fund" per se. The program is limited by appropriations of money from both the federal government and the respective state government. Thus, when state governments bow to fiscal pressure they sometimes reduce how much providers are paid or reduce the number of eligible beneficiaries to keep expenditures within limits. To some degree, individual eligibility, services covered, and amounts paid to providers vary from state to state. Obviously, this is fraught with political controversy, but the point here is that this program is a bit different from the risk pool concept associated with conventional insurance.

The Importance of Insurance to Providers

As discussed elsewhere in the book, insurance is important to provide a foundation permitting patients to have access to health insurance. In this chapter, the focus is more about how and why insurance is important to the providers. Insurance, more than any other source, provides the revenue used by healthcare providers to keep their businesses operating.

Budgeting Basics

As Brian develops his **budget**, he will keep in mind the following five points:

Budget
A statement that indicates financial administration for a set period of time. This is basically a guide to the organization's priorities.

1. *The organizational purpose:* What is the mission of the organization? Hope's mission is to consistently deliver compassionate, leading-edge healthcare to the people of coastal South Carolina. The wellness department's mission is to provide the latest in health news and information, along with programs, community health events, and a fully equipped health and fitness center to promote healthy lifestyles in the community. Brian, with input from his staff, needs to determine what activities they want to support financially and how well these activities fit with the missions of the organization and the department.
2. *Organizational goals:* What are the future-directed tasks to be completed? Brian has been told that his goal is to develop the wellness department to focus on the cardiovascular population. New budget line items should relate directly to this organizational goal.
3. *When the organization wants the goals to be accomplished:* What is the timeline? Brian is developing the budget for the upcoming year.
4. *Where the organization wants the staff to focus its time and energy:* What is the priority ranking of the goals? Staff input regarding priority of services would help Brian determine what cash outlays he should request in the budget.
5. *How well the manager accomplishes items 1 through 4 and stays within the budget.*

Managers, however, can only do the who, what, where, when, and how if they know what they can and cannot afford to do. An understanding of their **revenues** and **expenses** allows managers to help their employees meet organizational goals and fulfill the organization's mission. Knowledge of budgets—what they are, what they are used for, and how to develop and defend them—is key for healthcare managers. If managers are well informed about the cost of running a department and they know what is being asked of their department, they are better able to deliver a plan of action that responds to the who, what, when, where, and how.

Revenue
Income produced from providing goods or services.

Expense
Costs incurred by a unit's actions (associated with services provided) or overhead costs not directly related to generating revenue.

In the process of budgeting, it is essential to have a clear understanding of what the revenues will be before accepting the obligation to incur any particular expense. An administrator once said to his boss, "I have the expenses all figured out, now I need to come up with the revenue." This approach is exactly 180 degrees wrong; completely backward. It is critical to have an understanding of revenue first so the administrator will know what funds are available to pay for the planned expenditures. The caveat is that, like expenses, the revenue figure is the product of forecasting.

HOW TO GENERATE REVENUE

A healthcare organization's revenue depends on how many people are served and what they (or their insurance company) will pay for that service. In healthcare, there are multiple kinds of services, so an administrator must understand these points in terms of every kind of service to be provided. Then, using that information, the administrator can begin to project the revenue.

For example, if a department serves 1,000 people who use service "x" at a cost of $100 per unit of service, and 450 people who use service "y" at a cost of $150 per unit of service, then the projected revenue for this department will be (1,000 × $100) + (450 × $150) = $167,500.

However, it is important to understand the differential in service payments because payments may vary among insurance companies for the same service. Consider another example: Of a group of 1,000 people using service "x," 400 are covered by Sasnak Insurance, which pays $100 for that service, while 600 are covered by Aksarben Insurance, which only pays $75. Another group of 450 people uses service "y"; 300 of them are covered by Sasnak Insurance, which will pay $150 for the service, while the other 150 have Aksarben Insurance, which will only pay $100. So, what are the revenues for this department?

(400 × $100) + (600 × $75) + (300 × $150) + (150 × $100)
= $40,000 + $45,000 + $45,000 + $15,000
= $145,000

This is $22,500 less than the $167,500 in our earlier projection—a big difference—and it underscores the importance of knowing payment comes from multiple sources. Further, understanding that different payers will pay different amounts for the same or similar services, Brian will be able to forecast revenues much more accurately.

Brian needs to develop an annual operations budget that includes (1) anticipated revenue from future services and (2) expenses that reflect the activities necessary to provide those services. His budget is a written plan expressed in dollars that projects revenue (dollar amount earned from services provided) and expenses (resources needed to provide the services) for the upcoming year. Since Brian is responsible for adhering to the budget, he plays a significant role in its preparation and monitoring. Exhibit 11.2 illustrates the wellness department's operating budget from the previous year, which does not include the cardiovascular directive.

Note that, even though it is not included in this chapter, any budget would have supporting documentation behind it. For example, the revenue figures would each have a document describing the source of the revenue (payer), the amount, and the units of service

Exhibit 11.2
Wellness Department Operating Budget, 2018–2019

I. Revenue and Income	
Inpatient Charges	$425,000
Outpatient Charges	150,000
Fitness Center Dues	25,000
Continuing Education Conference	12,000
Community Education Programs	-22,000
Foundation Monies (Donations and Gifts)	12,500
Total Revenue	**$602,500**
II. Expenses	
Direct Expenses	
Salaries	$400,000
Honorarium for Continuing Education Conference	500
Equipment for Fitness Center	4,500
Materials and Supplies	62,000
Equipment Service Contracts	1,600
Advertising/Public Relations	600
Total Direct Expenses	**$469,200**
Indirect Expenses	
Employee Benefits (23%)	92,000
Administration (Allocated 2%)	28,000
Equipment Depreciation	1,200
Equipment Maintenance and Repairs	7,500
Custodial (Allocated 3%)	15,000
Total Indirect Expenses	**$143,700**
Excess of Revenues over Expenses	***($ 10,400)***

required to reach that budget goal. The services provided by the department for health education and wellness did not generate enough revenue to cover expenses (the department spent $10,400 more than it earned). Fortunately for Brian, the department's mission is defined as a community benefit and, thus, his department does not need to generate a **profit**. However, Brian should determine how to at least meet his expenses and, if possible, to generate an **excess of revenues over expenses** (i.e., make a profit).

Profit
In a for-profit organization, total income or cash flow minus expenditures.

Excess of revenue over expenses
In a nonprofit organization, the remaining cash after revenues minus expenses.

THE DIFFERENCES BETWEEN FOR-PROFIT AND NOT-FOR-PROFIT HOSPITALS

As you learned in chapter 1, hospitals began as charitable institutions to serve the community's poorest residents. Indeed, many churches organized and operated hospitals as part of their spiritual missions. The Catholic Church was particularly active in starting hospitals, as was the Methodist Church along with other denominations. Over time, hospitals not aligned with a church came into existence as charitable organizations with missions to serve the community. In the time when hospitals were just beginning—before the germ theory of medicine became an accepted fact—people of means received care in their homes. With the development of germ theory and the advancing science of medicine, hospitals transformed into healthcare providers, though they remained charitable organizations. Community leaders often served as both donors and stewards of these organizations that served the less well-to-do.

In short, hospitals became religious-affiliated or community-based institutions organized around missions focused on providing service to the community. The concept of operating "for profit" was not a part of the ethos: Hospitals were committed to providing health services as their primary mission, regardless of whether they made money. To state the obvious, however, "no margin, no mission." In other words, community hospitals had to make enough money to support their mission, but when they generated revenue in excess of expenses, the excess was reinvested into the organization, permitting it to continue and to expand its services. This is the definition of a not-for-profit hospital: The hospital uses revenues exceeding expenses to reinvest in the physical plant or to enhance services, thereby further advancing its mission.

In the last third of the twentieth century, entrepreneurs conceived of a way to make hospitals profitable for themselves and their investors. Corporations sold stock to generate capital to acquire hospitals. Owning several hospitals under one umbrella provided an opportunity. By consolidating the purchase and management of goods required to operate the business, and by consolidating functions such as human resources and payroll, chains of hospitals could create economies of scale that had the effect of reducing costs, thereby increasing the amount of revenue in excess of expenses. That revenue would be used for future investment to expand the business and also be dedicated as earnings for shareholders. This is "for profit." Hospital revenue in excess of expenses can reward investors through distribution of dividends and increases in stock value. In addition, it can be used to expand the business by acquiring more hospitals.

There are two primary differences between "not-for-profit" and "for-profit" hospitals. First, not-for-profit hospitals are tax exempt, which means they do not pay federal or state income taxes, nor local property taxes. In exchange for those exemptions, not-for-profit hospitals must demonstrate a community benefit, which is to say they must demonstrate they provide a positive value to the community in the form of charity care, community education, and support for other community service agencies. (Chapter 7 contains additional explanation of community benefits.) The second difference, and this one is more nuanced, is that not-for-profit hospitals reinvest revenue in excess of expenses in the services provided by

THE DIFFERENCES BETWEEN FOR-PROFIT AND NOT-FOR-PROFIT HOSPITALS *(CONTINUED)*

the organization. This can sometimes be difficult to distinguish from the habits of for-profit hospitals, which use profits to grow their businesses.

For-profit hospitals pay taxes—federal and state income taxes as well as local property taxes. As a result, they are under no legal obligation to provide community benefits such as community health education or support for community social service agencies. However, while they are not legally required to provide charity care, for-profit hospitals do provide some as a practical matter. The calculation of *how much* not-for-profit hospitals and for-profit hospitals actually spend on charity care is extraordinarily difficult because of varying accounting and business practices, but it seems the amount is roughly even (Bannow 2018).

The second difference is how revenues in excess of expenses—profits—are used by for-profit hospitals. For-profit hospitals are under no obligation to reinvest in the improvement of the organization. They can use all the profit to reward the shareholders. As a practical matter, however, for-profit hospitals do reinvest in the business to retain a competitive edge by improving the care they provide to their patients.

Examples of not-for-profit healthcare systems include Ascension, Cleveland Clinic, Mayo Clinic, Intermountain Healthcare, and literally thousands of others. Examples of for-profit healthcare organizations include HCA, Tenet Corporation, and Community Health Systems, along with many others. Owing to the history of hospital development, there are many more not-for-profit hospitals and health systems than for-profit counterparts. In 2018, 59 percent of the country's nearly 5,000 hospitals were not-for-profit; 21 percent were for-profit; and 20 percent were owned by state and local governments (American Hospital Association 2018).

The distinction between for-profit and not-for-profit hospitals is important for several reasons. First, there is a public policy debate about the level of community benefit provided by not-for-profit hospitals. The question is whether the community benefit justifies the favored tax status enjoyed by not-for-profit hospitals. The second reason for the importance in the distinction is also controversial: Are for-profit hospitals as committed to serving the community as their not-for-profit counterparts, or does that emphasis on service decline with the need to provide value to the shareholders? Finally, the remaining important distinction between the two types of hospitals is in the accounting mechanisms they use. Not-for-profit hospitals use a fund accounting system that identifies revenues and expenses associated with specific activities, while for-profit hospitals use a general ledger that reflects the overall business activity (Masters 2018). The key difference is that fund accounting focuses on accountability. This means that not-for-profit entities deal with funds that are restricted for a particular use. This enhances accountability on the activity associated with the fund: If it exceeds its resources, then a conscious decision to cross-subsidize the loss must come from a higher authority such as the board of trustees or its executive committee. For-profit entities have a single ledger that includes all the accounts for recording financial transactions, creating a greater emphasis on the single bottom line.

Statement of operations
A statement that shows the revenues, expenses, and net income of an organization.

Contractual allowance
The amount a provider discounts from the cost of service in exchange for treating a higher volume of patients.

Charity write-off
The cost of providing service to people who cannot pay, requiring the provider to take a financial loss.

Incremental budgeting
Creating a financial plan that is increased or decreased according to previous expenditures for a set period of time.

Zero-based budgeting
Creating a financial plan for a set period of time that requires each budget item to be justified according to the unit's goals.

Rolling budgeting
A financial plan that is reviewed and updated on a regular, ongoing basis, such as every month or quarter, to reflect recent activities.

As he prepares the budget, Brian should take into account factors that may affect demand for the wellness center's services. The growth of the retirement community along the beach area leads to an expected increase in demand for wellness programs for active seniors. Brian should remain realistic and project revenues and costs that are practical and a good fit with the organization as a whole. At the same time, he needs the wellness center to be ready to capture additional revenues (and incur additional costs) because of increased demand in the community.

He also should consider Hope's current economic status by referring to its **statement of operations** (see exhibit 11.3). Overall, the statement of operations indicates that Hope's growth reflects the population growth along the coast and that Hope is in a good position to develop new projects that meet its mission to the community. Its patient revenue growth is a reflection of its commitment to the cardiovascular center initiative and a positive response from the community. From 2015 to 2017, net patient service revenue (gross patient service revenue minus **contractual allowances** minus **charity write-offs**) and premium revenue earned from managed care prepaid contracts steadily increased because of service expansion. Other revenue (gift shop, cafeteria) and net assets (donor release of a restricted gift to unrestricted in operations) have increased because of the increase in patient volume and visitors and successful foundation efforts to generate more contributions. Expenses increased as well to respond to the growth initiative.

The Budgeting Process

Organizations typically use one of four different forms of budgeting for planning and control: incremental, rolling, activity-based, and zero-based. If Brian were to employ **incremental budgeting**, he would examine last year's operations budget and add or subtract a percentage, based on expenditures. Since he has been given the new growth directive, he would estimate what percentage budget increase the department would need to fulfill the organizational goal. An advantage to incremental budgeting is that it is time-efficient; however, it does not allow for a more in-depth evaluation of costs incurred and revenue sources.

Zero-based budgeting refers to building the department's budget starting from $0.00. Unlike with incremental budgeting, the manager does not refer to last year's budget. Rather, the process requires each budget item to be justified. If Brian were to use zero-based budgeting, he would, in essence, "forget" about last year and provide a detail of all the resources needed to accomplish the goals fully in the upcoming year.

Rolling budgeting refers to the development of an annual budget that is reviewed on a specified time frame (monthly or quarterly) and updated. A benefit of this practice is that the budget is continually revised to reflect recent activities; however, it is time-consuming. If Brian were to employ rolling budgeting for his department, he would estimate revenue and costs for the upcoming year and reevaluate the budget at monthly or quarterly intervals.

Exhibit 11.3
Hope Community Hospital Statement of Operations (in thousands)

Unrestricted Revenues, Gains, and Other Support			
	2019	**2018**	**2017**
Revenue			
Net patient service revenue	$ 84,250	$77,650	$65,750
Premium revenue	$ 9,800	$ 8,700	$ 7,500
Other revenue	$ 8,700	$ 8,078	$ 6,700
Net assets released from restrictions for operations	$ 300	$ 0	$ 0
Total Operating Revenues	**$103,050**	**$94,428**	**$79,950**
Expenses			
Salaries and benefits	$ 54,490	$49,750	$42,750
Medical supplies and drugs	$ 28,770	$25,650	$19,350
Insurance*	$ 8,300	$ 8,150	$ 7,950
Depreciation	$ 4,600	$ 4,430	$ 3,750
Interest	$ 1,850	$ 1,900	$ 1,825
Provision for bad debts	$ 1,600	$ 1,400	$ 1,100
Other expenses	$ 2,750	$ 2,500	$ 2,450
Total Operating Expenses	**$102,360**	**$93,780**	**$79,175**
Net operating income	$ 690	$ 648	$ 775
*Investment (nonoperating) income***	$ 3,800	$ 3,400	$ 2,500
Total All Revenues	**$106,850**	**$97,828**	**$84,450**
Excess of Revenues over Expenses	***$ 4,490***	***$ 4,048***	***$ 3,275***

*Hospitals need insurance, too! This represents payment of premiums for things like malpractice insurance, insurance against property loss due to catastrophe, and health insurance for employees.
**Investment income is considered separately because it is not income derived from operation of the hospital. It is from dividends and interest paid on investments. The separation permits the user to see actual net income separately from the operation of the enterprise to determine its profitability.

Activity-based budgeting
Creating a financial plan that focuses on the manager's allocating costs to each activity performed on behalf of the unit's responsibilities (e.g., patient care).

Activity-based budgeting involves allocating costs to each activity performed on behalf of the patient. Thus, instead of a budget that has a line item based on the department's costs (e.g., salaries, supplies), the budget item reflects the performance inputs and the costs associated with each activity (e.g., costs incurred to deliver the cardio exercise classes). Thus, Brian could classify activities as primary or secondary and those that added value to the patient and community and those that did not. Then, he could determine on which activities the department should spend more or fewer resources.

Defining Revenues and Costs

The focus of financial controls for managers in for-profit healthcare organizations is to generate profits for the stockholders or owners. In nonprofit healthcare organizations, the focus is to generate profits for reinvestment in the organization. Both goals rely on the management of revenues and expenses. As Hope is a nonprofit, Brian's budgeting process is not focused on growing profits; nonetheless, Hope must generate revenues and control costs to remain in business. The wellness department delivers community benefits through health-centered educational programs and fitness center activities. Hence, operating revenues are generated by inpatient and outpatient services, program fees, and fitness center dues. Other revenues include donations and the interest earned on donated funds.

Fixed costs
Expenses that will be incurred regardless of volume of activity or usage.

Variable costs
Expenses that will change as the volume of activity changes.

Direct costs
Expenses associated with a specific activity provided by a unit.

Indirect costs
Expenses that are not associated with a specific unit activity.

Brian also knows it is important to classify the costs of doing business so he can understand where costs may be controlled and where he can generate additional revenue. Costs may be fixed or variable, direct or indirect. A **fixed cost** is a cost that does not vary according to use, such as number of patients. For example, Brian and his staff are considering hiring exercise trainers to lead new cardio exercise classes at the fitness center. It does not matter whether 10 people or 50 people attend the cardio class; Brian needs to allocate resources to pay for the trainer. Therefore, the trainer's salary for the class is a fixed cost. Brian also plans to give each person attending the cardio exercise class a personal package of heart-healthy items. How many packages he puts together depends on the number of people in the class. Hence, the personal heart-healthy package cost is a **variable cost**: It will change as the volume changes. If Brian has 12 people in the class, he needs to purchase supplies for 12 packages. If he has 20 people in the class, he needs to purchase supplies for 20 packages.

Direct costs are those associated with an activity. **Indirect costs** are those not associated with a specific activity. To determine whether costs are direct or indirect, Brian may ask, "If this specific something did not exist, would the cost for leasing the current facility that would house the program still exist?" For example, "If this exercise class did not exist, would the costs for running the wellness department still exist?" If the answer is "yes," it is an indirect cost. If the answer is "no," the cost is direct. To illustrate, the cost of exercise mats is a direct, variable cost to the wellness department. The number of mats needed varies according to the number of center attendees, and the cost would not exist if the exercise center did not exist. To further illustrate, indirect costs (e.g., electricity needed for lights and air-conditioning) are associated with the hospital as a whole and may be prorated by time allocated to specific departments. They are costs that cannot be specifically attributed to an individual project. See exhibit 11.4 for an illustration of costs that pertain to the wellness department.

Classifying costs associated with the wellness department allows Brian not only to know what is being spent and why, but also to explain and justify his budget. If he budgets for new equipment, he can explain why his department needs that particular piece of equipment to fulfill the goal. Projected usage and the acquisition of items may enhance patient care and attract new patients to the hospital. It is particularly important that Brian have a very clear understanding of his fixed costs, both indirect and direct. These numbers will

Exhibit 11.4
Cost Classifications for Hope Wellness Department

	Direct	Indirect
Fixed	Brian's salary	Custodial contracted services (allocated portion)
Variable	Heart-healthy packages	Repairs of equipment in fitness center

help set a minimum baseline for financial performance because these are costs that must be covered regardless of the volume of services his unit generates.

Also, if Brian classifies costs as direct and fixed, indirect and fixed, direct and variable, and indirect and variable, he gains an understanding of the cost allocations to his department, which helps him determine whether these allocations are fair. Brian can determine fairness of the allocated costs only if he is aware of the actual versus allocated costs to the department. Last year, his department was responsible for 3 percent of Hope's custodial care expenses. As he plans for the upcoming year's growth initiative, he may find that his department needs to assume responsibility for a larger allocation of the custodial care costs. This should be reflected in the proposed budget.

With the budget information referenced here and the program planning created by Brian and his staff, he will be well equipped to prepare, propose, and defend the budget for the wellness department. He will become knowledgeable about the cost of running a department; he will know what is being asked of the wellness department employees; and his department will be better able to deliver a plan of action that responds to the who, what, when, where, and how for Hope Community Hospital.

Conclusion

This chapter offered students a rudimentary understanding of how healthcare organizations are financed and how they budget—that is, plan—to manage their resources. The budget represents a statement of how the organization will achieve its mission. The distribution of resources reflects an organization's important priorities. Understanding both sides of the equation—revenues and expenses—is essential to producing an effective budget. Thus, because insurance payments are a frequent source of revenue, it is helpful to understand how various types of insurance work. Likewise, understanding how much it costs to deliver a service is indispensable to crafting and following a budget.

Mini Case Study: Developing the Budget for the Dialysis Center

Gabe Richards, a dialysis center unit supervisor, reviewed his previous two years of budgeting for the center. He noted budgeted and actual expenses. Then he subtracted the difference. In some areas, he had budgeted more than he had spent. In other areas, he had budgeted less. Look at Gabe's notes in exhibit 11.5. As he prepares the budget for the upcoming fiscal year, what factors should he consider?

EXHIBIT 11.5
Budget Expenses for Dialysis Unit Staff Operations (Physicians Not Included)—Gabe's Notes

Previous Year					
	Salaries	*Professional Development*	*Materials and Supplies*	*Equipment Expensed*	*Total*
Spent	$1,233,041.57	$ 34,446.10	$241,001.66	$21,246.66	$1,529,735.99
Budgeted	$1,246,870.00	$ 66,528.00	$235,000.00	$21,000.00	$1,569,398.00
Difference	$ (13,828.43)	$(32,081.90)	$ 6,001.66	$ 246.66	$ (39,662.01)

Current Year					
	Salaries	*Professional Development*	*Materials and Supplies*	*Equipment Expensed*	*Total*
Spent	$1,425,052.20	$58,800.00	$250,000.00	$23,000.00	$1,756,852.20
Budgeted	$1,534,548.00	$68,400.00	$248,000.00	$22,500.00	$1,873,448.00
Difference	$ (109,495.80)	$ (9,600.00)	$ 2,000.00	$ 500.00	$ (116,595.80)

Projected Year					
	Salaries	*Professional Development*	*Materials and Supplies*	*Equipment Expensed*	*Total*
Spent					
Budgeted					

Gabe had anticipated being able to operate fully staffed for the current year; however, the dialysis center was understaffed. How is this reflected in the budget?

Mini Case Study Questions

1. Considering what has happened in the past two years and knowing that the goal is to have the center fully staffed, fill in the budget numbers for salaries, professional development, material and supplies, and equipment for the projected year.
2. What increase, if any, would you propose for the center?
3. Why did you propose what you proposed?
4. Do you think you could defend your budget effectively?

Points to Remember

- Understanding sources of revenue is the foundation of effective budgeting.
- Different payers may very well pay different amounts for the same service.
- Budgets should reflect the mission of the organization.

- Direct costs are costs directly associated with the activity presented in the budget; indirect costs are those that would need to be paid whether the activity existed or not, usually prorated across multiple departments in an organization, such as air-conditioning for the facility.
- Variable costs are those costs that change because of expenses related to the activity being presented in the budget; fixed costs are those that are not sensitive to the volume of activity in the program.

Challenge Yourself

1. With reference to the budget presented in exhibit 11.2, construct an incremental budget for the wellness center. What percentage increase/decrease did you select? Defend your choice. Now, with reference to your budget, construct a rolling budget. What are the advantages of using an incremental budget for planning? What are the advantages of using a rolling budget?
2. Offer three examples of direct and indirect costs in a healthcare facility. Why is it important to differentiate between the two?
3. Refer to the following list and identify whether the cost is fixed or variable. If you were trying to contain costs, which set of costs would you try to reduce first? Why?
   - Costs of tongue depressors
   - Costs of occupational therapists' salaries
   - Costs of contracted per patient occupational therapists' salaries
   - Costs of rent for the wellness center's exercise site

For Your Consideration

1. Research what percentage of the average hospital budget is funded by Medicare and by Medicaid. What are these figures? Why are they important?
2. Find an example of a healthcare organization's budget. Get the mission statement for that same organization. How does the budget support the mission statement?

References

American Hospital Association (AHA). 2018. *AHA Hospital Statistics: 2018*. Chicago: AHA.

Bannow, T. 2018. "Charity Care Spending Flat Among Top Hospitals." *Modern Healthcare*. Published January 6. www.modernhealthcare.com/article/20180106/NEWS/180109941.

Masters, T. 2018. "The Major Accounting Differences Between Profit and Not-for-Profit Organizations." Published June 27. https://smallbusiness.chron.com/major-accounting-differences-between-profit-non-profit-organizations-26257.html.

CHAPTER 12

HUMAN RESOURCE MANAGEMENT

Important Terms

- Age Discrimination in Employment Act, 1967
- Americans with Disabilities Act, 1990
- Civil Rights Act, 1991
- Civil Rights Act, Title VII, 1964
- Discrimination
- Equal Employment Opportunity Act, 1972
- Equal Employment Opportunity Commission (EEOC)
- Human resource management
- Job description
- Occupational Safety and Health Act, 1970
- Organizational fit
- Performance evaluation
- Pregnancy Discrimination Act, 1978
- Retention
- Sexual harassment
- Termination
- The Joint Commission
- 360 evaluation
- Uniformed Services Employment and Reemployment Rights Act, 1994

Learning Objectives

After reading this chapter, you will be able to do the following:

➤ Define basic principles of federal laws regarding human resources

➤ Describe employee rights and responsibilities in the healthcare environment

➤ Describe the issue of sexual harassment in the workplace

➤ Evaluate the significance of organizational fit in hiring

- Explain the job description role in the hiring process
- Identify retention and discuss current retention issues in healthcare organizations
- Describe the performance evaluation process
- Explain the HR termination process and consider key factors involved in the process

Case Study: Professional Behavior

Dr. Dorothy Daunt, chair of Medical University's biology department, had just met with Roberta Smith, who was studying to become a physical therapist. Roberta had earned her bachelor's in health services management and knew the courses would help her attain her career goals of opening a clinic and employing speech therapists, occupational therapists, and physical therapists to provide therapy. Roberta's goal was not only to provide the best-quality care that rehabilitative services had to offer, but also to recharge the patients' minds and spirit. She was planning to name the clinic "Full Motion Innovations," and she was working hard to make certain her dream could be a reality.

In her undergraduate healthcare management and healthcare law and ethics classes, she had been introduced to laws and ethical principles pertaining to students' and employees' rights and responsibilities. From these teachings she knew she needed to report what had been happening in one of her classes, so she had made the appointment with Dr. Daunt.

More than 12,000 students, all preparing for careers in medicine, attend the university, and all are required to take Dr. Charles Fox's course, Cell Biology. The students are studying to become physical therapists, occupational therapists, radiology technologists, physicians, nurses, pharmacists, and other professionals within the medical field. Hence, Roberta was a student in Dr. Fox's class.

Dr. Fox shows more than 200 cell slides per class, and the students need to remember each one. Dr. Fox slips in an X-rated slide—always a nude woman in a suggestive, sexual pose—before he shows "important" slides.

Roberta had already voiced objections to this practice. She spoke to the professor and requested he use different surprise slides. She recommended using pictures of babies or people skiing on snowy slopes or impressive sunset panoramas. However, Dr. Fox defended his practice by saying the nude pictures work. "They get the students' attention, and the students will remember what a real cancer slide looks like."

During the meeting with Dr. Daunt, Roberta explained that she found the pictures of nude women offensive and intimidating. "How would you like to be trying to memorize what a cancer cell looks like when the professor pops in a slide like that? I sometimes get a stomachache just thinking about having to come to class." She asked Dr. Daunt to stop Dr. Fox from showing the nude slides in class.

Dr. Daunt promised Roberta she would follow up. After Roberta left the office, Dr. Daunt called the university's human resources (HR) and legal departments. She wanted to review university policy regarding such behavior before she spoke with Dr. Fox. She was concerned the professor might be in violation of sexual harassment laws. Last, she pulled Dr. Fox's file and noted that his annual reviews were positive. He had been in her department for two years, and she knew him to have an excellent publication record. His research area was pancreatic cancer and pain management, and his work was nationally recognized. His service work to the cancer community was exemplary. She knew little about his teaching, but had heard comments that some students did not like him. The phone rang for her conference call with Legal and HR. As she picked up the receiver, she wondered why some intelligent people showed little sense. She knew that showing nude pictures in class was not right. How had Medical University gotten stuck with this guy?

Introduction

In chapter 10, we discussed ethics and laws concerning respect for people as they work in healthcare organizations. Some of the laws presented in chapter 10 are repeated here as we discuss employee rights and responsibilities in the healthcare workplace, focusing on the role of managers as they hire and supervise staff, and create opportunities for their employees' professional development. The purpose of this book is not to provide comprehensive human resource management information; instead, it is to provide information so that you—as a future healthcare manager—have a working understanding of your professional responsibilities when you participate in the hiring process and supervision.

To accomplish this, the chapter is divided into four sections. First, we discuss employee rights and responsibilities. Second, we revisit a subject introduced in chapter 6 regarding sexual harassment in the workplace. Third, we introduce the importance of hiring candidates who are the best fit for the organization, because it is just as critical to hire a person who will perform well in the specific department as it is to hire someone qualified and competent. Last, we discuss retention and performance appraisals as we examine what managers should focus on to keep their excellent hires working in the department.

Rights and Responsibilities of Healthcare Organizations and Employees

Human resource management
The management of activities related to healthcare employees.

Healthcare is a business, and like every other business it needs good management to keep it running smoothly, especially when it comes to **human resource management**—the management of activities related to healthcare employees. Good management creates an environment that is conducive to employees doing their work well. As in any other business, healthcare organizations must comply with federal and state laws regarding employees' rights and responsibilities. For example, the code of ethics of the American College of Healthcare Executives (ACHE 2017) serves as the standard of conduct for healthcare managers. Among its directives, it advises managers to "comply with all laws and regulations pertaining to healthcare management in the jurisdictions in which the healthcare executive is located or conducts professional activities."

Laws pertaining to employee rights include equal opportunity, which are in sync with the ACHE code pertaining to executives' responsibilities to their employees. According to ACHE (2017), healthcare executives' responsibilities include the following:

A. Creating a work environment that promotes ethical conduct;
B. Providing a work environment that encourages a free expression of ethical concerns and provides mechanisms for discussing and addressing such concerns;
C. Promoting a healthy work environment, which includes freedom from harassment, sexual and other, and coercion of any kind, especially to perform illegal or unethical acts;
D. Promoting a culture of inclusivity that seeks to prevent discrimination on the basis of race, ethnicity, religion, gender, sexual orientation, age or disability;
E. Providing a work environment that promotes the proper use of employees' knowledge and skills; and
F. Providing a safe and healthy work environment.

Promoting a culture of inclusivity that seeks to prevent **discrimination** on the basis of race, ethnicity, religion, gender, sexual orientation, age, or disability means employees have the legal right *not* to be discriminated against on the basis of any non-job-related factor just listed. For example, in adherence to the Pregnancy Discrimination Act of 1978, if an employee is expecting or has just delivered a baby, the organization must keep her position open the same amount of time it would have for an employee who was on leave because of illness. Consider the case of *Byrd v. Lakeshore Hospital* (1994). Miranda Byrd worked as a receptionist at Lakeshore Hospital, and when she was pregnant she used her earned sick time for pregnancy-related illnesses. Lakeshore terminated her position and explained she was let go because her job performance had been unsatisfactory. The court ruled that Lakeshore unlawfully discriminated because it terminated Byrd for taking pregnancy-related sick leave while affording sick leave to non-pregnant, temporarily disabled workers (*Byrd v. Lakeshore Hosp.*, 30 F.3d 1380, 1383 [11th Cir. 1994]).

Discrimination
Prejudice or unjust treatment of people based on group characteristics rather than individual merit.

Equal opportunity also applies to race. In 2013, Hurley Medical Center in Michigan settled a case with the **Equal Employment Opportunity Commission (EEOC)** because it complied with parents who requested their infant not be cared for by an African-American nurse. Assignment of employees based on customer racial preferences violates Title VII of

Equal Employment Opportunity Commission (EEOC)
The US government agency that enforces federal employment discrimination laws.

the Civil Rights Act of 1964 (EEOC 2013). As part of the settlement, Hurley Medical Center signed a five-year agreement with EEOC to provide internal training about inclusion and nondiscrimination; it also agreed to offer community educational initiatives with community youth through high school career days at the medical center. Cober, the director of the EEOC field office, made the following statement (EEOC 2013):

> This case exemplifies the EEOC's commitment to stop and remedy employment discrimination. It is important for the public to know that the EEOC is ever vigilant in our efforts to root out discrimination in the workplace. Assignments of caregivers according to their race and based on customer preference is against the law period and will not be tolerated. We commend Hurley Medical Center for their willingness to resolve this matter in a comprehensive way that will have a lasting positive effect in the Flint/Genesee community.

Equal opportunity also pertains to age, specifically workers older than 40. The EEOC sued Hawaii Healthcare Professionals for age discrimination because it terminated an office coordinator who looked "like a bag of bones" and "sounded old on the telephone" (EEOC 2012). The coordinator's performance reviews indicated she was a "thorough and efficient worker," and Park, the regional attorney for the EEOC in this case, said that (Fastenberg 2012)

> what makes this case especially appalling is the flagrant disregard for a worker's abilities, coupled with disparaging ageist remarks and thinking.

Hawaii Healthcare Professionals was ordered to pay the complainant more than $190,000 (EEOC 2012).

A brief description of other labor laws appears in exhibit 12.1.

The case study at the beginning of this chapter presents an issue that represents the importance of effective human resource management. It also illustrates why a manager should understand basic tenets of equal opportunity laws. Dr. Fox has rights as an employee of Medical University, but he also has responsibilities. And, Dr. Daunt knows that Dr. Fox is exemplary regarding his research, though he seems (apparently) to be deficient in other areas. While considering her potential plan of action, Dr. Daunt must balance his rights with his student Roberta's rights and to ensure Dr. Fox meets his responsibilities. Dr. Daunt's call to HR and Legal is a first step to ensure she understands the basic principles of federal laws regarding employment. It also enables the HR and legal experts to counsel her on ways to address the issue.

Healthcare managers are not expected to know all the details about each and every law, but an understanding of the basic principles of employees' rights and responsibilities is key to effectively addressing issues such as Dr. Fox and his teaching techniques. In this

Exhibit 12.1
Labor Laws and Subject Matter

Labor Law and Website for More Information	Subject Matter
Age Discrimination in Employment Act, 1967 www.eeoc.gov/laws/statutes/adea.cfm	Prohibits age discrimination in employment for those 40 years or older.
Americans with Disabilities Act, 1990 www.eeoc.gov/eeoc/history/35th/1990s/ada.html	Prohibits discrimination in employment, public services, accommodations, and telecommunications for those with disabilities.
Civil Rights Act, Title VII, 1964 www.eeoc.gov/laws/statutes/titlevii.cfm	Prohibits discrimination in employment on the basis of sex, race, color, national origin, and religion. This applies to organizations with 15 or more employees.
Civil Rights Act, 1991 www.eeoc.gov/eeoc/history/35th/1990s/civilrights.html	Contained provisions regarding the right to a trial and the receipt of damages in cases of intentional discrimination.
Equal Employment Opportunity Act, 1972 www.eeoc.gov/eeoc/history/35th/thelaw/eeo_1972.html	Contained the provision that the Equal Employment Opportunity Commission may sue in federal courts if there is reasonable cause to believe employment discrimination occurred based on race, color, religion, sex, or national origin.
Equal Pay Act, 1963 www.eeoc.gov/laws/statutes/epa.cfm	Mandates pay equity to both men and women who work in the same organization and do similar work.
Family and Medical Leave Act, 1993 www.dol.gov/whd/regs/statutes/fmla.htm	Mandates job-protected and unpaid leave for up to 12 weeks during any 12-month period for qualified medical and family reasons.
Genetic Information Nondiscrimination Act, 2008 www.eeoc.gov/laws/types/genetic.cfm	Prohibits discrimination in employment based on an employee's genetic information.
Occupational Safety and Health Act, 1970 www.epa.gov/laws-regulations/summary-occupational-safety-and-health-act	Mandates worksite safety for employees.
Pregnancy Discrimination Act, 1978 www.eeoc.gov/laws/statutes/pregnancy.cfm	Prohibits discrimination in employment based on pregnancy.
Rehabilitation Act, 1973 www.eeoc.gov/laws/statutes/rehab.cfm	Prohibits discrimination in employment based on disabilities.
Uniformed Services Employment and Reemployment Rights Act, 1994 www.justice.gov/servicemembers/uniformed-services-employment-and-reemployment-rights-act-1994-userra	Prohibits discrimination of veterans in civilian employment, protecting their seniority, status, and salary.

case, take, for example, the student Roberta. She is a graduate student, studying to become a physical therapist, and she has reported that the professor engages in behavior that gives her a stomachache as he shows slides of nude women in class. Is this **sexual harassment**? Consider your answer to this as we discover the topic more in depth.

Sexual harassment
The illegal practice of unwelcome sexual behavior in the workplace.

In chapter 6, we discussed sexual harassment in the workplace with reference to the "#MeToo" Movement. We also described a 2014 survey of women who were assistant professor–level clinical scientists and who had received career development awards form the National Institutes of Health; when asked if they had experienced sexual harassment, 30 percent said that they had (Jagsi et al. 2016). EEOC (2018a) defines sexual harassment as the following:

> Unwelcome sexual advances, requests for sexual favors, and other verbal or physical conduct of a sexual nature constitute sexual harassment when this conduct explicitly or implicitly affects an individual's employment, unreasonably interferes with an individual's work performance, or creates an intimidating, hostile, or offensive work environment.

Managers in healthcare settings should be aware of the potential consequences of staff members' behaviors. Sexual harassment is a form of sex discrimination that violates Title VII of the Civil Rights Act of 1964. Any organization that employs 15 or more people is subject to this law. In 2011, the EEOC resolved more than 12,500 sexual harassment charges in the United States. The persons who made the charges and other aggrieved parties received $52.3 million in monetary benefits (EEOC 2018b). Sexual harassment is not only illegal, but it can also cost an organization money that could be put to better use.

A study on sexual harassment in medical training indicated that about 59 percent of medical trainees had experienced at least one form of harassment during their training (Fnais et al. 2014). In 2015, the Association of American Universities conducted a survey about sexual assault and misconduct on 27 college campuses. About 48 percent of the respondents reported they had experienced some form of sexual harassment, and about 30 percent defined the harassment as their being subjected to sexual remarks or insulting or offensive jokes or stories (Cantor et al. 2015).

The following circumstances apply to sexual harassment (EEOC 2018a):

1. The victim as well as the harasser may be a woman or a man. The victim does not have to be of the opposite sex.
2. The harasser can be the victim's supervisor, an agent of the employer, a supervisor in another area, a coworker, or a nonemployee.
3. The victim does not have to be the person harassed but could be anyone affected by the offensive conduct.

4. Unlawful sexual harassment may occur without economic injury to or discharge of the victim.

5. The harasser's conduct must be unwelcome.

In the case study, Dr. Daunt's conference call is an important step in addressing the situation. She can relate the student's description of the slide pictures as unwelcome and offensive, and she can note Roberta's stomachaches. Moreover, she could relate how Roberta had proposed an alternative teaching method she would not consider offensive (i.e., Dr. Fox using photos of babies and other innocuous scenes). During the conversation among Dr. Daunt, HR, and Legal, they could determine whether any information could be construed as evidence that Dr. Fox's actions are creating an intimidating and hostile classroom environment. The call also allows for discussion regarding potential plans of action to address the situation.

The EEOC recommends that organizations such as Medical University in the case study have a formal, written policy for employees regarding sexual harassment. The EEOC also encourages training employees in what sexual harassment is, what to do if they suspect sexual harassment, and what the effective complaint or grievance process is to address harassment concerns. In addition, the organization should communicate the disciplinary options that would face a confirmed harasser. Depending on the scope and severity of the action, punishment could include verbal or written reprimand, suspension, demotion, or dismissal.

Now, back to the case study. Do you view it as an example of sexual harassment?

This case is true; the events really did happen (the names of the place and people were changed to protect their identities). The outcome was that Dr. Daunt, in consultation with HR and Legal, concluded this was indeed an example of sexual harassment by Dr. Fox. She met with Dr. Fox in his office and explained she had been informed he was showing slides of nude women in sexually suggestive poses in class. Then, she stopped talking and listened. He explained the importance of his showing something to disrupt the class so the students would pay attention to the particularly important slides, and he defended the use because those slides had worked in the past. However, upon his reflecting about his conversation with a female student, he had come to realize this practice was not appropriate. From now on, he would show slides of impressive views of places around the world, such as the Taj Mahal in India and Old Faithful geyser in Yellowstone National Park, to disrupt the class so students would pay close attention to the next slide.

He also apologized for not having realized this sooner. He was reported to have stated, "I was so focused on the outcome of the students' learning what to look for in the slide, I forgot to treat all of my students with respect."

Dr. Daunt followed up with Roberta within two weeks of her conversation with Dr. Fox, and Roberta reported that Dr. Fox was now showing slides of travel sites. She also thanked Dr. Daunt for her response to her concerns and noted that she was satisfied with the outcome.

After the incident, Dr. Fox and the other faculty and staff at Medical University attended sexual harassment training, and Dr. Fox received a verbal reprimand for his behavior. No further complaints regarding Dr. Fox have occurred since the event.

Hiring the Best Fit

Over the course of their careers, healthcare professionals can expect to work at different sites in different positions. These job changes may be due to work performance, a pursuit of lifelong learning and new challenges, and appealing career opportunities. However, each time competent staff members leave to work elsewhere, it is costly for the organization they leave behind.

A survey of more than 10,000 healthcare facilities found that job turnover rates in healthcare averaged more than 19 percent a year (Compdata 2015). The survey also found that place of work influenced turnover: People working in long-term care were more likely to leave their jobs (the voluntary turnover rate in that field was 19 percent), while employees working in medical groups were the least likely to leave (voluntary turnover rate was 10 percent) (Compdata 2015).

Each of these departures is expensive. While there are savings incurred (the money that would have been expensed on salary and benefits), the department is not fully staffed, and other personnel must make up the difference by increasing their workload. Thus, while the organization saves some money because of the open position, it also faces costs: paying short-term employees, paying overtime to regular employees to complete all the necessary work, and paying any costs associated with a search. For example, replacing a registered nurse costs, on average, more than $36,000 (Lewin Group 2009), and replacing a hospital's entire staff would cost more than 5 percent of its total annual budget (Waldman et al. 2004). In addition, turnover is time-consuming, as new staff must be hired, introduced to the facility and new coworkers, and trained to follow the procedures of their new workplace.

Organizational fit An employment candidate's qualification for the position advertised and ability to work well with others in the specific work environment.

Two critical factors for healthcare managers to consider during the hiring process are (1) the need to hire a person qualified for the position advertised and (2) the need to hire someone who will perform well in the specific work environment. Building a team of staff members who possess the knowledge, skills, and abilities to do their jobs well and who work well together enables a department to perform well. The goal of recruitment is to find the person who meets the specific job requirements and who is the best **organizational fit**. Dr. Fox may be an excellent researcher and may be highly involved with professional service; however, his behavior as a teacher was called into question in his specific work environment.

Job description A document that clearly defines the tasks, duties, responsibilities, and performance standards associated with a position.

Fottler (2015) proposed that a **job description** may be used to clearly define the tasks, duties, responsibilities, and performance standards associated with a position. The use of a job description may enhance a candidate's awareness of expectations pertaining to specific job requirements. The following box shows the job description for Dr. Fox's position. In the announcement, the description clearly states that the professor is expected to teach, conduct research, and participate in professional service. Specific to Roberta's concern, the description also states that the professor is expected to exhibit professional behavior.

POSITION ANNOUNCEMENT
Tenure Track Faculty in Cell Biology

Minimum Education/Experience: A PhD in Biology, Biochemistry, or a Biology-related field, such as Molecular Biology or Genetics, with training in cancer research is required, as well as at least one year of appropriate postdoctoral research experience. The successful candidate will have a strong record of scholarly achievements. Qualifying degrees must be received from appropriately accredited institutions.

Special Instructions to Applicant: Applicants must submit a cover letter, curriculum vitae, contact information for at least three references, and statements of research interests and teaching experience/philosophy. We will ask top candidates to have three reference letters sent to the Search Committee Chair via e-mail within seven (7) days of notification. Official transcript and original hard-copy reference letters are required upon employment. Inquiries regarding this position may be directed to Search Committee Chair or the Lead Administrative Associate.

Review of applications will begin in September. Job is open until filled.

Job Duties: The Department of Biology invites applications for a nine-month tenure-track position at the Assistant Professor level with expertise in Cell Biology. Qualified applicants who have the potential to contribute to innovation in cancer research are encouraged to apply. The successful candidate will establish a strong record of scholarly achievements, be expected to establish a vigorous, externally funded research program, and actively engage in mentoring graduate student research. The successful candidate will also be expected to teach graduate students effectively in the classroom. Candidates are expected to engage in university, community, and professional service. The Department of Biology supports a diverse, professional, interdisciplinary faculty. Extensive opportunities for research collaboration exist both within the department and across the university. The Department of Biology is committed to enriching the lives of students, faculty, and staff by providing a diverse, professional academic community where the exchange of ideas, knowledge, and perspectives is an active part of living and learning. The department seeks to create an environment that fosters the recruitment and retention of a diverse student body, faculty, staff, and administration and works to increase diversity and access to higher education for groups underrepresented in the medical professions by building an environment that welcomes, celebrates, and promotes respect for diversity.

Past research supports the practice of hiring based on a candidate's good fit with the organization as well as his or her good fit for the position (Bowen, Ledford, and Nathan 1991; Lam, Huo, and Chen 2018; Yu 2014). That is, the candidate should have the credentials and knowledge for the position, *and* should possess qualities that are in sync with the organizational culture. Moreover, person–organization fit influences how well an individual will perform at work because the better the fit, the more satisfied a person will be regarding work, which in turn will influence her performance (Farooqui and Nagendra 2014). Thinking back to the hiring of Dr. Fox in our case, the question emerges of whether behavioral expectations should have been emphasized more during the interview process. Alternatively, the hiring team could have underscored the importance of fit with the organization. However, even if the hiring team had emphasized a culture of professionalism, Dr. Fox still might have exhibited the behavior Roberta described. No hiring system is perfect.

Nonetheless, the takeaway from Bowen, Ledford, and Nathan's (1991) and Farooqui and Nagendra's (2014) research is the importance of a good fit between individual and job and between individual and organization. There are advantages for the person and for the organization to selecting candidates whose values match the organization's culture. These advantages include higher reported job satisfaction (Adkins and Caldwell 2004; Kristof 1996), positive work performance (Hoffman and Woehr 2006; Kristof 1996), and less turnover (Chatman 1991; O'Reilly, Chatman, and Caldwell 1991).

A hiring misstep may result in extra work and additional stress for the manager and the other staff members throughout the person's employment. The manager must also spend more of her time on corrective action plans and disciplinary options. In the case study, Dr. Daunt met with Roberta and arranged for the meeting with the HR and legal departments. She met with Dr. Fox, followed up with him and the student, and supervised Dr. Fox's subsequent in-class behavior. She also directed efforts for the in-house sexual harassment training. If Roberta had filed a formal complaint with the EEO/Affirmative Action office on campus, Dr. Daunt could have been involved in an EEO hearing. She spent extra time and effort because a member of her team was behaving inappropriately.

This incident also had positive outcomes. Dr. Fox came to understand that the slide show was unacceptable; he stated he had learned from his mistake. Part of Dr. Daunt's responsibilities as chair was to supervise and lead the departmental members to become better professionals. This incident provided an excellent opportunity for Dr. Fox's professional development as an instructor.

To determine whether a qualified candidate also demonstrates fit with the organization, consider having the search committee assess the following:

1. Review the position advertisement and job description.
2. Screen applicant files to ensure each candidate's qualifications meet the job specifications.

3. Participate in the interview process.
4. Evaluate each candidate's strengths and weaknesses.
5. Contact each candidate's references.
6. Advise the administration regarding candidate selection preferences.
7. Continually work with an HR representative throughout the process.

Another important factor concerns training about an appropriate hiring process. When the hiring team conducts interviews, they should know what they can and cannot ask a candidate. They may ask questions about a candidate's past job and educational experiences, and questions regarding the candidate's ability to perform the specific job advertised. They may not ask questions about the candidate's age (unless the specific job has an age requirement), family status (e.g., married, divorced, single, parent), credit status, physical or mental disabilities unrelated to job performance, political affiliation, race, or religion. The initial applicant screening is used to determine whether the applicant meets the job qualifications; the face-to-face interview allows the recruiting team members to meet candidates, and vice versa. The candidate should use the interview time to assess whether the organization is a good fit for her. Given that employees will spend at least 40 hours per week at a job, good fit is important to both the organization and the candidate.

A challenge specific to hiring in the healthcare industry is the ongoing healthcare labor shortage. Sportsman (2007) describes it as a challenge of finding and retaining competent people during an overall shortage of competent healthcare professionals. The healthcare industry is experiencing and will continue to experience a deficit of nurses, pharmacists, technicians, and therapists (Keeler et al. 2018; Leider et al. 2018; Shi and Singh 2013; Vandyk et al. 2017). These shortages exacerbate the hiring challenge. Recruitment teams seek the best person with the best fit for the position, but find themselves in a highly competitive environment. As a result, healthcare organization managers who are able to hire people should also be concerned about keeping the people they have hired. The focus is on retaining, motivating, and helping staff members develop professionally, work well, and enjoy their work.

Retention and Performance Appraisals: The Importance of Feedback

Retention refers to keeping good staff at an organization. As mentioned earlier, turnover is costly in terms of the time spent to replace a staff member and the dollars spent to advertise, review applications, and interview candidates. Effective managers look into why good staff members leave their organization and what encourages them to stay. The reasons someone

Retention
The keeping of employees at an organization.

leaves may highlight what can be done to keep other valued employees. Donoghue and Castle (2007) found that registered nurses, licensed practical nurses, and nursing assistants often left their positions in nursing homes because of the work environment; the primary reasons for their departures were understaffing and the organizations' deficiency citations—that is, citations by state licensing agencies for restraining residents or for the prevalence of residents' pressure ulcers.

As healthcare managers, we have an ongoing responsibility to hire the most competent and committed healthcare professionals. However, with the current labor shortage, this responsibility has become a challenge. Hence, employee retention is essential to organizational success, and key to this goal is creating and sustaining a work environment that meets The Joint Commission's standards.

Joint Commission
A not-for-profit accrediting agency that assesses an organizations' ability to meet standards of performance in key healthcare operations.

The **Joint Commission** is a not-for-profit accrediting agency that assesses healthcare organizations according to standards of performance in key healthcare operations, such as infection control and patient treatment. The Joint Commission reviews hospitals; home care organizations; hospices; long-term care facilities; behavioral healthcare, substance abuse, and mental health programs; ambulatory care centers; and independent laboratories. Its review is focused on quality assurance, and its mission is (Joint Commission 2018)

> to continuously improve the safety and quality of care provided to the public through the provision of healthcare accreditation and related services that support performance improvement in healthcare organizations.

Other characteristics of retention strategies include

1. a focus on the positive recognition of staff members' accomplishments,
2. a compensation process that is linked to staff members' work performance,
3. a culture of mutual respect,
4. a competitive package that includes leave time for vacation and holidays,
5. opportunities for professional training and development,
6. a commitment by leaders to provide the resources necessary to meet accreditation agencies' standards, and
7. a commitment by managers to implement the organization's retention strategy.

Research indicates that the best managers follow a strategy that values their employees, meets employees' personal and practical needs (i.e., salary, work schedule, vacation time); provides rewards and recognition when appropriate; allows for professional advancement; provides compelling reasons the employees should be part of the organization; and links compensation with **performance evaluation** (Bassi and McMurrer 2007; Fibuch and Ahmed 2015; Gering and Conner 2002; Vatwani and Hill 2018). Linking pay increases with performance is related to lower turnover of top performers, as the employees see firsthand that merit matters (Nyberg, Pieper, and Trevor 2016).

Performance evaluation The process of reviewing employees' work behavior and efforts.

Performance evaluations can be formal or informal. For example, saying, "Nice work explaining that procedure to the new technician today," is an example of informal, immediate feedback. Feedback is critical to good leadership, helping managers develop close relationships with staff members and helping staff assess their work performance. Managers should stay in regular contact with each employee (Gratto and McConnell 2008; Harter and Adkins 2015). These interactions allow managers and employees to identify and address potential problems and provide a manager with opportunities to notice and praise an employee for work well done.

Formal performance evaluations should be undertaken on a regular basis. Typically, they are held annually with each staff member to provide feedback regarding performance, to review performance standards, and to offer guidance on the employee's goals for the upcoming year. Effective performance evaluations include overall assessment of the employee's strengths and weaknesses, recommendations for improvement in performance, and information that is the basis for compensation, promotions, or corrective actions. Exhibits 12.2 and 12.3 at the end of this chapter show performance appraisals used by Portneuf Medical Center (PMC) in Pocatello, Idaho, for a practice director and for an office manager who reports to the practice director. The appraisals include a detailed job description, performance expectations, an assessment of the employees' progress toward the goals set during last year's review, and the employees' plans for the upcoming year. They also include information to which the supervisor (the vice president of medical practices for the practice director, and the practice director for the office manager) may refer when making promotion and salary decisions.

An important part of the performance evaluation is a face-to-face meeting between the manager and the employee to discuss the evaluation. The manager should establish a meeting atmosphere that allows for interaction between both the manager and the employee. This makes the employee a participant in the process and enables her to discuss her accomplishments over the past year, the challenges she faced, and the objectives and goals she anticipates. The manager's job is to deliver a performance appraisal that identifies strengths and weaknesses, shows the employee that she is valued (if this is indeed the case), and motivates her to improve performance. To do so, the manager should use a copy of the job description; pertinent reviews of the employee's performance from other staff members; a copy of the previous year's review, including the goals stated; and any other information about the specific employee's performance for the time period under review.

360 evaluation A review process in which the supervisor, the employee, and staff members who work with the employee assess the work behavior and efforts of an employee.

Another option is the **360 evaluation**. This type of review incorporates evaluation from an employee's superiors, colleagues, and subordinates. Palmer and Loveland (2008) note that 360 reviews may yield a more accurate and valid assessment overall by providing the manager with information from many sources, thereby negating individual biases. The manager, however, needs to be mindful that some evaluations submitted in this process may not be objective. Furthermore, Palmer and Loveland (2008) note that group ratings are more legally defensible than individual ratings on some issues, such as discrimination.

Termination Considerations

Along with recognizing, developing, and promoting talented employees, managers also shoulder the responsibility of firing staff. An employee who has consistently failed to meet expectations, failed to perform according to corrective plans, or engaged in a fireable offense may be subject to **termination**. If the manager has the facts and documentation to support such a decision and has followed the protocol for working with the employee to correct the poor performance, she should not wait for the annual formal performance evaluation (Thompson 2007). Observation, documentation, corrective plan action development with the employee, and follow-up should all be part of the process for the manager, the poorly performing employee, and an HR representative. The exception to this protocol is any behavior that warrants immediate dismissal, such as a hospital employee firing a weapon at the hospital.

Termination
End of an employee's contract with a company.

Bucking (2008) offers ten steps to follow when an employee's performance may warrant termination:

1. **Know the facts.** Speak to all parties involved and listen to the information they share.
2. **Review the documents.** The supervisor should review the file of the employee in question to determine whether the employee's past reviews have consistently been poor, average, or outstanding. This review could indicate whether the incident is an anomaly or a reflection of consistent underperformance. A review of other employees' files allows the supervisor to note whether similar behaviors have occurred with others and to ascertain whether employees are being treated fairly.
3. **Create new documents.** Ensure that documentation presents an honest and direct record of the events.
4. **Be aware of the electronic scourge.** Bucking (2008) advises supervisors that electronic records are not informal communications that disappear. Treat electronic communications as though they were formal writings.
5. **Tell the truth.** Be honest with the employee and other pertinent parties. It is not easy to let someone go from his employment. Be honest with the person being fired.

6. **Do not be gratuitously cruel.** There is no need for a person who is being fired to be treated in a cruel manner. If the decision has been made to terminate employment, then the manager should do so without engaging in a debate or argument with the employee.
7. **Conduct the termination respectfully.** Be polite and conduct the termination meeting without an audience. There is no need to fire someone in front of other employees. If possible, an employee should not be fired on a date that is special to her. For example, firing someone on her birthday should be avoided. Furthermore, the day of the week the firing occurs is worthy of consideration. Some universities have a policy against firing employees on a Friday. The concern is that the employee may not be able to contact the HR office to ask questions about their employee rights until the following Monday, and the two-day wait may be too stressful for the terminated employee.
8. **Have backup.** If possible, the manager should have a witness present during the termination meeting. This witness, however, should not be a coworker (see item 7). Rather, a representative from HR or another supervisor should be present.
9. **Pay all compensation due.** The employee earned the compensation; she should receive it.
10. **Think about other agreements or commitments.** If the employee has a company laptop, for example, the employee should be reminded to return it. Also, an HR representative can be the one to discuss severance agreements; he or she could also offer a business card so the employee can make future contact if there are questions.

Conclusion

At the beginning of this chapter, we met student Roberta and Department Chair Daunt, who were forced to deal with Dr. Fox's teaching techniques. Roberta, with knowledge she had gained from her undergraduate healthcare management and healthcare law and ethics classes, knew she should report Dr. Fox's behavior. In turn, Dr. Daunt, as Dr. Fox's supervisor, worked with the human resources and legal departments to ensure that she ethically and legally handled the situation appropriately.

This chapter next featured a discussion of employees' rights and responsibilities, along with laws that define what is and is not acceptable behavior at work. We then turned our attention to the importance of hiring, retention, and performance appraisals to ensure that the people with the best fit for the position and who perform well remain and professionally grow at their workplace. Last, we elaborated on the need for managers to, at times, terminate employees, and provided some advice on how best to handle this potentially difficult task. Throughout this chapter, we emphasized that it is important to understand rights and responsibilities when hiring and supervising staff.

Mini Case Study: Social Media and Human Resources

Elena Chernyakova was admitted to Northwestern Memorial Hospital in Chicago in 2013 for intoxication. Dr. Vinaya Puppala, a physician who was not providing care for Chernyakova, came to her hospital room, photographed the patient, and posted the photos on Instagram and Facebook with the hashtags #bottle #service #gone #bad (Abramson 2013; Le Mignot 2016; Weineke 2013). In 2016, Chernyakova initiated a lawsuit against Puppala. Northwestern made the following statement in response (Le Mignot 2016):

> Our first priority is to address the health needs of the patients we are privileged to serve—and to do so within an environment of care that protects and upholds their right to privacy. The allegations detailed in this complaint indicate this person was acting entirely on [her] own and had no treatment relationship with the plaintiff. Any invasion of privacy at the hands of our trusted health personnel or extended care team of training fellows is unacceptable and not indicative of the Patients First culture of Northwestern Memorial Hospital, which has zero tolerance for exploitation of private health information, including photography.

Mini Case Study Questions

1. What employee responsibilities did Puppala violate in this mini case?
2. What would you recommend Northwestern do regarding its working relationship with Puppala? Explain your reasoning.
3. How does hiring according to person–organization fit play into your answers to questions 1 and 2?

Points to Remember

- Hiring the best qualified candidate who is also the best fit for the organization is important as a manager makes decisions that are in the best interest of the employers and the workplace.
- Sexual harassment is not to be tolerated, and human resources and legal department personnel will partner with a supervisor to handle such situations appropriately.

- Retention is key, not only to keep the best employees and thus provide quality patient care, but also because of the cost associated with hiring and training new staff members.
- Performance evaluations offer managers opportunities to acknowledge employees' excellent work as well as provide overall assessment of the employees' strengths and weaknesses.

Challenge Yourself

1. The Age Discrimination in Employment Act of 1967 prohibits age discrimination for workers 40 years or older. In the example discussed earlier in the chapter, Hawaii Healthcare Professionals was ordered to pay a complainant in an age-discrimination suit more than $190,000 (EEOC 2012).

   Consider yourself in the position of a manager in the Hawaii Healthcare Professionals organization. What should have been done when the disparaging remarks were made against the office coordinator? How would you ensure that such an event not occur in your future workplace?
2. Thinking back to the case study from the beginning of the chapter, what would you have recommended that the hiring team ask Dr. Fox during his interview to assess his level of professionalism? Keep in mind the questions that are and are not legally allowed during an interview.
3. Offer suggestions to a manager who is dealing with a sexual harassment allegation pertaining to one of his employees against another. Whom should the manager contact, and what should the manager discuss with the employee who has made the charge?

For Your Consideration

Portneuf Medical Center in Pocatello, Idaho, provided the practice director job description and performance appraisal in exhibit 12.2 (at the end of this chapter). PMC also provided exhibit 12.3 (at the end of this chapter), which is the job description and performance appraisal used for an office manager who reports to the practice director. Compare the information in both performance appraisals. What is similar about them? What is different? Why do you think there is such commonality between the two? What do the differences between the essential job functions indicate about the differences in performance expectations, duties of the position, and seniority? Explain, for example, the different responsibilities associated with the essential job function of financial acumen. How does this function statement show the different responsibilities of each position?

Exercise 12.1 Identifying Sexual Harassment

JinMing Sue was hired to work as an HR representative at Medical University in Oklahoma. During his employee orientation, Harvin Fairchild, an HR senior benefits counselor, asked JinMing to review the EEOC sexual harassment guidelines.

Harvin said, "JinMing, welcome to the HR office. I am so glad you are working with us now. One of your responsibilities will be to serve as the EEOC liaison. As part of your orientation, please read the following cases and decide what issue(s) should be addressed and what decisions you would make in each case. When you are through, we'll go over the examples and talk about them. Oh, I am so glad that I don't have to do this anymore! Welcome aboard."

JinMing opened the case book and began to read.

Case 1: Maintenance Matters

Bill Jackson and Nils Larsen have worked together as groundskeepers at Medical University for more than 20 years and are highly respected. They designed and planted a prayer garden for families of patients, complete with strategically placed benches where family members can sit and partake of the natural beauty during a potentially stressful time. The landscaping of Medical University's campus has often received praise, thanks to the gardening expertise Bill and Nils have brought to the job. If the nurses knew of a patient who had not had any visitors, they let one of the groundskeepers know. The patient would receive a bouquet of freshly cut flowers from the grounds to brighten her or his hospital room.

Several months ago, Florence Brighton was hired as an additional groundskeeper. It quickly became obvious that Bill and Nils did not approve of Florence. They told other people in the department, "Florence can't do the work and was only hired because she's a woman." The two of them conducted a campaign emphasizing Florence's shortcomings, got into arguments with her, and urged the nurses to complain about her to their boss, Hane Hightower.

After several weeks of this behavior, Bill and Nils requested a meeting with Hane. At the meeting, they contended that Florence was not carrying her fair share of the workload, and they resented having to do her work. They said that if Florence didn't leave, they would.

Case 2: The IT Training

Betty Summerton is the supervisor of Medical University's X-ray department. Sean Hartzog is a single male X-ray technologist. The university has purchased a new piece of X-ray equipment that requires intensive information technology (IT) training. Betty has asked Sean to be the team leader for the technologists regarding the equipment. Sean is smart and good with one-on-one communication. He would have made an excellent teacher. Everyone knows that once he is trained, the other technologists will become proficient with the machine in no time. Sean will make sure the technologists are well trained on the new machine before he allows them to work with it. The IT trainer is Cindy Barton, and she has met with Sean on two occasions to discuss the machine. Betty has learned that Cindy has asked Sean out on a date, and that Sean has accepted.

Case 3: Physical Therapy Squared

Danielle Thompson is a physical therapist who is efficient, good natured, and a compassionate caregiver. She has been working at Medical University for five months. Danielle has come to see Sharon, an HR staff member. She tells Sharon that within a month of her first day at the hospital, her supervisor, Ken, began making odd comments when they were alone. Then, he put his arm over her shoulder when they were working with a patient. He also patted her rear end. This has happened three times. Each time, Danielle told Ken to stop and not do it again. But each time, Ken just laughed it off and told Danielle that she was too reserved. The day before, Ken had reminded Danielle that her six-month probationary review was coming up. "He told me I needed to get a good review from him, and then he patted my rear again!" Danielle took a journal from her lab coat pocket. "Here," she said as she gave the journal to Sharon. "It's all in there. Will you help me, please?"

JinMing reviewed the cases and wrote a paragraph for each that addressed what he thought was the problem, options to help provide solutions, and, with reference to the options, his recommendations for addressing the problem. If you were JinMing, what would you have written?

Exercise 12.1 Questions

1. Identify the problem for each case.
2. Offer a list of options that might address the problem.
3. Recommend a solution to the problem you identified.

References

Abramson, A. 2013. "Chicago Doctor Accused of Posting Photos of Intoxicated Patient." ABC News. Published August 20. https://abcnews.go.com/US/chicago-doctor-sued-photographing-hospitalized-intoxicated-woman/story?id=20003303.

Adkins, B., and D. Caldwell. 2004. "Firm or Subgroup Culture: Where Does Fitting In Matter Most?" *Journal of Organizational Behavior* 25 (8): 969–78.

American College of Healthcare Executives (ACHE). 2017. *Code of Ethics*. Amended November 13. www.ache.org/about-ache/our-story/our-commitments/ethics/ache-code-of-ethics.

Bassi, L., and D. McMurrer. 2007. "Maximizing Your Return on People." *Harvard Business Review* 85 (3): 115–23.

Bowen, D., G. Ledford, and B. Nathan. 1991. "Hiring for the Organization, Not the Job." *Academy of Management Executives* 5 (4): 35–51.

Bucking, J. 2008. "Employee Terminations: 10 Must-Do Steps When Letting Someone Go." *Supervision* 69 (5): 11–13.

Byrd v. Lakeshore Hosp., 30 F.3d 1380 (11th Cir. 1994).

Cantor, D., B. Fisher, S. Chibnall, R. Townsend, H. Lee, C. Bruce, and G. Thomas. 2015. *Report on the AAU Campus Climate Survey on Sexual Assault and Sexual Misconduct*. Association of American Universities. Published September 21. www.aau.edu/sites/default/files/%40%20Files/Climate%20Survey/AAU_Campus_Climate_Survey_12_14_15.pdf.

Chatman, J. 1991. "Matching People and Organizations: Selection and Socialization in Public Accounting Firms." *Administrative Science Quarterly* 36 (3): 459–84.

Compdata. 2015. "Rising Turnover Rates in Healthcare and How Employers Are Recruiting to Fill Openings." Published September 17. www.compdatasurveys.com/2015/09/17/rising-turnover-rates-in-healthcare-and-how-employers-are-recruiting-to-fill-openings-2.

Donoghue, C., and N. Castle. 2007. "Organizational and Environmental Effects on Voluntary and Involuntary Turnover." *Health Care Management Review* 32 (4): 360–69.

Equal Employment Opportunity Commission (EEOC). 2018a. "Facts About Sexual Harassment." Accessed May 21. www.eeoc.gov/eeoc/publications/fs-sex.cfm.

———. 2018b. "Sexual Harassment Charges." Accessed May 21. www.eeoc.gov/eeoc/statistics/enforcement/sexual_harassment.cfm.

———. 2013. "Hurley Medical Center Agrees to Settle EEOC Race Discrimination Case." Published September 26. www.eeoc.gov/eeoc/newsroom/release/9-26-13e.cfm.

———. 2012. "Court Orders Hawaii Healthcare Professionals and Its Owner to Pay over $190,000 for Age Discrimination." Published July 19. www.eeoc.gov/eeoc/newsroom/release/7-19-12.cfm.

Farooqui, S., and A. Nagendra. 2014. "The Impact of Person Organization Fit on Job Satisfaction and Performance of the Employees." *Procedia Economics and Finance* 11: 122–29.

Fastenberg, D. 2012. "Worker Debra Moreno Wins $193,000 in Age Discrimination Lawsuit." Published July 25. www.huffingtonpost.com/2012/07/25/worker-debra-moreno-wins-_n_1701287.html.

Fibuch, E., and A. Ahmed. 2015. "Physician Turnover: A Costly Problem." *Physician Leadership Journal* 2 (3): 22–25.

Fnais, N., C. Soobiah, M. Chen, E. Lillie, L. Perrier, M. Tashkhandi, S. Straus, M. Mamdani, M. Al-Omran, and A. Tricco. 2014. "Harassment and Discrimination in Medical Training: A Systematic Review and Meta-Analysis." *Academic Medicine* 89 (5): 817–27.

Fottler, M. D. 2015. "Job Analysis and Job Design." In *Human Resources in Healthcare: Managing for Success*, edited by B. J. Fried and M. D. Fottler, 143–80. Chicago: Health Administration Press.

Gering, J., and J. Conner. 2002. "A Strategic Approach to Employee Retention." *Health Care Financial Management* 56 (11): 40–44.

Gratto, L. J., and C. R. McConnell. 2008. *Management Skills for the New Health Care Supervisor*, 5th ed. Boston: Jones & Bartlett Publishers.

Harter, J., and A. Adkins. 2015. "What Great Managers Do to Engage Employees." *Harvard Business Review*. Published April 2. https://hbr.org/2015/04/what-great-managers-do-to-engage-employees.

Hoffman, B. J., and D. J. Woehr. 2006. "A Quantitative Review of the Relationship Between Person–Organization Fit and Behavioral Outcomes." *Journal of Vocational Behavior* 68 (3): 389–99.

Jagsi, R., K. Griffith, R. Jones, C. Perumalswami, P. Ubel, and A. Stewart. 2016. "Sexual Harassment and Discrimination Experiences of Academic Medical Faculty." *Journal of the American Medical Association* 315 (19): 2120–21.

Joint Commission. 2018. "About The Joint Commission." Accessed May 24. www.jointcommission.org/about_us/about_the_joint_commission_main.aspx.

Keeler, H., T. Sjuts, K. Niitsu, S. Watanabe-Galloway, P. Mackie, and H. Liu. 2018. "Virtual Mentorship Network to Address the Rural Shortage of Mental Health Providers." *American Journal of Preventive Medicine* 54 (6): S290–S295.

Kristof, A. L. 1996. "Person–Organization Fit: An Integrative Review of Its Conceptualizations, Measurement, and Implications." *Personnel Psychology* 49 (1): 1–49.

Lam, W., Y. Juo, and Z. Chen. 2018. "Who Is Fit to Serve? Person–Job/Organization Fit, Emotional Labor, and Customer Service Performance." *Human Resource Management* 57 (2): 483–97.

Leider, J., F. Coronado, A. Beck, and E. Harper. 2018. "Reconciling Supply and Demand for State and Local Public Health Staff in an Era of Retiring Baby Boomers." *American Journal of Preventive Medicine* 54 (3): 334–40.

Le Mignot, S. 2016. "Suit: Northwestern Hospital Physician Posted Pics of Intoxicated ER Patient Online." CBS Chicago. Published April 21. https://chicago.cbslocal.com/2016/04/21/suit-northwestern-hospital-physician-posted-pics-of-intoxicated-er-patient-online/.

Lewin Group. 2009. "Evaluation of the Robert Wood Johnson Wisdom at Work: Retaining Experienced Nurses Research Initiative." Published January. www.rwjf.org/content/dam/farm/reports/evaluations/2009/rwjf41981.

Nyberg, A., J. Pieper, and C. Trevor. 2016. "Pay-for-Performance's Effect on Future Employee Performance: Integrating Psychological and Economic Principles Toward a Contingency Perspective." *Journal of Management* 42 (7): 1753–83.

O'Reilly, C. A., J. A. Chatman, and D. F. Caldwell. 1991. "People and Organizational Culture: A Profile Comparison Approach to Assessing Person–Organization Fit." *Academy of Management Journal* 34 (3): 963–75.

Palmer, J. K., and J. M. Loveland. 2008. "The Influence of Group Discussion on Performance Judgments: Rating Accuracy, Contrast Effects, and Halo." *Journal of Psychology* 142 (2): 117–30.

Shi, L., and D. Singh. 2013. *Essentials of the U.S Health Care System*, 3rd ed. Burlington, MA: Jones & Bartlett Learning.

Sportsman, S. 2007. "The Human Resources Function in Hospitals." In *Managing Human Resources in Health Care Organizations*, edited by L. Shi, 185–223. Sudbury, MA: Jones & Bartlett.

Thompson, J. 2007. "The Strategic Management of Human Resources." In *Introduction to Health Care Management*, edited by S. B. Buchbinder and N. H. Shanks, 265–301. Burlington, MA: Jones & Bartlett.

Vandyk, A., J. Chartrand, E. Beke, L. Burlock, and C. Baker. 2017. "Perspectives from Academic Leaders of the Nursing Faculty Shortage in Canada." *International Journal of Nursing Education Scholarship* 14 (1): 286–97.

Vatwani, A., and C. Hill. 2018. "Examining Factors, Strategies, and Processes to Decrease Physical Therapy Turnover Rates in Acute Care Hospitals: A Review of the Literature." *Journal of Acute Care Physical Therapy* 9 (1): 11–18.

Waldman, J., F. Kelly, S. Aurora, and H. Smith. 2004. "The Shocking Cost of Turnover in Health Care." *Health Care Management Review* 29 (1): 2–7.

Weineke, D. 2013. "Social Media Rule #1: Shed Your Idiots Now." Useful Arts. Published September 5. http://usefularts.us/2013/09/05/elena-chernyakova-vinaya-puppula/.

Yu, K. 2014. "Person–Organization Fit Effects on Organizational Attraction: A Test of an Expectations-Based Model." *Organizational Behavior and Human Decision Processes* 124 (1): 75–94.

EXHIBIT 12.2
PMC Performance Appraisal Form: Practice Director's Annual Review

Portneuf MEDICAL CENTER Be well.	JOB DESCRIPTION AND PERFORMANCE EVALUATION FORM			
	Employee Name			
	Position Title:	Practice Director	**Effective Date:**	04/2015
	Department:	Medical Practice	**Last Revision:**	04/2015
	Review Responsibility:	Vice President Medical Practices	**FLSA Status:**	Exempt

Position Summary: Accountable for the financial health and overall stability of multiple specialties, potentially in multiple geographic locations. Responsible for staffing decisions; setting and achieving production targets for physicians and other Allied Health Professionals; and work schedules for the practices as well as staff, physicians and other Allied Health Professionals. Responsible for ensuring vendor and support department performance meets expectations, including revenue cycle. Recommends additions, changes or deletions of service offerings based upon community need, ability to deliver, and financial viability. Participates in physician recruiting activities, including interviewing, onboarding and mentoring programs. Creates budgets for assigned specialties and performs regular financial reviews with the Vice President of Medical Practices. Works closely with the Vice-President of Medical Practices to ensure the provision of comprehensive departmental compliance, patient satisfaction, and performance improvement.

Minimum Qualifications:

- Education and/or experience equivalent to a bachelor's degree is required, with a working understanding of accounting principles, as well as excellent communications skills and financial proficiency.
- Must have at least five years of experience in the medical field with previous medical practice management or leadership background. At least three years of managerial experience required.
- Must have experience working directly with physicians, staff, patients and external entities.

Essential Job Functions:

- **Data Analytics:** Ability to create data, analyze results, derive conclusions and recommend improvement activities and priorities.
- **Financial Acumen:** Ability to read and analyze financial data in order to prioritize activities that improve the financial health of the practice as well as set annual budgets.
- **Communication:** Ability to effectively communicate vertically and horizontally throughout the organization and externally to patients and other stakeholders.
- **Leadership:** Ability to inspire others and the credibility to enlist action.
- **Process Improvement:** Ability to utilize a scientific approach to problem solving utilizing scientific method, lean, Six Sigma, etc.

Knowledge, Skills and Abilities:

- Demonstrate sound judgment, patience and maintain a professional demeanor at all times
- Ability to work in a busy and stressful environment
- Organizational skills and the ability to prioritize
- Computer skills: Word, Excel, Outlook, Electronic medical records software
- Strong interpersonal verbal and written communication skills
- Creativity, problem analysis and decision making
- Ability to work varied shifts

Exhibit 12.2
PMC Performance Appraisal Form: Practice Director's Annual Review *(continued)*

Work Positions & Activities *N = Not at all 0-10% O = Occasionally (10-35%) F = Frequently (35-66%) C = Continually (67-100%)*	
1. Lift (floor to waist)	
a. Up to 10 pounds (sedentary)	F
b. 11-20 pounds (Light)	O
c. 21-50 pounds (Medium)	O
d. 51-100 pounds (Heavy)	N
e. >100 pounds (Very Heavy)	N
2. Lift (over head)	
a. Up to 10 pounds (sedentary)	O
b. 11-20 pounds (Light)	O
c. 21-50 pounds (Medium)	O
d. 51-100 pounds (Heavy)	N
e. >100 pounds (Very Heavy)	N
3. Patient Transfer: (weight per employee)	
a. <50 pounds	N
b. >50 pounds	N
c. >100 pounds	N
d. >150 pounds	N
4. Carry	
a. Up to 10 pounds (sedentary)	F
b. 11-20 pounds (Light)	O
c. 21-50 pounds (Medium)	O
d. 51-100 pounds (Heavy)	N
e. >100 pounds (Very Heavy)	N
5. Push or pull	
a. Up to 10 pounds (sedentary)	O
b. 11-20 pounds (Light)	O
c. 21-50 pounds (Medium)	O
d. 51-100 pounds (Heavy)	O
e. >100 pounds (Very Heavy)	N
6. Climb (stairs) - climb & descend	O
7. Reach	F
8. Stoop or bend	O
9. Crouch	O
10. Kneel	O
11. Handle or feel	F
12. Talk	C
13. Hear	C
14. See	C
15. Sit (continuous)	
a. 30 minutes	F
b. 60 minutes	F
c. 1-3 hours	F
d. 3-6 hours	O
16. Walk	F
17. Stand (continuous)	
a. 30 minutes	O
b. 60 minutes	N
c. 1-3 hours	N
d. 3-6 hours	N
18. Repetitive activities (continuous)	
a. 30 minutes	O
b. 60 minutes	O
c. 1-3 hours	N
d. 3-6 hours	N
Mental Demands *(Y = Yes or N = No)*	
a. Alertness	Y
b. Precision	Y
c. Analytic ability	Y
d. Problem Solving	Y
e. Memory	Y
f. Communication	Y
g. Creativity	Y
h. Concentration	Y
i. Judgment	Y
j. Imagination	Y
k. Initiative	Y
l. Patience	Y
Work Environment *(Y = Yes or N = No)*	
a. Inside work	Y
b. Outside work	N
c. Noise	Y
d. Vibration	N
e. Wet/Humid	N
Hazard Exposure/risk of bodily illness/ injury	
a. Mechanical	O
b. Electrical	O
c. Explosives	N
d. Burns	N
e. Chemicals	N
f. Fumes/Gases/Odors	N
g. Toxic waste	N
h. Frequent travel	N
i. Long/irregular hours	N
j. Cramped/confined work area	N
k. Moving machinery	N
l. Ionizing radiation	N
m. Strong magnetic fields	N
n. Biochemical hazards/waste	Y
o. Blood borne pathogens	N
p. TB Mask Fitting	N

(continued)

Exhibit 12.2
PMC Performance Appraisal Form: Practice Director's Annual Review *(continued)*

Section 1 – Hospital Wide Performance Areas

Check the rating that most closely matches the behavior. Comments or examples of specific behavior should be added to explain or illustrate the job behavior. Ratings must be supported by comments.

3 – High or Exceeds Standard(s): Clearly outstanding; always exceeds job requirements and expectations. Performance role model for others providing an exceptional contribution.
2 – Mid or Meets Standard(s): Solid contributor. Understands duties and consistently meets standards, policies and practices. Generally needs little oversight with a little room to grow to become a high performer.
1 – Below Standard(s): Understands duties and may meet minimal standards, policies or practices. Performance issues are identified and the employee is actively working on them; continued improvement is needed.

Lives the values: Professionalism and Continuous Improvement	**Overall Rating** 3 ☐ 2 ☐ 1 ☐
HIGH: Values diversity and embraces ideas from others. Stays current with knowledge through learning; Approaches situations and problems with a fresh perspective; Adapts to change with a positive attitude. Recognizes failure, apologizes and tries again; **MID:** Willing to listen to others ideas. Has a solid Knowledge of hospital policies and procedures. Understands innovation however may sometimes lean towards staying the course. Goes with and supports change when implemented; Will apologize when recognized; **LOW:** Can be stuck on 'the way we do things here' mentality. Does not keep current in field; May point out problems or poke holes at the ideas of others. May also make changes without input/discussion or thinking of ripple effects of actions. Resists change and/or feedback. Does not consistently apologize.	
Supervisor comments:	

Lives the values: Ownership, Integrity and Ethics	**Overall Rating** 3 ☐ 2 ☐ 1 ☐
HIGH: Is accountable for their actions, expectations, and outcomes. Is honest with him/herself and others; is loyal even to those not present. Treats others with respect; does not gossip; Approaches conflict directly, privately, and with a desire to improve the relationship. Always behaves ethically and honestly; Accepts responsibility for own decisions and actions. **MID**: Is mostly accountable for their actions, expectations, and outcomes. Is honest with others; is generally loyal. Treats others with respect; Deals with conflict and resolves issues. Solid person with no significant issues; **LOW:** At times this person attempts to deflect or avoid being accountable. Tends to say what others want to hear. Can be passive aggressive or overtly disruptive interpersonally. Is not consistently honest, respectful and/or loyal in word and deed.	
Supervisor comments:	

Lives the values: Communication and Problem Solving	**Overall Rating** 3 ☐ 2 ☐ 1 ☐
HIGH: Approaches every individual with caring and concern. Takes the time to listen; seeks to put other's needs before their own. Connects with others to relieve their stress, anxiety and resolve their concerns; Goes outside comfort zone; Finds appropriate individual(s) if outside scope of services. **MID:** Practices active listening. Restates or paraphrases while communicating for understanding. Is usually seen as sincere in their interpersonal relationships; Fosters understanding and has minimal misunderstandings and conflicts. Generally solves problems. **LOW:** Tends to listen with the intent to reply, not to understand. Seems to knows what they will say before others finish. Filters through their life experiences, their frame of reference; May not 'get' or acknowledge how others are feeling. Solves issues if confronted or required.	
Supervisor comments:	

Exhibit 12.2 PMC Performance Appraisal Form: Practice Director's Annual Review *(continued)*

Lives the values: Personal Engagement	**Overall Rating** 3 ☐ 2 ☐ 1 ☐
HIGH: Adds joy and enriches life at PMC. Is happy; recognizes the good around us; Works hard, and takes time off to recharge. Celebrates personal success as well as the success of others; is involved in employee celebration events; knows others in some measure outside of work. **MID:** Is a positive person. Contributes to PMC; May need to make more time to recharge. Celebrates the success of others; could be seen as needing to open up a little more or show more enthusiasm. May miss some employee celebrations; Relationships and/or interactions are generally work related in nature. **LOW:** Is seen as indifferent or not a positive person. Does their job and no more; looks to get things done and off the to-do pile. Does not consistently thank and/or recognize the efforts/success of others. May dampen excitement and enthusiasm. Not interested in staff and/or hospital outside of work relationship.	
Supervisor comments:	

Lives the values: Teamwork	**Overall Rating** 3 ☐ 2 ☐ 1 ☐
Coordinates efforts at every opportunity. Recognizes need for others. Trusts others and engenders their trust. Faces challenges by working with others. Collaborates, and coordinates improvement. Adds synergy and completes assignments. **MID:** Committed to improving performance of work unit and organization. Is generally trustworthy; eventually deals with challenges. Sometimes delays others. Solid team player however may not consistently demonstrate amazing teamwork. **LOW:** Tendency to micro-manage. May spend too much time on less critical issues delaying the team. Trust may be shaky at times. May meddle in non-important details; Deals with work or challenges if confronted or reminded. Gives appearance of team work but lacks consistently demonstrated substance.	
Supervisor comments:	

Lives the values: Service - Every Patient Every Time	**Overall Rating** 3 ☐ 2 ☐ 1 ☐
Consider how the individual ensures that patient care and/or customer service is the highest priority. How well does this individual model, teach and consistently demonstrate AIDET, MANAGING UP, KEY WORDS AT KEY TIMES and WORLD CLASS CARE EVERY PATIENT EVERY TIME?	
Supervisor comments:	

Lives the values: Organizational Accountability	**Overall Rating** 3 ☐ 2 ☐ 1 ☐
Is highly productive; completes assignments timely or communicates delays; Attendance is consistent. Looks for strengths, is optimistic; empowers people. Demonstrates a caring attitude. Integrates safety and safety guidelines into their work; Looks for and promotes patient and staff safety. Knows and consistently follows departmental and hospital policies and procedures; Completes licensing, education, competencies and other requirements in a timely manner. Knowledge and ability to respond to emergency preparedness procedures and to report safety issues (e.g. employee injury, patient safety, variance and equipment failures).	
Supervisor comments:	

(continued)

Exhibit 12.2
PMC Performance Appraisal Form: Practice Director's Annual Review *(continued)*

Section 2 – Essential Job Functions

Essential Job Function/Standard	Overall Rating 3 ☐ 2 ☐ 1 ☐
Data Analytics: Ability to create data, analyze results, derive conclusions and recommend improvement activities and priorities. **HIGH**: Uses data on a daily basis to drive decisions; Data is posted and updated daily; Employees understand the data being presented and have a high-level of trust in its meaning; A combination of graphs and tables are used; When computerized data is not available, uses manual charting to tell the story; **MID:** Data is posted and is mostly kept current; Team members are aware of the data and can connect their own role to the success of the group; **LOW:** Data is not readily available to team members, accurate or up-to date; Improvement activities appear sporadic and not tied to clear metrics; Blames the lack of data on others or the source as not trustworthy.	
Supervisor comments:	

Essential Job Function/Standard	Overall Rating 3 ☐ 2 ☐ 1 ☐
Financial Acumen: Ability to read and analyze financial data in order to prioritize activities that improve the financial health of the practice as well as set annual budgets. **HIGH**: Can clearly articulate the financial position and accurately project the following month or period; Can build an accurate and meaningful budget and meet expectations; Effectively communicates expenses and accurately reflects accruals; Is trusted by physicians to directly communicate profit and loss variances; **MID:** Can clearly articulate the financial position of the practices for the prior month, explaining variances (both positive and negative) and can project the following month with moderate accuracy; Understands and utilizes ratios in analyzing financial reports to find opportunities; Understands and participates in accurals; Can effectively communicate profit and loss statements to physicians with some guidance; **LOW:** Unable to explain variances in the financial statements; Unable to initiate improvement activities without reviewing financial statements with an executive or member of the finance team; Inaccurate or missing expense accruals.	
Supervisor comments:	

Essential Job Function/Standard	Overall Rating 3 ☐ 2 ☐ 1 ☐
Communication: Ability to effectively communicate vertically and horizontally throughout the organization and externally to patients and other stakeholders. **HIGH**: All team members can clearly articulate how their individual role ties to the Mission, Vision and Values of the practice; Goals are visible as is progress towards those goals; Stakeholders in the practice are aware of the goals and are included in improvement activities; Teaches others how to effectively communicate with patients and other guests; **MID:** Can clearly articulate the goals, current state and barriers to team members and stakeholders; Effectively solicits help from other departments and/or vendors as applicable; Can share information in a succinct but meaningful way; Can tell meaningful stories to engage others; Written communications are free from gramatical and/or spelling errors **LOW:** Team members have no clear connection with the work they do and the Mission, Vision, Values; Communications may cause confusion and require clarification from others; Communcations with patients does not likely result in the de-escalation of issues.	
Supervisor comments:	

Exhibit 12.2
PMC Performance Appraisal Form: Practice Director's Annual Review *(continued)*

Essential Job Function/Standard	**Overall Rating** 3☐ 2☐ 1☐
Leadership: Ability to inspire others and the credibility to enlist action. **HIGH**: Team members actively participate in improvement activities; Gets their hands dirty and periodically walks in the shoes of each team member; Leads by example even when it's difficult; Rewards and recognizes individual contributors with thank you notes and other forms of recognition; Teaches to missed opportunities; **MID:** Regular rounding with purpose; Mostly leads by example; Takes accountability for results; Team members are often asking what more can be done to improve the patient journey; **LOW:** Accountability for positive results but may lay blame for negative outcomes; Spends majority of time in the office and/or in meetings; Team members are complacent and satisfied with the current state.	
Supervisor comments:	

Essential Job Function/Standard	**Overall Rating** 3☐ 2☐ 1☐
Process Improvement: Ability to utilize a scientific approach to problem solving utilizing scientific method, lean, Six Sigma, etc. **HIGH**: Uses a consistent improvement methodology that yields demonstrated results; Team members understand the approach and actively use the methodology at every level; With all improvement efforts, the methodology is clearly followed and results are consistent; **MID:** Uses a consistent improvement methodology in most cases; Results are fairly consistent; Improvements are made rapidly and impact is quickly measured; Improvements that do not yield positive results are mostly reflected and improved upon; Most team members can talk to the methodology used and actively participate in improvement efforts; **LOW:** Results are sporadic and not typically sustained; Improvement efforts take considerable time to implement and frequently involve re-work; Improvements are leadership driven with little involvement from team members.	
Supervisor comments:	

(continued)

EXHIBIT 12.2
PMC Performance Appraisal Form: Practice Director's Annual Review *(continued)*

Section 3 - INDIVIDUAL/HOSPITAL GOALS

GOALS AGREED UPON BY EMPLOYEE AND SUPERVISOR	OVERALL RATING		
1. Inpatient Satisfaction Scores	3☐	2☐	1☐
2. AIDET Leader Validation Completed	3☐	2☐	1☐
3.	3☐	2☐	1☐
4.	3☐	2☐	1☐

OVERALL PERFORMANCE SCORE FROM MATRIX: ______________ *(attach matrix to evaluation)*

OVERALL PERFORMANCE CATEGORY FROM MATRIX: ☐ Exceeds ☐ Meets ☐ Below

MERIT INCREASE: As a part of the annual evaluation process review, Administration will review available budgetary resources and decide any percentages for an Exceeds or Meets overall rating. Merit increases usually are effective starting with the full first pay period in July.

EMPLOYEE COMMENTS:

EMPLOYEE ACKNOWLEDGMENT: This is to acknowledge that I have reviewed the above information and the attached job description. I understand that I should ask my immediate supervisor if I have questions regarding this information. I also understand that PMC may modify or alter the job description if in its sole judgment, it no longer serves the best interests of the patients or hospital.

Employee Signature Date

SUPERVISOR ACKNOWLEDGMENT: This is to acknowledge that I have reviewed the above information with the employee. I have included a copy of the evaluation matrix and the required annual competencies for this individual.

Direct Supervisor Date Human Resources (as needed) Date

Exhibit 12.3
PMC Performance Appraisal Form: Office Manager's Annual Review

Portneuf Medical Center Be well.	JOB DESCRIPTION AND PERFORMANCE EVALUATION FORM			
	Employee Name			
	Position Title:	Office Manager	**Effective Date:**	1/1/2015
	Department:	Medical Practices	**Last Revision:**	10/27/2016
	Review Responsibility:	Practice Director	**FLSA Status:**	Non Exempt

Position Summary: To provide operational support services, assisting the practice to deliver exceptional patient care and service with a high degree of reliability. The operational support services include, but are not limited to: Assures staffing levels match that of patient demand; Ensures work standards are being followed and exceptions are highlighted as improvement opportunities; Manages supplies and other materials to ensure no disruption to patient or team member flows; Performs daily audits to ensure charge capture processes are working effectively and accurately represent the work performed. Conducts daily huddles with team members in order to facilitate staff engagement, continuous improvement activities, and timely & accurate communication. This position represents an active member of the team and as such will be called upon to step into any clinic functions he/she is qualified/licensed to perform.

Minimum Qualifications:

- Associate Degree in Healthcare Administration or related field or equivalent experience
- Minimum of five years experience working in a medical office environment; one to two years supervisory experience preferred. (Equivalent educational experience may be considered.)

Essential Job Functions:

- Analyze results, derive conclusions and recommend improvement activities and priorities.
- Read financial data in order to prioritize activities that improve the financial health of the practice.
- Effectively communicate vertically and horizontally throughout the organization and externally to patients and other stakeholders.
- Inspire others and the credibility to enlist action.
- Utilize a scientific approach to problem solving utilizing scientific method, lean, Six Sigma, etc.

Knowledge, Skills and Abilities:

- Demonstrate sound judgment, patience and maintain a professional demeanor at all times
- Ability to work in a busy and stressful environment
- Organizational skills and the ability to prioritize
- Computer skills: Word, Excel, Outlook, Electronic medical records software
- Strong interpersonal verbal and written communication skills
- Creativity, problem analysis and decision making
- Ability to work varied shifts

(continued)

EXHIBIT 12.3
PMC Performance Appraisal Form: Office Manager's Annual Review *(continued)*

Work Positions & Activities *N = Not at all 0-10% O = Occasionally (10-35%)* *F = Frequently (35-66%) C = Continually (67-100%)*	
1. Lift (floor to waist)	
a. Up to 10 pounds (sedentary)	F
b. 11-20 pounds (Light)	O
c. 21-50 pounds (Medium)	O
d. 51-100 pounds (Heavy)	N
e. >100 pounds (Very Heavy)	N
2. Lift (over head)	
a. Up to 10 pounds (sedentary)	O
b. 11-20 pounds (Light)	O
c. 21-50 pounds (Medium)	O
d. 51-100 pounds (Heavy)	N
e. >100 pounds (Very Heavy)	N
3. Patient Transfer: (weight per employee)	
a. <50 pounds	N
b. >50 pounds	N
c. >100 pounds	N
d. >150 pounds	N
4. Carry	
a. Up to 10 pounds (sedentary)	F
b. 11-20 pounds (Light)	O
c. 21-50 pounds (Medium)	O
d. 51-100 pounds (Heavy)	N
e. >100 pounds (Very Heavy)	N
5. Push or pull	
a. Up to 10 pounds (sedentary)	O
b. 11-20 pounds (Light)	O
c. 21-50 pounds (Medium)	O
d. 51-100 pounds (Heavy)	O
e. >100 pounds (Very Heavy)	N
6. Climb (stairs) - climb & descend	O
7. Reach	F
8. Stoop or bend	O
9. Crouch	O
10. Kneel	O
11. Handle or feel	F
12. Talk	C
13. Hear	C
14. See	C
15. Sit (continuous)	
a. 30 minutes	F
b. 60 minutes	F
c. 1-3 hours	F
d. 3-6 hours	O
16. Walk	F

17. Stand (continuous)	
a. 30 minutes	O
b. 60 minutes	N
c. 1-3 hours	N
d. 3-6 hours	N
18. Repetitive activities (continuous)	
a. 30 minutes	O
b. 60 minutes	O
c. 1-3 hours	N
d. 3-6 hours	N
Mental Demands *(Y = Yes or N = No)*	
a. Alertness	Y
b. Precision	Y
c. Analytic ability	Y
d. Problem Solving	Y
e. Memory	Y
f. Communication	Y
g. Creativity	Y
h. Concentration	Y
i. Judgment	Y
j. Imagination	Y
k. Initiative	Y
l. Patience	Y
Work Environment *(Y = Yes or N = No)*	
a. Inside work	Y
b. Outside work	N
c. Noise	Y
d. Vibration	N
e. Wet/Humid	N
Hazard Exposure/risk of bodily illness/ injury	
a. Mechanical	O
b. Electrical	O
c. Explosives	N
d. Burns	N
e. Chemicals	N
f. Fumes/Gases/Odors	N
g. Toxic waste	N
h. Frequent travel	N
i. Long/irregular hours	N
j. Cramped/confined work area	N
k. Moving machinery	N
l. Ionizing radiation	N
m. Strong magnetic fields	N
n. Biochemical hazards/waste	Y
o. Blood borne pathogens	N
p. TB Mask Fitting	N

Exhibit 12.3
PMC Performance Appraisal Form: Office Manager's Annual Review *(continued)*

Section 1 – Hospital Wide Performance Areas

Check the rating that most closely matches the behavior. Comments or examples of specific behavior should be added to explain or illustrate the job behavior. Ratings must be supported by comments.

3 – High or Exceeds Standard(s): Clearly outstanding; always exceeds job requirements and expectations. Performance role model for others providing an exceptional contribution
2 – Mid or Meets Standard(s): Solid contributor. Understands duties and consistently meets standards, policies and practices. Generally needs little oversight with a little room to grow to become a high performer.
1 – Below Standard(s): Understands duties and may meet minimal standards, policies or practices. Performance issues are identified and the employee is actively working on them; continued improvement is needed.

Lives the Values: Professionalism and Continuous Improvement	Overall Rating 3 ☐ 2 ☐ 1 ☐
HIGH: Values diversity and embraces ideas from others. Stays current with knowledge through learning; Approaches situations and problems with a fresh perspective; Adapts to change with a positive attitude. Recognizes failure, apologizes and tries again; **MID:** Willing to listen to others ideas. Has a solid knowledge of hospital policies and procedures. Understands innovation however may sometimes lean towards staying the course. Goes with and supports change when implemented; Will apologize when recognized; **LOW:** Can be stuck on 'the way we do things here' mentality. Does not keep current in field; May point out problems or poke holes at the ideas of others. May also make changes without input/discussion or thinking of ripple effects of actions. Resists change and/or feedback. Does not consistently apologize.	
Supervisor comments:	

Lives the Values: Ownership, Integrity and Ethics	Overall Rating 3 ☐ 2 ☐ 1 ☐
HIGH: Is accountable for their actions, expectations, and outcomes. Is honest with him/herself and others; is loyal even to those not present. Treats others with respect; does not gossip; Approaches conflict directly, privately, and with a desire to improve the relationship. Always behaves ethically and honestly; Accepts responsibility for own decisions and actions. **MID**: Is mostly accountable for their actions, expectations, and outcomes. Is honest with others; is generally loyal. Treats others with respect; Deals with conflict and resolves issues. Solid person with no significant issues; **LOW:** At times this person attempts to deflect or avoid being accountable. Tends to say what others want to hear. Can be passive aggressive or overtly disruptive interpersonally. Is not consistently honest, respectful and/or loyal in word and deed.	
Supervisor comments:	

Lives the Values: Communication and Problem Solving	Overall Rating 3 ☐ 2 ☐ 1 ☐
HIGH: Approaches every individual with caring and concern. Takes the time to listen; seeks to put other's needs before their own. Connects with others to relieve their stress, anxiety and resolve their concerns; Goes outside comfort zone; Finds appropriate individual(s) if outside scope of services. **MID:** Practices active listening. Restates or paraphrases while communicating for understanding. Is usually seen as sincere in their interpersonal relationships; Fosters understanding and has minimal misunderstandings and conflicts. Generally solves problems. **LOW:** Tends to listen with the intent to reply, not to understand. Seems to knows what they will say before others finish. Filters through their life experiences, their frame of reference; May not 'get' or acknowledge how others are feeling. Solves issues if confronted or required.	
Supervisor comments:	

(continued)

EXHIBIT 12.3
PMC Performance Appraisal Form: Office Manager's Annual Review *(continued)*

LIVES THE VALUES: PERSONAL ENGAGEMENT	OVERALL RATING 3 ☐ 2 ☐ 1 ☐
HIGH: Adds joy and enriches life at PMC. Is happy; recognizes the good around us; Works hard, and takes time off to recharge. Celebrates personal success as well as the success of others; is involved in employee celebration events; knows others in some measure outside of work. **MID:** Is a positive person. Contributes to PMC; May need to make more time to recharge. Celebrates the success of others; could be seen as needing to open up a little more or show more enthusiasm. May miss some employee celebrations; Relationships and/or interactions are generally work related in nature. **LOW:** Is seen as indifferent or not a positive person. Does their job and no more; looks to get things done and off the to-do pile. Does not consistently thank and/or recognize the efforts/success of others. May dampen excitement and enthusiasm. Not interested in staff and/or hospital outside of work relationship.	
Supervisor comments:	

LIVES THE VALUES: TEAMWORK	OVERALL RATING 3 ☐ 2 ☐ 1 ☐
HIGH: Coordinates efforts at every opportunity. Recognizes need for others. Trusts others and engenders their trust. Faces challenges by working with others. Collaborates, and coordinates improvement. Adds synergy and completes assignments. **MID:** Committed to improving performance of work unit and organization. Is generally trustworthy; eventually deals with challenges. Sometimes delays others. Solid team player however may not consistently demonstrate amazing teamwork. **LOW:** Tendency to micro-manage. May spend too much time on less critical issues delaying the team. Trust may be shaky at times. May meddle in non-important details; Deals with work or challenges if confronted or reminded. Gives appearance of team work but lacks consistently demonstrated substance.	
Supervisor comments:	

LIVES THE VALUES: SERVICE - EVERY PATIENT EVERY TIME	OVERALL RATING 3 ☐ 2 ☐ 1 ☐
Consider how the individual ensures that patient care and/or customer service is the highest priority. How well does this individual model, teach and consistently demonstrate AIDET, MANAGING UP, KEY WORDS AT KEY TIMES and WORLD CLASS CARE EVERY PATIENT EVERY TIME?	
Supervisor comments:	

LIVES THE VALUES: ORGANIZATIONAL ACCOUNTABILITY	OVERALL RATING 3 ☐ 2 ☐ 1 ☐
Is highly productive; completes assignments timely or communicates delays; Attendance is consistent. Looks for strengths, is optimistic; empowers people. Demonstrates a caring attitude. Integrates safety and safety guidelines into their work; Looks for and promotes patient and staff safety. Knows and consistently follows departmental and hospital policies and procedures; Completes licensing, education, competencies and other requirements in a timely manner. Knowledge and ability to respond to emergency preparedness procedures and to report safety issues (e.g. employee injury, patient safety, variance and equipment failures).	
Supervisor comments:	

EXHIBIT 12.3
PMC Performance Appraisal Form: Office Manager's Annual Review *(continued)*

SECTION 2 – ESSENTIAL JOB FUNCTIONS

ESSENTIAL JOB FUNCTION/STANDARD **OVERALL RATING** 3 ☐ 2 ☐ 1 ☐

Data Analytics: Analyze results, derive conclusions and recommend improvement activities and priorities.
HIGH: Shares data with team on a daily basis; Frequently re-evaluates data being shared to determine relevance to the team; When data is not available electronically – he/she will create it; **MID:** Visual boards used to share data are creative and staff understand how they impact data; Data is mostly kept current; Team members are clear on the goals of the practice; Team members can use the data to focus their efforts; **LOW:** Data is not readily available to team members, accurate or up-to date; Blames the lack of data on others or the source as not trustworthy.

Supervisor comments:

ESSENTIAL JOB FUNCTION/STANDARD **OVERALL RATING** 3 ☐ 2 ☐ 1 ☐

Financial Acumen: Read and analyze financial data in order to prioritize activities that improve the financial health of the practice.
HIGH: Leverages staffing ratios to appropriately manage staffing to patient demand; Evaluates medical supplies and other materials for cost savings; **MID:** When asked, can determine how many staff members should be working to match demand but may not always flex staffing without assistance; reviews daily charges and with reasonable accuracy match charges to the work performed; Can quickly identify supply or material charges that are excessive; **LOW:** Does not flex staff appropriately creating excess and/or short-staffed situations; Unable to match charges to work performed with proficiency; Expense anomalies are largely unnoticed.

Supervisor comments:

ESSENTIAL JOB FUNCTION/STANDARD **OVERALL RATING** 3 ☐ 2 ☐ 1 ☐

Communication: Effectively communicate vertically and horizontally throughout the organization and externally to patients and other stakeholders.
HIGH: All team members can clearly articulate how their individual role ties to the goals of the practice; Goals are visible as is progress towards those goals; Stakeholders in the practice are aware of the goals and are included in improvement activities; Teaches others how to effectively communicate with patients and other guests; **MID:** Can clearly articulate the goals, current state and barriers to team members and stakeholders; Effectively solicits help from Practice Administrator and others as applicable; Can share information in a succinct but meaningful way; Can tell meaningful stories to engage others; **LOW:** Team members have no clear connection with the work they do and the practice goals; Communications may cause confusion and require clarification from others; Communcations with patients does not likely result in the de-escalation of issues.

Supervisor comments:

(continued)

EXHIBIT 12.3
PMC Performance Appraisal Form: Office Manager's Annual Review *(continued)*

ESSENTIAL JOB FUNCTION/STANDARD	OVERALL RATING 3 ☐ 2 ☐ 1 ☐
Leadership: Inspire others and the credibility to enlist action. **HIGH**: Team members actively participate in improvement activities; Leads by example even when it's difficult; Rewards and recognizes individual contributors in the daily huddle and provides accurate scouting reports for Practice Administrator; **MID:** Frequently walks in the shoes of each team member; Mostly leads by example; Escalates issues timely while there is momentum behind improvement efforts; Consistently looking for ways to improve the patient journey and team member job satisfaction; **LOW:** May lay blame for negative outcomes; Spends majority of time in the office and/or in meetings; Complacent and satisfied with the current state.	
Supervisor comments:	

ESSENTIAL JOB FUNCTION/STANDARD	OVERALL RATING 3 ☐ 2 ☐ 1 ☐
Process Improvement: Utilize a scientific approach to problem solving utilizing scientific method, lean, Six Sigma, etc. **HIGH**: Frequently tries new solutions that are targeted to improve specific aspects of the practice; Sees failure as a learning opportunity and does not fear it; Consistently demonstrates a willingness to try new approaches; With all improvement efforts, the methodology is clearly followed; **MID:** Uses a consistent improvement methodology in most cases; Results are fairly consistent; Improvements are made rapidly and impact is quickly measured; Improvements that do not yield positive results are mostly reflected and improved upon; Most team members can talk to the methodology used and actively participate in improvement efforts; **LOW:** Results are sporadic and not typically sustained; Improvement efforts take considerable time to implement and frequently involve re-work; Improvements have little involvement from team members.	
Supervisor comments:	

Exhibit 12.3
PMC Performance Appraisal Form: Office Manager's Annual Review *(continued)*

Section 3 - Individual/Hospital Goals

GOALS AGREED UPON BY EMPLOYEE AND SUPERVISOR	Overall Rating		
1. Inpatient Satisfaction Scores	3☐	2☐	1☐
2. AIDET Leader Validation Completed	3☐	2☐	1☐
3.	3☐	2☐	1☐
4.	3☐	2☐	1☐

OVERALL PERFORMANCE SCORE FROM MATRIX: ____________________ *(attach matrix to evaluation)*

OVERALL PERFORMANCE CATEGORY FROM MATRIX: ☐ Exceeds ☐ Meets ☐ Below

MERIT INCREASE: As a part of the annual evaluation process review, Administration will review available budgetary resources and decide any percentages for an Exceeds or Meets overall rating. Merit increases usually are effective starting with the full first pay period in July.

EMPLOYEE COMMENTS:

EMPLOYEE ACKNOWLEDGMENT: This is to acknowledge that I have reviewed the above information and the attached job description. I understand that I should ask my immediate supervisor if I have questions regarding this information. I also understand that PMC may modify or alter the job description if in its sole judgment, it no longer serves the best interests of the patients or hospital.

Employee Signature　　Date

SUPERVISOR ACKNOWLEDGMENT: This is to acknowledge that I have reviewed the above information with the employee. I have included a copy of the evalaution matrix and the required annual competencies for this individual.

Direct Supervisor　　Date　　Human Resources (as needed)　　Date

CHAPTER 13

STRATEGIC PLANNING AND MARKETING

Important Terms

- Ancillary services
- Competitive advantage
- Covered lives
- Employer-sponsored insurance
- HCAHPS scores
- Health literacy
- Health promotion
- Medical staff privileges
- Mission statement
- Provider network
- Scenario planning
- Social marketing
- Strategy development
- Strategy implementation
- SWOT analysis: Strengths, Weaknesses, Opportunities, and Threats
- Tactical (operating) plan
- Values statement
- Vision statement

Learning Objectives

After reading this chapter, you will be able to do the following:

- ➤ Perform a SWOT analysis
- ➤ Discuss several different planning models
- ➤ Understand the difference between strategy identification and strategy implementation
- ➤ Understand the importance of organizational mission, vision, and values
- ➤ Explain the difference between a strategic plan and an operating plan

- Distinguish between strategy and marketing
- Understand key markets for healthcare providers
- Understand important communication techniques in marketing

Case Study: Wellbe Hospital—What Should We Do?

Wellbe Hospital is located in the rural community of Derricksville, which has a population of approximately 6,000. Like many small towns throughout the rust belt, Derricksville has seen more prosperous times. The oil industry, once a staple of the local economy, has long since migrated to places that still have oil. Likewise, the milling industry, formerly the other large player in the local economy, has completely collapsed. Today, the pride of the community's economic development effort is a new Super 8 Inn and a Walmart. Many people in the community are now relieved they no longer need to drive 30 miles to buy basic things like socks.

Derricksville's population once was 15,000. Having lost the bulk of its economic base, the largest employers are now the school district and the hospital. The surrounding counties are, likewise, seemingly at economic nadirs. There are no major communities, nor even major highways, in this region. In addition, there are no major economic development activities underway. In short, the four-county region that comprises the core of Wellbe's market is a significantly depressed area.

Over the past decade, the region has seen an influx of African-Americans. While this group represents a very small percentage of the population, it has grown by approximately 40 percent. The white population, in proportional terms, has decreased only slightly, reflecting the fact that minorities make up less than 5 percent of the population in the four-county area. The total population among these four counties has, over the last five years, declined by approximately 3,600 people—a slide of about 1.8 percent.

As the local economy withered during the last 20 years, large employers either shuttered their doors or left for greener pastures. Increasingly, young people growing up in Derricksville, believing there is no economic opportunity there, are reluctant to stay after finishing high school. Many do not pursue a college education, but leave the community for better economic opportunities elsewhere or for life in the military.

In a nutshell, the number of employers has declined, the number of employed people has declined, and so, too, has the number of residents with commercial health insurance. In addition, the community has lost a substantial portion of its population between the ages of 17 and 64. The proportion of the population aged 60 and older is growing, which has a significant long-term impact. Exhibit 13.1 demonstrates the problem.

Wellbe Hospital is a typical small community hospital. Licensed for 100 beds, it successfully staffs around 50. This means the hospital's license from the state permits it to have 100 beds (and patients), but for a variety of reasons (e.g., diminished need, inability to recruit

Exhibit 13.1 Wellbe Hospital Market Population Distribution, Years 2000, 2010, and 2020, by Selected Age Group

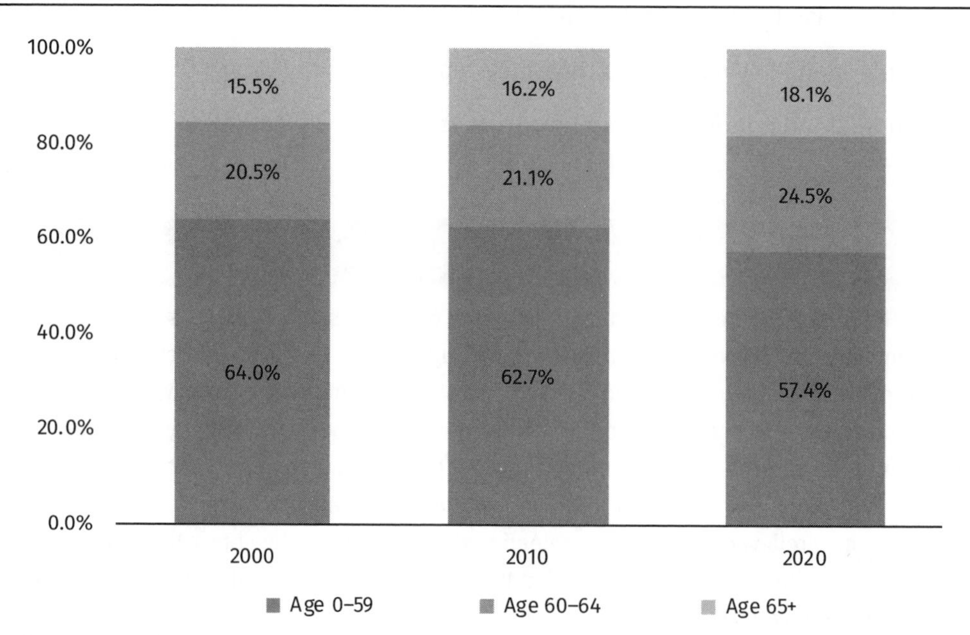

appropriate staff) the hospital operates at half its capacity, or "staffs" only 50 beds. From 2012 to 2017, total admissions dropped from 3,453 to 2,465. In 2017, the payer mix was 58.4 percent revenue from Medicare, 22.8 percent revenue from Medicaid, and 18.8 percent revenue from those patients with commercial insurance coverage. Wellbe enjoys strong loyalty from the people who know it; however, that is a diminishing number given the population trends in the region.

The administration at Wellbe is experienced; the CEO has been in the job for 12 years. His senior staff—including the chief financial officer, chief nursing officer, and the vice president for human resources—are all people he recruited to their jobs, and they all have been in place for at least five years. When the CEO first arrived, Wellbe was in dire financial straits. But because of his management acumen, the CEO is credited with "saving" the hospital. Unafraid to make tough decisions, he reduced staffing to 3.4 full-time equivalent employees per staffed bed, from nearly 4.25. Likewise, he has called on Wellbe's foundation to provide funds for some necessary expenditures. So far, Wellbe's "wall-to-wall" union staff has accepted management's explanations for the cuts and not threatened to strike.

The nursing staff is very competent. Indeed, the hospital enjoys a reputation in the community for having a caring staff. People generally appreciate that the hospital knows its limits and sticks to providing routine care well and avoiding advanced procedures that exceed its capabilities. This is partly a necessity, as an aging medical staff has created vacancies in key subspecialties. There is adequate primary care in the community, but a group of internal medicine physicians has had a quarrelsome relationship with the hospital. This is critical given the referral patterns from these physicians to subspecialists. Virtually no one wants this physician group to start sending—referring—its patients to specialists outside of Wellbe Hospital. Thus, many doctors are concerned about the state of relations between the hospital and this physician group. In addition, both recruitment and retention of certain types of physicians is problematic.

In particular, resources for general surgery (procedures on the abdomen and digestive tracts) are a major concern. One senior surgeon recently retired, and two others left the community for more robust practice opportunities elsewhere. The hospital has recruited only one new surgeon, and she has yet to gain the full confidence of referring doctors. Likewise, the sole urologist in town has announced his retirement, and the otolaryngologist (ear, nose, and throat specialist) is departing for a better opportunity. While the primary orthopedic surgeon is very competent, his bedside manner is somewhat gruff in the eyes of patients. He splits his practice between Wellbe and another hospital. His partner, with a smaller patient load, does the same, but spends most of his time in a competitor hospital. Some doctors complain about the hospital recruiting inept physicians; some members of the community wish the hospital would end the "turnstile" nature of the medical staff.

The nearest competitor hospital is 25 miles to the west. Located in the county seat, it is a medium-sized community hospital and has been successful in luring significant orthopedic business away from Wellbe because of the outstanding reputation of one of its local orthopedic surgeons. In addition, a major integrated delivery system associated with an academic health center has opened a hospital approximately 35 miles away to the south and west, in Shaleville. While local residents are resentful of the origins of this—it was an outgrowth of the closure of a community hospital—it offers high-quality care and access to one of the nation's leading medical centers. The impact of this institution on Wellbe is unclear. Finally, to the north, just beyond Wellbe's market area, is a larger community served by two hospitals, one of which is a major tertiary care center. While these hospitals do not compete with Wellbe in its primary market, they both seem to be gaining some market share at the market fringes. Wellbe has an alliance with the cancer center at the larger of these two hospitals, but otherwise has no major alliances with any other provider. There are no competitors, nor much population, to the east.

Introduction

It would seem that Wellbe Hospital is in a difficult situation. Imagine you are a new staff analyst there charged with coordinating the development of a strategic plan. Throwing up your hands and screaming, "I give up!" is not an option. As a healthcare leader, your job is to ensure the availability of good-quality healthcare to the people of Derricksville and the surrounding area. Note the term *good-quality healthcare*. To provide this, Wellbe Hospital needs to find a **competitive advantage** relative to its competitors and prospective competitors in the region (Porter 1985). As mentioned in the case study, Wellbe "knows its limits" and avoids taking on patients with complex conditions it is not capable of treating, or who

Competitive advantage
A set of attributes that puts a company in a favorable or superior business position.

Mission statement
An enduring statement of purpose defining what an organization does, whom it serves, and how it does it.

Vision statement
A statement identifying a specific desired future state of an organization; usually an inspiring goal for the organization many years into the future.

Values statement
A statement defining an organization's culture. It expresses values that are important and that guide the organization's work and its interactions with patients, the community, and employees.

need specialized medical procedures it is not able to perform. Thus, your job in planning for Wellbe's future is to sort out the kinds of medical services the Derricksville community requires and match those with the hospital's capabilities. The hospital and its medical staff will have to refer out any procedures beyond their expertise. The hospital must maximize the things it *can* do well and use those skills to address the community's needs.

So how do you go about doing all that? Begin at the beginning. Ask, Why is the hospital here? What should it be doing in the future? What does it, as an organization, care about? Exhibit 13.2 shows a simplified conceptualization of what a strategic planning process might look like. We will follow this model for Wellbe Hospital throughout this chapter.

Mission, Vision, and Values

Every hospital has a **mission statement**; most have **vision** and **values statements** as well. These represent the core of the hospital's being, its reason for existing, its ambitions for the future, and the principles that govern how it does its work.

Why are the mission, vision, and values (MVV) important in the planning process? The three reasons are as simple as the terms themselves. First, an organization cannot plan for the future if it does not have a clear understanding of what it does and why. If you do not know who you are, how can you define who you will be and how you can get there? Second, if an organization does not have a vision for its own future then how does it know what path to take to get there? In the immortal words of Zig Ziglar, "If you aim at nothing, you will hit it every time" (Ziglar 1976). Finally, without values—that is, without a moral compass—the work has no meaning. Values are the core of the character of an organization.

Exhibit 13.2 Example of a Strategic Planning Process

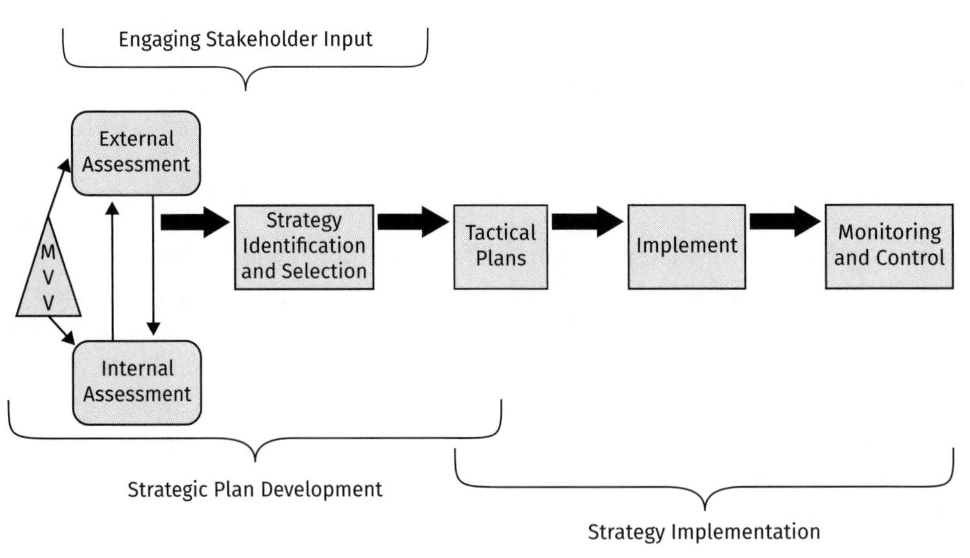

Note: MVV = Mission, vision, and values.

If a cancer center has been successful at saving lives, but then covers up a radiation mistake that cost the lives of others, has it produced ethically valuable work to the best of its capability? Why should potential patients trust that center? The MVV concept at the core of a planning effort is essential to determining an organization's future direction. As you will see, however, while the MVV is foundational, there is much more to an effective planning effort (Ginter, Duncan, and Swayne 2013). This is the first step in **strategy development**. Using appropriate planning tools to develop a thorough understanding of the organization's capabilities and its place in the larger community is the next step.

Strategy development
The part of the planning process in which the organization assesses its internal and external environments and begins to match capability with opportunity to lay the foundation for a strategic plan.

Planning Tools and Their Use

Strategic planning in a healthcare organization setting is a complex function. Healthcare is a unique enterprise that marries business principles with the often-conflicting mission of serving the community by caring for patients regardless of their ability to pay. For that reason, the planning process needs to account for both: It must recognize and acknowledge the obligation the organization has to the community while laying the groundwork to ensure adequate resources remain to sustain and grow the organization.

Some organizations, notably hospitals and large multidisciplinary clinics, will have in-house planning departments. Many other organizations do not have the resources to coordinate planning next to their day-to-day functions and regard such an internal office as a luxury. Regardless, organizations frequently retain consultants to assist with the planning process. The level of a consultant's involvement will vary based on an organization's need and its capacity to do the work, which will depend on issues such as in-house planning staff, analysts, and budget. Some organizations will retain a consultant to do everything from research and analyze data, facilitate stakeholder interaction, and write the final planning document. Others may just want someone to facilitate a focus group among managers. Still others may engage the services of an outside expert to facilitate a more extensive planning retreat. The essential point is that outside expertise is a resource healthcare organizations routinely employ to develop a strategic plan. In this chapter you will learn about some tools that can be applied to the planning process, but understand this is only a sample framework and a basic introduction.

There are many frequently used planning tools to help an organization develop a strategic plan, such as SWOT or the BCG Matrix, discussed later. To produce an effective plan for the future, the organization needs to have a thorough understanding of itself beyond its MVV. It will need to drill down on operational details to understand clearly what it does well, what it can do better, and where it might have additional potential or capacity.

Likewise, an organization must look to the outside world to understand where it fits in the external environment. No organization—particularly health services organizations such as hospitals—exist on an isolated island free from all the encumbrances of their earthly environment. The organization is a symbiotic element of the larger community: It affects, and is affected by, the larger community it serves. Therefore, it is essential that an organization also have a thorough understanding of its external environment and the community it serves (Harris 2018).

Exhibit 13.3
Conceptual Model of a SWOT Analysis

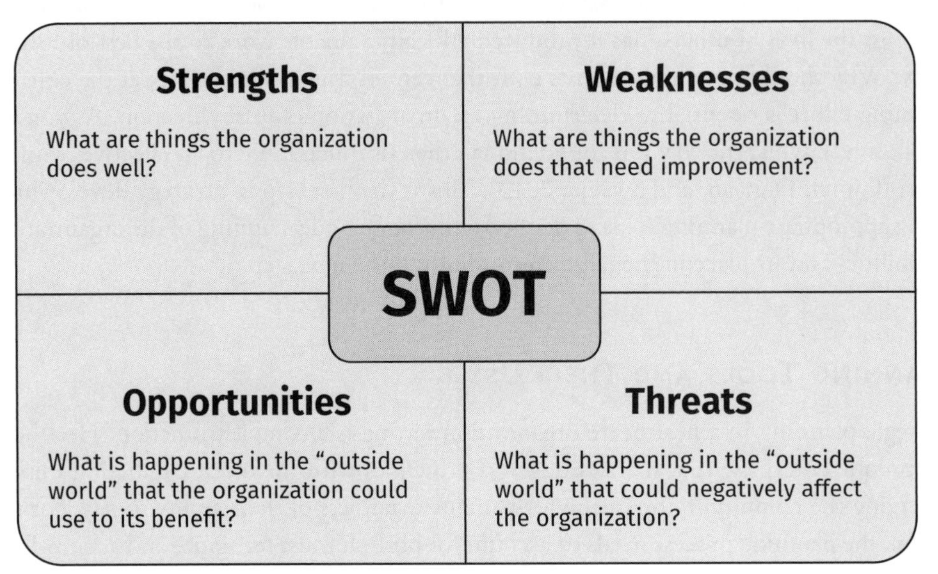

Strengths
What are things the organization does well?
Weaknesses
What are things the organization does that need improvement?
SWOT
Opportunities
What is happening in the "outside world" that the organization could use to its benefit?
Threats
What is happening in the "outside world" that could negatively affect the organization?

Here is a sample of some of the more frequently used tools and a brief description of each to give you a better understanding of how an organization might approach the process of ferreting out all of the internal and external data it needs to develop an effective strategic map to the future.

SWOT
Stands for strengths, weaknesses, opportunities, and threats. A basic tool of internal and external assessment that any organization can use as part of its strategic planning.

SWOT Analysis: First developed in 1965 by Albert Humphrey at the Stanford Research Institute, this is a process used to identify an organization's Strengths, Weaknesses, Opportunities, and Threats (Humphrey 2005). More specifically, **SWOT** is a relatively simple analytical framework used to assess the capabilities of an entity (in this case, a hospital) for factors both internal (the strengths and weaknesses) as well as external (the potential opportunities and threats). Once an organization matches its internal assessment with its external assessment, it should be able to sharpen its focus on projects that will facilitate its growth (Ginter, Duncan, and Swayne 2013). Exhibit 13.3 provides a model of a SWOT.

Boston Consulting Group Matrix

The Boston Consulting Group (BCG) developed a strategic analysis that compares an organization's market share with the anticipated growth of its market over the next five years (BCG 1973). The BCG Matrix is sometimes referred to as a *portfolio analysis tool* because it can be used to analyze the market progress of an entire organization, a division or other business unit of a company, or an individual product or service. While it has tremendous flexibility, it requires that the user understand the existing market share of the organization and have the ability to make an informed projection about the market's future. Perhaps the most novel, and most fun, aspect of

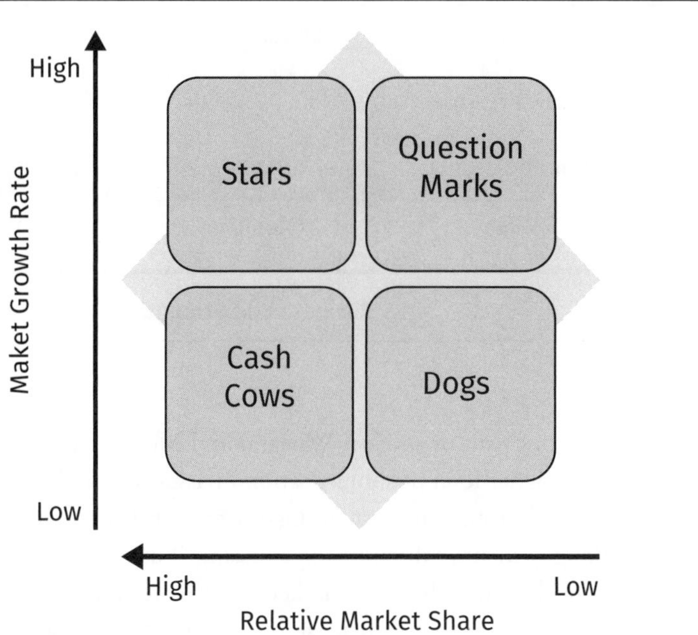

Exhibit 13.4 Boston Consulting Group Matrix Model

the BCG Matrix are the names it uses to characterize its outcomes: Stars, Question Marks, Cash Cows, and Dogs (Hambrick, MacMilan, and Day 1982). Exhibit 13.4 provides a graphic example.

In this framework, "Stars" are products, services, organizations, or business units that have a high relative market share in a market that is growing; "Cash Cows" are those entities that have a high share of their market, but in a market that displays little growth. Conversely, "Question Marks" (sometimes called "Problem Children/Child") are those with low market share in an expanding market, while "Dogs" are what you might expect: organizations with low market share in a no-growth or slow-growth market (Wayland and McDonald 2016).

In a business sense, the aspiration would be to develop strategies that would move Question Marks to Stars by capturing greater market share. Likewise, an organization would want to divest itself of Dogs or transform them into Cash Cows, again by capturing greater market share. Market growth rate is not something a business can necessarily control, so altering that variable is not a realistic option.

General Electric Matrix

The General Electric (GE) Matrix, also known as the GE/McKinsey Matrix (because GE developed it in concert with the consulting firm McKinsey and Company) is similar to the BCG Matrix, but is slightly more complex. A nine-box tool used to assess market attractiveness and business strength, it is flexible like the BCG Matrix in that it can be applied to an entire company, a division, or a single product or service (Jurevicius 2014). It also can be

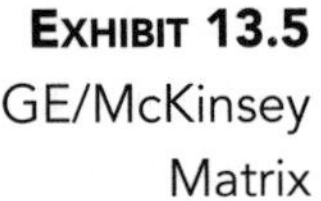

Exhibit 13.5
GE/McKinsey Matrix

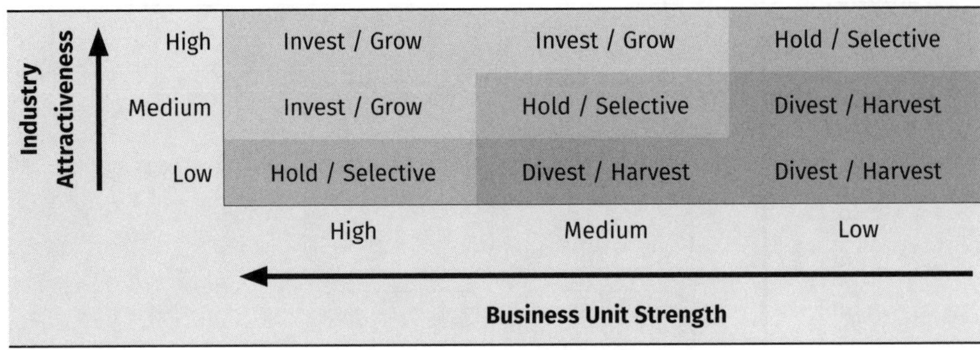

used to analyze more than one unit or service (Wayland and McDonald 2016). However, the GE Matrix demands a higher level of sophistication in assessing market attractiveness and business strength, and a thorough understanding of what constitutes "attractiveness" is an absolute necessity, along with strict discipline in assessing "business strength."

"Attractiveness" considers such things as market growth rate and size, industry profitability, variability of demand, and other similar factors. Each factor is weighted and then used to calculate the market's attractiveness. "Business Strength" requires the user to examine market share, growth in market share, profit margins relative to competitors, and similar factors. Then, the user performs another calculation before plotting the results in the nine-box grid (Quick MBA 2010). The formulas provide a quantitative basis by which to make a decision regarding the future of the business or product subject to the analysis. See exhibit 13.5 for a graphic display of the GE /McKinsey Matrix.

A Closer Look at Wellbe Hospital

Before we begin the planning process for Wellbe Hospital, let us examine its MVV statements:

- *Mission:* Wellbe Hospital is committed to providing quality healthcare services to the residents of our community, with an emphasis on personal attention, compassion, and respect.
- *Vision:* Our vision is to continually exceed the expectations of those we serve by working together as a team, dedicated to a process of never-ending improvements.
- *Values:* The health, safety, and satisfaction of our patients are extremely important to our staff. When you seek our help, you can rest assured that you have a say in your care and will be treated with the respect you deserve.

It is clear that Wellbe Hospital is committed to the people of the local community; desires to always exceed expectations by continually improving; and values treating patients with respect. What you do *not* see here is an ambition to grow into a regional or national healthcare system. Nor do you sense an interest in becoming a more research-focused, academic organization that would contribute to medical knowledge by conducting research and educating future physicians. Furthermore, you do not see an expression of interest in expanding the breadth of its services. What the MVV statements *do* say, basically, is that Wellbe is a good community hospital desiring to improve continually the care it provides to the residents of its community and to treat those patients respectfully as individuals, not as another clinical exercise. This is critical to understand at the beginning of the planning process as it helps set some boundaries on the outcomes. It would make little sense, in the shadow of the MVV as stated, to plan for advanced cardiac surgery, to initiate tertiary services like organ transplants, or to attempt to open a medical school, as examples.

SWOT Applied to Wellbe

As noted earlier, it would be possible to apply several strategic planning tools to the situation at Wellbe Hospital. For the purposes of this chapter, we will use SWOT analysis. Both the BCG and the GE/McKinsey models are advanced tools that require much more data than available here and more analytical rigor than appropriate for this book.

SWOT encompasses both an internal and an external element. The internal assessment element consists of evaluating the hospital's strengths and weaknesses; the external assessment is about opportunities and threats (Ginter, Duncan, and Swayne 2013). The process begins with an internal assessment so users can develop a clear picture of their organization's current status.

Wellbe's Strengths and Weaknesses

Strengths and weaknesses are inherently internal to an organization. They are, respectively, things the organization does well and the areas where it needs to improve. These have nothing to do with what a competitor may be doing, for example. They are only about one's own organization, in this case Wellbe Hospital. To assess strengths and weaknesses, consider elements like these:

- Organizational performance
- Financial condition
- Strategic performance
- Clinical capabilities

- Physical plant
- Quality of personnel

The case at the beginning of the chapter paints a pretty bleak picture of Wellbe's circumstances. There are, however, some positive elements in the complicated mosaic. What are they? If you read the facts carefully, you should see at least some of the strengths and weaknesses listed in exhibit 13.6. But how do you know whether to characterize a factor as a strength or a weakness? For example, why is "declining volume in orthopedic surgery" a weakness—an internal factor within Wellbe's control—if it is seemingly the result of the nearby hospital's good reputation in orthopedics? It is considered internal, and a weakness, because in this case Wellbe *can* determine its own fate by recruiting a good orthopedic surgeon (or two) who could turn the tide. The same concept is applicable to all the weaknesses: Wellbe Hospital can address them itself, regardless of the behavior or capability of a competitor.

One very important caveat about the conclusions shown in exhibit 13.6: In reading the facts of the case, different people might draw several different conclusions regarding strengths and weaknesses. Indeed, that is why it is important to engage various stakeholders in the process: to provide multiple perspectives and obtain a more comprehensive picture of the organization. Thus, this exhibit may not be exhaustive of all of Wellbe Hospital's strengths and weaknesses. This is but a representation of what those strengths and weaknesses might look like based on one person's reading of the case.

Completing our internal assessment means we are only half done with the SWOT analysis. The next step is the external assessment.

EXHIBIT 13.6
Internal Assessment Results for Wellbe Hospital

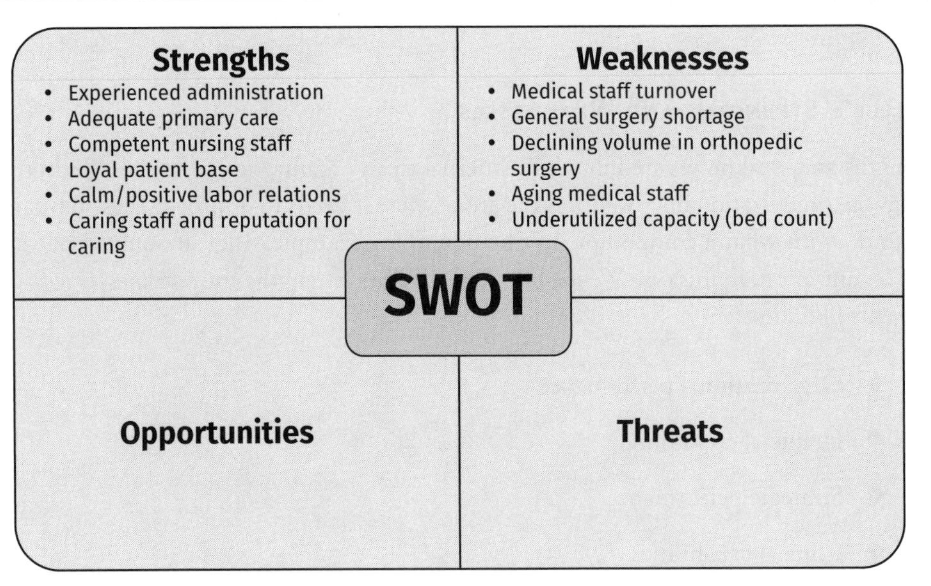
Strengths
• Experienced administration
• Adequate primary care
• Competent nursing staff
• Loyal patient base
• Calm/positive labor relations
• Caring staff and reputation for caring
Weaknesses
• Medical staff turnover
• General surgery shortage
• Declining volume in orthopedic surgery
• Aging medical staff
• Underutilized capacity (bed count)
SWOT
Opportunities
Threats

Wellbe's Threats and Opportunities

Threats and opportunities are inherently external to an organization. These are events and conditions in the external environment that could affect an organization's future, but over which the organization has no control. To assess threats and opportunities, examine such elements as the following:

- Market demographics
- Reimbursement trends
- Other healthcare organizations' activities
- Merger and acquisition trends
- Government regulations
- Local economy

When reviewing what is happening in the larger community, consider what factors can be an opportunity for the hospital. What is happening that might be a threat? Review exhibit 13.7.

Consider the threats first. Clearly, the local economy is a significant problem. The case study described the almost complete demise of local business and the decline in the number of commercially insured patients. This means the hospital is more reliant on public

Exhibit 13.7 Internal and External Assessment Results for Wellbe Hospital

SWOT

Strengths	Weaknesses
• Experienced administration • Adequate primary care • Competent nursing staff • Loyal patient base • Calm/positive labor relations • Caring staff and reputation for caring	• Medical staff turnover • General surgery shortage • Declining volume in orthopedic surgery • Aging medical staff • Underutilized capacity (bed count)
Opportunities	**Threats**
• Shaleville market • Geriatric population • Women's health • Outlying clinics • Recruitment of younger medical staff • Mergers and acquistions; alignment	• Local economy • Aging population • Stagnant population growth • Affordable Care Act • Mergers and acquisitions; alignment • Regional competition

insurance for compensation and, in particular, is increasingly dependent on Medicaid, which does not pay very well compared to either Medicare or commercial insurance. Compounding this problem is the fact that the population—and the economic base—are not growing. If anything, they are shrinking. We can see in exhibit 13.1, for example, that the portion of the population ages 0 to 59 is shrinking relative to the overall population. As a whole, the local population is aging, and that will become a significant threat to Wellbe Hospital for an unsettling reason: We know that the hospital is heavily reliant on Medicare, and Medicare patients are, by definition, mostly senior citizens. That means their life expectancy is relatively short, so the hospital will lose Medicare reimbursement as those residents pass away. Even as the portion of the population ages 60 to 64 has increased slightly, this will only delay the inevitable, because the 0-to-59 portion is shrinking. In the long term, this will increase the hospital's reliance on Medicaid, and it will come to occupy a larger share of the hospital's overall revenue. In addition, mergers and acquisitions are a "threat" because surrounding hospitals may gradually align with one another to strengthen their own competitive advantage relative to Wellbe. (This is also an opportunity because Wellbe might be able to align itself with another hospital or group of hospitals to preserve the integrity of the services it provides to the people of Derricksville.) Finally, the reimbursement mechanisms called for in the Affordable Care Act, specifically those that emphasize preventable readmissions and quality of care, could be a threat to Wellbe because the hospital does not yet have the capacity to meet the demands of that statute.

Now, let us look at the opportunities, for despite all these challenges Wellbe does have some chances to thrive in this environment. First, it could take advantage of the resentment toward the new hospital in Shaleville by locating a clinic there. Second, the geriatric nature of the population suggests Wellbe could profit from an intensified focus on specialized services for the elderly that are reimbursable under Medicare. Third, Wellbe has the opportunity to rebuild a younger medical staff by recruiting younger physicians and incentivizing them to stay in the immediate area. In addition, women's health can be an interesting opportunity: Women tend to make household care decisions, so appealing to their particular, specialized medical needs could have an impact beyond the target market (Matoff-Stepp et al. 2014). Women are also an important market in this particular case because they are expected to outlive their male counterparts. Finally, aligning with another organization is an opportunity that could provide Wellbe with the necessary tools to fill some of the gaps previously described.

The Planning Process

Now that you have conducted a basic SWOT analysis, you just need to write the planning memo matching those outcomes to the hospital capabilities and tell everyone involved to move ahead, right? Wrong. As tidy as that sounds, if an executive did that, the plan would never get off the ground.

Simply documenting the components of a SWOT analysis, as you did for Wellbe Hospital, is often the easy part of the process. You were able to take a shortcut of sorts in developing the SWOT for Wellbe Hospital in this book. The process of developing a SWOT in an actual setting is much more complicated, because for a plan to succeed, it needs to engage multiple groups of stakeholders.

Chapter 5 introduced the concept of stakeholders. These are people who have a vested interest in an organization's success. There are internal and external stakeholders, and engaging both groups in the planning process greatly increases the chances of successfully implementing a strategic plan. When stakeholders feel they have been engaged in the process, they are much more likely to support the planning group's decisions. Thus, groups like physicians, patients, patients' families, board of trustee members, managers, and others all should be included in the planning process. Accomplishing this is complicated because of the schedules of the people involved. In addition, some stakeholders may be more closely involved with the enterprise than others, which means their perspectives will likely be much better informed and more nuanced than the views of those with a more distant relationship. Exhibit 13.8 depicts stakeholder relationships to a hospital. The person leading the planning process will need to find different ways of engaging each group of stakeholders (Bonnafous-Boucher and Rendtorff 2016). The next sections will explore various methods.

Questionnaires

Questionnaires are a useful tool for gathering relatively simple, direct information. Using a questionnaire permits the questioner to, partly, direct the respondent's thoughts about

Exhibit 13.8
Relative Relationship of Stakeholders to a Hospital

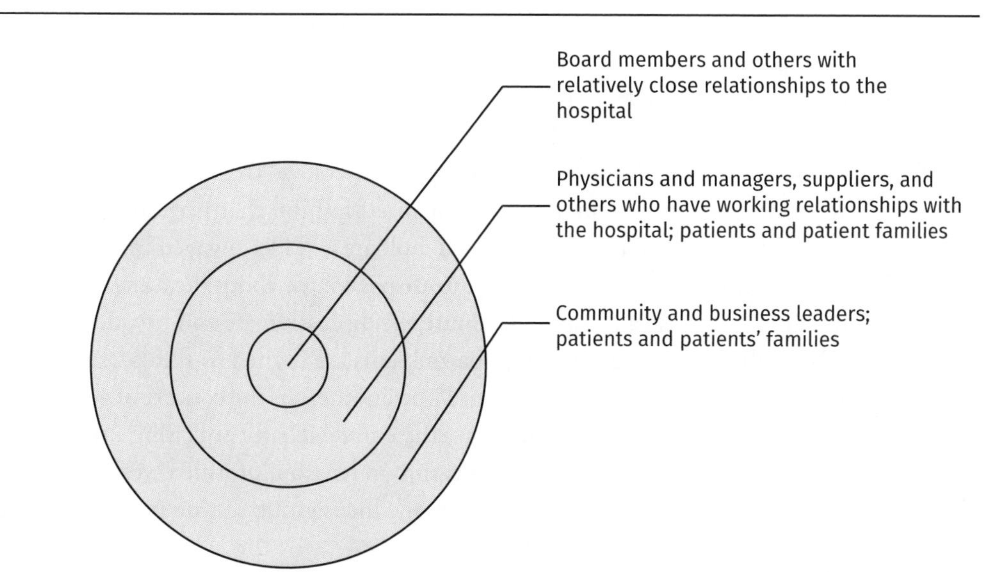

an organization. For example, if you ask, "What are the strengths of Wellbe Hospital," you might include a list of predetermined answers from which the respondent should select. That would narrow the respondent's choices and plant the seeds for ideas that the respondent might otherwise not have identified.

The second useful benefit of a questionnaire is that it lets you quantify data to make a more compelling case. For example, based on questionnaire responses you might be able to say something like "60 percent of community stakeholders favor an expansion of geriatric services in Derricksville." A questionnaire can also include open-ended questions to spur additional thinking from the respondent. While such questions yield answers that are not as easily quantified, they have value in yielding new or different perspectives. Using a questionnaire helps build consensus around certain initiatives. Likewise, it may reveal a strong difference of opinion, suggesting the absence of a consensus that should give rise to significant doubt about including that item in the strategic plan.

Questionnaires also are useful for obtaining planning information from a large group, such as community leaders. Often, the questionnaire will be deployed near the end of the planning process, for two reasons: First, in developing the questionnaire, you may want to include information or insights gained from working with managers or board members. Second, doing it near the end of the process provides an opportunity to adjust the pool of recipients. In other words, based on knowledge gleaned from those with a close understanding of the organization, the planner may want to expand (or less frequently, reduce) the group of questionnaire respondents.

Focus Groups

Focus groups are another useful tool for obtaining information from groups of people who may share similar perspectives, such as physicians or managers. Focus groups can also gather members from different stakeholder groups, which may make for a more robust discussion. Even within a single group of stakeholders, individuals may have differing ideas about the best future course for the organization, which is perfectly okay. The idea behind a focus group is to assimilate information in a semipersonalized fashion that permits developing consensus around planning initiatives. Again, stakeholders will feel engaged in the process.

The person leading the focus group must be dispassionate about the outcome, never expressing an opinion but instead helping facilitate the discussion around broader themes (Kruger and Casey 2015). During the group, participants are invited to speak freely while maintaining a civil and respectful attitude toward one another. In the context of a strategic plan for a hospital, the focus group provides an efficient vehicle for soliciting input from stakeholders who are close enough to the organization to have an informed, vested interest in its future. You may even want to host more than one focus group session per stakeholder group to engage still more people in the process.

Individual Interviews

An individual interview is the best way to elicit detailed information and perspective, but it is also the most time-consuming. That is why this tool should be reserved for use with individuals who have the closest involvement with the hospital, such as board members, the chief of the medical staff, the CEO, the chief operating officer, and other members of the C-suite. These people, because of their important role in hospital operations, have the closest relationship with it and, thus, have the most informed view of the organization. Their help and input will be critically important as the hospital moves further into the planning process. People occupying important stakeholder roles also will appreciate the individualized attention, and there is much to gain from what they have to say.

One critically important point regarding the entire planning process, however, is that some questionnaire respondents, focus group participants, and individual interviewees may have a disinclination toward change, as we discovered in the chapter on change leadership. In other words, some people may fear that a strategic plan will take the organization in a direction that threatens their status, and so their opinions during a SWOT analysis may serve to protect their own limited interests. The good news, though, is that soliciting input from many people, and eliciting a comprehensive picture of an organization using internal and external assessments, will counteract these kinds of biases. If the planning group properly structures how it conducts the SWOT analysis, the final product will satisfy multiple perspectives.

Strategy Identification and Selection

The next step in the process is to identify a strategy that (1) makes the most effective use of the hospital's strengths to address fully its opportunities, (2) minimizes the impact of any threats, and (3) improves on areas with weak performance. Again, a single person cannot be responsible for this whole process. For practical reasons, this *part* of the process typically does not engage as many stakeholders or stakeholder groups as the initial SWOT. But it can be managed by a working group familiar with all facets of the hospital as well as the SWOT analysis. Keep in mind that this is one of several possible planning models to follow. There may be instances where draft plans or ideas are circulated broadly to various stakeholders to keep the dialogue dynamic and to continue to engage stakeholders and solicit their support for the final product.

In general, the next step of the process is asking several questions:

1. *Are the assumptions correct?* The beginning conversation at this juncture should seek to validate (or invalidate) some of the assumptions that were part of the SWOT. For example, the SWOT identifies an opportunity in the Shaleville market. The theory behind seeing this as an opportunity is the belief that the community is resentful of the new hospital because it put the local hospital out

of business. Conversely, however, that new hospital can provide state-of-the-art care through its affiliated academic health center. And it has another powerful advantage: a recognizable brand associated with high-quality care. With these factors in mind, is it realistic to think a small community hospital like Wellbe can successfully compete against the behemoth? This could be a bit like David challenging Goliath. It would take a miracle to succeed.

Challenging the existing thinking that created the SWOT is a form of validation. Creating a plan based on faulty assumptions will not be useful to Wellbe; but creating a plan based on *reasonable* assumptions improves the chances of success. Therefore, it is worth spending the time to conduct a rigorous review and to challenge assumptions.

2. *What is feasible for us?* For example, if we assumed Wellbe Hospital could recruit some new general surgeons within the next six months, the planning group may want to consider that idea in depth. How long would the recruitment process actually take? What goes into that process? Realistically, how long would it take a surgeon to relocate from an existing practice to Derricksville? Why would they want to do so? What incentive can the hospital (legally) provide to induce them to come? Is it feasible—realistic—to believe the hospital could entice a new surgeon to come to the community in half a year? The answer to this question will affect the amount of revenue Wellbe can project to gain from a new surgeon joining the community.

3. *How can we move toward our vision?* Recall Wellbe Hospital's vision statement from earlier in the chapter: "Our vision is to continually exceed the expectations of those we serve by working together as a team, dedicated to a process of never-ending improvements." Remember, the vision statement defines how the hospital will look in the future, and the strategic planning process determines a road map the organization can follow as it attempts to meet its mission while striving to achieve its vision.

   How should Wellbe apply what it has learned in its SWOT analysis as it moves toward becoming a hospital that "continually exceed[s] the expectations" of its patients while seeking "never-ending improvements"? Focusing on geriatric services might be just the thing that addresses this issue. Likewise, successfully recruiting (and retaining) new general and orthopedic surgeons would be an improvement.

Scenarios and Targets

In this phase of the strategy identification and selection process, the team should raise additional questions:

- What should our financial targets be?
- What resources are/will be available?
- What are some of the multiple scenarios that may play out?

Scenario planning is an attempt to create a virtual reality of a particular assumption to think through clearly and carefully if the assumption is reliable. For example, if Wellbe assumed a clinic in Shaleville would be profitable, then considering that possibility in detail would be necessary. The people engaged in the planning process would need to consider virtually every possibility of things that could go right or wrong to create a workable scenario.

Scenario planning
A planning tool that provides a structured way to think about the future and how things might unfold that could affect an organization's well-being.

Continuing with our example, working with the assumption that Wellbe Hospital moves ahead with opening the Shaleville Clinic, what would the estimated costs be? What would the one-time costs be, and what would the ongoing operating costs be? What equipment would be necessary? How many examination rooms would be needed? Would it be possible to open a small clinic that could grow later if it proves it can work? What revenues would the clinic generate? What would the anticipated payer mix be? How long would it be before the clinic becomes profitable? Answering these questions requires a careful study of both the cost and revenue questions. The team needs to balance its desire to grow and be successful with the reality of how establishing a clinic really works. In short, the team needs to develop a scenario that, conceptually, establishes the clinic and projects costs and revenue (Krentz and Gish 2000). Indeed, the team may want to develop two or three alternative scenarios and test the underlying assumptions with other stakeholders.

The same concept applies to the recruitment of one or more general or orthopedic surgeons. How long would it take to get a surgeon in place? How much money would it take to recruit a candidate to Derricksville? Keep in mind there are legal limits on how much a hospital can do to accomplish this goal; this is not professional athletics, so there are no signing bonuses. Once the surgeon arrives, how long would it take to outfit an office? Can that time be shortened? By how much and at what cost? What can the hospital do to help the surgeon gain the confidence of those physicians from whom the surgeon's referrals will come? How much time will pass before the surgeon has a full patient load and is able to generate revenue for the hospital? Again, the team will want to explore several alternative scenarios to answer as accurately as possible these complex questions.

Keep in mind that this process would take place over an extended period of time, involve multiple stakeholders, and apply to a host of possible initiatives. For example, the planning team may want to have a similar conversation about the focus on geriatrics mentioned earlier as a potential opportunity. Likewise, the team may want to subject the potential women's health initiative to the same scrutiny.

Some decisions will surface from this process. Wellbe Hospital may decide it is more important to recruit a pair of orthopedic surgeons than one more general surgeon. Based on the analysis, it may also decide to forgo a women's health initiative while enhancing geriatric services.

These elements will all be compiled into an overall strategic plan. The plan will include financial targets based on historical performance as well as assumptions based on the initiatives to be included. It also will include a market analysis, showing how adopted initiatives will change the market. A strategic plan is a comprehensive document that will set priorities, focus energies and resources, and guide organizational decision-making for the term of the plan. If done correctly, it should also serve as a rallying point for employees to work toward improving the organization. In short, the strategic plan should not be a document that goes on a shelf once completed, but rather is a road map to the future, with widely engaged and energized stakeholder groups who use it to work toward common ends (Ginter, Duncan, and Swayne 2013).

There may be other kinds of plans that accompany the strategic plan such as a facilities plan, a fund-raising plan, and a capital improvement plan, but those are beyond the scope of this book.

Strategy Implementation: Moving Forward

As the strategy development phase winds down, the organization will move toward the next phase: **strategy implementation**. At this point, stakeholders have been engaged in shaping the various strategic initiatives incorporated into the plan. Depending on the level of stakeholder engagement facilitated by the planning leadership team, stakeholders may have had the opportunity to provide affirmative support for preliminary drafts of the plan or its initial ideas. The next step is implementing the strategic plan by preparing smaller plans that lead to the strategic objectives. Refer back to exhibit 13.2 for a visual depiction of where this falls in the planning process.

Strategy implementation
The part of the planning cycle in which the organization attempts to operationalize the strategic plan to meet its strategic goals.

Tactical (operating) plan
Shorter-term, smaller-scale, specific plan intended to carry out the larger goals of the strategic plan. Departments or divisions develop these plans focused on annual objectives. Examples include an operating plan, marketing plan, and fund-raising plan.

Recall that the strategic planning process considers an organization's external and internal elements, attempting to match the various strengths and opportunities and mitigate the weaknesses and threats as it considers the health of the organization for the next three to five years. The next phase of planning delineates specific steps the organization must take to meet its strategic objectives.

These are **tactical plans**, also sometimes called **operating plans**. Various departments within the organization will develop tactical plans to spell out their goals for the coming year. Note that these are generally one-year plans, compared to the strategic plan's three-to-five-year period. The other distinguishing characteristic of an operating plan is its department-level focus, meaning that it deals only with a single department or division and relies on an annual budget that reflects the strategic plan. Thus, the department charged with opening the Shaleville clinic in our example will include both projected expenses and revenues in its annual budget. Given that it may take time to produce revenue, the operating plan for this department unit in the first year of the strategic planning period will most likely show a loss for the Shaleville initiative.

Planning Summary

The organization is now at that phase where "the rubber hits the road," in a manner of speaking. Obviously, there is more to meeting the goals of a strategic plan than developing an operating plan. The critical element now becomes implementing the plan through executing management functions: carrying out the activities that will help meet the operating plan objectives and, ultimately, satisfy the strategic plan's intentions. Execution is what the rest of this book is about, so discussion beyond a mention here would be redundant. Chapter 9 addresses how to get things done, covering the final "Monitor and Control" element from exhibit 13.1. Suffice it to say that all the planning in the world will not matter if the organization does not have sufficient execution to monitor and control its allocation of resources.

The concepts presented here as separate and discrete activities are, indeed, different from one another. Most often, however, these activities do not fall neatly within a designated time frame. Frequently, one activity will overlap with another, as shown in exhibit 13.2. Seldom does an organization totally complete, for example, the tactical and operational planning process without partly beginning to implement the strategic plan. As you encounter this process in the real world, be prepared for it not to be as tidy as in a textbook.

Finally, the strategic planning concepts listed in this chapter are not exhaustive. Many other successful and widely used models can facilitate change in organizations. Some of these are referred to as large-scale interventions. Examples include Future Search and Appreciative Inquiry. Widely used to facilitate change in organizations and larger communities, these specialized techniques require additional, specific training (Janoff and Weisbord 2010; Whitney and Trosten-Bloom 2010).

Marketing

Marketing and strategic planning are frequently considered together. A field of study unto itself, marketing is an important tactical tool an organization can employ to support its strategic goals. It is largely about communicating and "packaging" an organization's features so they appeal to different groups of customers. For example, to grow its emergency services, a hospital might run billboards that display live wait times for its emergency room.

Marketing describes, in part, the "processes for creating, communicating, delivering, and exchanging offerings that have value for customers" (American Marketing Association 2013). Healthcare organizations can, and do, take a number of different approaches to this function. It is a multipronged challenge. The messaging and organizing offerings that have value to customers is a form of a tactical plan supporting the broader organizational goals and objectives identified in the strategic planning process.

In the case of a hospital like Wellbe, marketers would first ask the question: Who are the customers? This will have a complex and multifaceted answer. Patients, physicians, payers, and the public are all customers and potential customers of any healthcare organization (Cellucci, Wiggins, and Farnsworth 2014). Even a small physician practice will draw customers from all these groups, including other physicians. After all, that doctor's colleagues constitute referral sources.

Let us look at each of these groups of customers in more detail.

Patients

Patients are most certainly customers. Indeed, part of the consumer-driven healthcare movement is to view "patients" less as patients and more as customers. The distinction is subtle but important: The term *patient* connotes a person who is relatively passive in the exchange with healthcare professionals, whereas "customers" actively interact with the provider and the healthcare system. Almost gone are the days when caregivers were offended by the use of the term *customer* in favor of *patient*.

Marketing a hospital to the customer known as the patient can be a particularly awkward challenge. Most prospective patients of a hospital do not really want to go there—or any hospital for that matter. Frequently, a trip to the hospital is a result of something bad in the customer/patient's life. Thus, marketing needs to speak to improving the prospective patients' perceptions of what will happen to them. The idea that health systems and providers are selling "health" is an amorphous concept: What *is* health?

The definition depends on the person. A young mother would think differently about the health of her infant than her aged grandmother would perceive her own health. Given the wide differences in what it means to people, can any healthcare organization actually sell *health*? The concept is far more dependent on how people care for themselves than on what any healthcare system or provider can do. Indeed, traditional providers and health systems did not develop as a way to keep people healthy. Instead, they are trained and designed to treat people who are ill or injured. That is one of the challenges of our healthcare system: It evolved primarily to address the needs of the acutely ill, not as a proactive mechanism to help customers achieve and maintain good health.

However, the healthcare system as we know it is undergoing a transformation. The focus on population health and rewarding health systems for keeping people healthy is starting to change how some health systems operate. There is a much greater focus on *prevention* than there has been historically. This means that hospitals and health systems can, in their marketing efforts, talk about not only repairing what is wrong, but also supporting customers' efforts to stay well. There are, in effect, two kinds of marketing taking place here. First is the need to tell the patients that your organization can provide the best care for acute purposes. Second, the organization must sell itself as a neighborhood institution that helps the community stay healthy.

One element changing how healthcare organizations market themselves is the increased level of transparency in the system. For example, customers can now compare, at least on some measures, a hospital's success rates in certain areas thanks to the online publication of scores on the Hospital Consumer Assessment of Healthcare Providers and Systems (HCAHPS) survey. Pronounced "H-caps" and also known as the CAHPS Hospital Survey, this is a survey instrument and data collection methodology for measuring patients' perceptions of their hospital experience. While many hospitals have long collected information on patient satisfaction for their own internal use, until HCAHPS there was no national standard for collecting and publicly reporting information about patient experience of care that allowed consumers to make valid comparisons across hospitals locally, regionally, and nationally. For example, now a potential customer can find hospitals near their zip code and examine comparisons for several categories related to patient care. An expectant mother can see the percentage of unnecessary cesarean sections by hospital; a cancer patient can see which hospital is better at providing appropriate radiation care; and so forth. Potential patients can also find information from patient surveys that may be helpful in guiding their decision. When confronted with the need to use a hospital, a consumer, at least in theory, can shop for better quality thanks to HCAHPS data (CMS 2015). As a result, hospitals are now increasingly focused on ways to improve patient care so they can enjoy higher scores and a competitive advantage.

As a whole, the Internet has greatly facilitated the consumer movement in healthcare. While patients can now compare **HCAHPS scores**, as we have seen (Al Ghamdi and Moussa 2012), hospitals and healthcare systems have taken advantage of the digital trend by creating websites to inform consumers of locations, affiliated physicians, services, quality rankings, and much more (Ford et al. 2012). In recent years, healthcare systems have taken this initiative even further by maintaining a presence on social media sites such as Facebook and LinkedIn. The underlying message from all these healthcare marketing initiatives is "We can provide you high-quality care when you need it." In short, the marketing efforts focus the attention of patients and prospective patients on two of the three elements of the iron triangle referenced in chapter 2, quality and access.

HCAHPS scores
Results on the Hospital Consumer Assessment of Healthcare Providers and Systems survey, the first national, standardized, publicly reported survey of patients' perspectives on hospital care.

The second part of a healthcare organization's marketing message will be discussed later in "The Public" section, when we explore the concept of social marketing.

Physicians

A hospital or integrated health system has another class of customers beyond the people referred to as patients. To a large degree, even though the healthcare system is evolving in ways that partially diminish this point, physicians remain hospital "customers," too. Independent, private-practice physicians in urban and suburban areas generally can choose from more than one hospital where they may obtain **medical staff privileges**—that is, the facility to use when referring their patients for hospital care. To that end, hospitals provide all manner of amenities to entice physicians to choose them, such as private lunchrooms and convenient parking places. Once a physician applies for and receives medical staff privileges at a particular hospital, he or she can admit patients there. To be clear, the amenities are not the only reason a physician may choose to admit to a particular hospital, but a physician's decision about hospital affiliation is important.

Medical staff privileges
Permission to practice in the hospital granted to physicians who pass the hospital's credentialing process. Physicians already granted privileges at the hospital frequently oversee this process; it is a form of peer review and acceptance.

In addition to affecting physicians, the concept of medical staff privileges also affects patients. Consider the example of a patient who was concerned about a development in his eye; it was generating pus, which made it difficult for him to see. He was able to visit his primary care physician on short notice, and she diagnosed an infection requiring hospital-level care, probably intravenous antibiotics. When the patient indicated a preference for a particular hospital because he had experience there and was confident about the quality of care he would receive, the physician told him she did not have staff privileges there and, thus, could not admit him there. He would need to go to the hospital with which she was associated, thus making the patient's choice of hospital irrelevant.

As we discussed in chapter 3, the healthcare system is evolving with regard to this erstwhile relationship. Physician practices and hospitals are increasingly binding together to form larger integrated healthcare entities. In many cases, this takes the form of hospital ownership of physician practices. The closely integrated relationship also can take the form of a contract between a physician practice and a hospital. In addition, payment mechanisms, such as bundled payments that compensate each episode of care with a single lump sum, also affect the physician–hospital relationship. Regardless of how, the relationship between the physician and the hospital is changing. Physicians increasingly are linked to hospital patient information systems that improve the sharing and transfer of patient records. This is also "the tie that binds" in a sense, because it makes it difficult for either party to abandon their respective role. It would be expensive and time-consuming for the physician to leave this arrangement for another hospital or system, and a hospital terminating a physician practice would lose revenue because the physicians would no longer be able to admit there.

Hospitals are dependent on physicians, just as physicians are dependent on hospitals. In many ways, the hospital is the physician's workspace. This is particularly true for a wide variety of specialists who perform invasive procedures. Cardiologists use the catheterization ("cath") lab; orthopedic surgeons, neurosurgeons, general surgeons, and cardiothoracic surgeons all use the operating rooms; and many of these same doctors use the hospital's labs and imaging services. Primary care physicians often use patient rooms and a variety of a hospital's **ancillary services**.

Ancillary services
Services provided by a hospital that are incidental to patient care, such as imaging and laboratory services. Clinicians use these services for both inpatients and outpatients.

The mutually beneficial relationship between physicians and hospitals, however, can also create tension. Physicians traditionally have argued that the hospital administration will not spend the resources physicians need to do their jobs properly. Conversely, hospital leadership will at times argue that physicians are too demanding in their requests for more space, staff support, and diagnostic equipment. The art of leadership is not only to prevent this cross-tension from spiraling out of control, but also to use the best thinking from both sides to improve the quality of care for the patient. Indeed, physicians' concern for their patients is something the hospital tries to address by maintaining a high-quality staff that can support the physicians in their work. This is a key point in hospital marketing efforts aimed at physicians. The amenities are not about the better parking place or the semiprivate lunchroom per se. Instead, they are about improving the physicians' ability to care for their patients by making access to the hospital and its workings more convenient.

Payers

Marketing for a healthcare organization not only needs to target patients to create awareness and consumer confidence, and to target physicians to promote quality. It also needs to address payers, as being part of a payer's network is essential to getting consumers. Said another way, patients whose insurance does not include your hospital will most likely not go to your hospital for services.

As discussed in chapter 11, there are several types of insurance. The discussion here will focus primarily on commercial insurance, of which **employer-sponsored insurance** is the most common type. The companies that create and sell these commercial plans constitute important markets for any healthcare organization. Insurance plans negotiate with a health system to obtain a discount on the provider's traditional charges and fees in exchange for ensuring a large population of patients will come to the health system for care. From the system's perspective, negotiation with commercial insurers aims to maximize revenue by obtaining both the assurance of patients and an appropriate fee for caring for them (Reinhardt 2009).

When marketing to commercial payers, a healthcare organization needs to convey two messages: (1) that it has the capacity to care for the **covered lives** the payer represents in its health plan, and (2) that the payer will receive good value for its money, with care costs that are competitive with the rest of the market. Private insurance plans negotiate with healthcare providers to bring those providers into their **provider network**. The agreement for a provider to be in a health plan's network centers on availability and cost. Again, the relationship is awkwardly symbiotic: A health plan needs providers to care for the covered lives it represents, while a provider needs patients covered by the health plan for whom to care so it can generate revenue.

Public insurance plans—Medicare, Medicaid, and the Children's Health Insurance Program (CHIP)—work somewhat differently. While the provider must be approved by either the Centers for Medicare & Medicaid Services (federal agency overseeing Medicare) or the state agency that oversees Medicaid and CHIP to receive payment for services rendered,

Employer-sponsored insurance
Insurance plans for which the employer pays part of the premium for the benefit of the employees and sometimes their family members. The primary way Americans obtain health insurance.

Covered lives
The number of people and dependents enrolled in a particular health plan. There is no standard term for such a person, as they may be referred to as beneficiary, member, insured, subscriber, or the like.

Provider network
A list of hospitals, doctors, and other providers with whom a health plan has contracted and who, therefore, are contractually obligated to provide care for the covered lives in the health plan at a negotiated payment rate.

there is no negotiation as to payment. A provider may choose to be a participant in Medicare, for example, but the reimbursement they will receive is established by Medicare and is not subject to negotiation (MedicareResources.org 2015). Medicaid works similarly by publishing a fee schedule—a list of payments that is determined by the state government (Medicaid.gov 2017).

Marketing to these public entities is slightly different than marketing to private insurance companies. To maximize payments, a healthcare organization might be inclined to engage in a bit more puffery about the value of its services when negotiating with a private insurer. But there is no need for that with public sector insurance, as there is no chance of obtaining higher payment rates.

The Public

For the public at large, a healthcare organization must take a broader approach. In this case, the organization wants to demonstrate to the community that it is a full partner in that community and is an active citizen with positive impact and merit. It also may seek to build on and amplify the awareness and confidence image it projects with patients. The best way to accomplish both goals is through actually being an active citizen and furthering initiatives like **health literacy** and **health promotion** (Cellucci, Wiggins, and Farnsworth 2014).

Health literacy
The degree to which one has and understands health information essential to making informed health decisions.

Health promotion
Activities designed to influence individual behaviors that affect personal health.

In helping to advance health literacy, a healthcare organization might undertake an active campaign to disseminate accurate, helpful information that would guide people in making important health-related decisions. This information could be about vaccination against flu, measles, shingles, and other preventable diseases. The organization could also disseminate information about the relationship of excess weight to diabetes, heart disease, high blood pressure, and a variety of cancers. This kind of public service would help establish the healthcare organization as a useful member of the community that cares about the overall health of the local population.

Health promotion seeks to alter individual behaviors. Indeed, it is almost an animation of health literacy. Examples include "quit smoking" campaigns and messages about avoiding dangerous or illegal drugs. Public interventions such as communitywide weight-loss challenges also fall under this broad heading of "health promotion." In short, health promotion seeks to change the behavior of individuals for the benefit of both them and the community at large.

Social marketing
The creation, communication, and delivery of information, events, and programs to influence individual behavior for the benefit of both the individual and the community as a whole.

Closely tied to this is the concept of **social marketing**, which attempts to influence groups and communities as a whole. (This is not the same as social *media*, which will be discussed later.) Both health promotion and social marketing incorporate a public health message. Thus, communicating the health benefits of diet and exercise to raise individual awareness of these behaviors will have (hopefully) both an individual and community outcome: Individuals change their behavior to eat better and exercise more, which results in the improved health status of the community overall (Cellucci, Wiggins, and Farnsworth 2014).

One of the keys to a successful social marketing campaign is to start with groups that are "ready for action" (Kotler, Roberto, and Lee 2002). Social marketing is fraught with challenges: Its effectiveness is difficult to measure; it may be focused on effects rather than causation; it is difficult to get people to change long-held beliefs and habits; and it lacks clarity and has too many definitions (Andreasen 2006).

Despite these challenges, healthcare organizations will find support when they undertake social marketing promotions. While progress may be difficult to measure, the broader image of being an engaged community citizen is a valuable profile for any healthcare organization.

A brief note about the difference between social *marketing* and social *media*. Many if not most healthcare organizations now maintain a presence on social media outlets such as Facebook, LinkedIn, Instagram, and the like. The kind of messaging the healthcare organization undertakes on its social media platform(s) can be as wide-ranging as the types of healthcare organizations themselves. Social media may be used to promote a specific provider, facility, or treatment. It may likewise be used to educate and provide a degree of health promotion or even social *marketing*. However, just because a healthcare organization chooses to use social media to extend its identity or message does not, by itself, indicate the organization is engaged in social marketing.

Marketing Summary

As you can see, marketing for a healthcare organization or provider is a multilayered proposition. A healthcare system must speak to patients, physicians, payers, and the public at large. While each group may receive a message emphasizing a slightly different aspect of the organization, the overall message must be consistent and cohesive to support the organization's image and reputatation. If one stakeholder group senses it is getting a different message than other stakeholder groups, it will brandish the notion that the healthcare organziation is "speaking out of both sides" of its mouth. For that reason, healthcare marketers need to be creative problem solvers in order to shape just the right message with just the right emphasis for each specific stakeholder group.

Conclusion

Strategic planning and marketing go hand in hand even though they are not quite the same things. Planning requires examination of the "big picture" for an organization. Where does it fit in the external environment? What are its internal capabilities? What strengths does it have that match the community's needs? A strategic plan generally covers a three- to five-year period. It becomes difficult to make assumptions for a time period extending beyond five years.

Marketing is a way to help implement a plan. It calls for a more detailed look at who the customers are and what kinds of services they may need or want. In the case of a healthcare organization, it generally will have a handful of different "markets": physicians, patients, payers, and the public. Certainly, these stakeholder groups will be considered in the strategic planning, but communicating with them in detail and in ways specific to their needs is the marketer's function.

This chapter provided an introductory look at both functions. To be fully conversant in either one will require further study.

Mini Case Study: Expanding into the Suburbs

The following is a press release taken from a real hospital:

The Medical University Hospital of South Carolina (MUSC) has received approval for its Certificate of Need (CON) to build a new hospital in Dorchester County. The state Department of Health and Environmental Control (DHEC) granted the approval. DHEC is the state body that must issue a CON before certain types of health care acquisitions, expansions and creation of new facilities are allowed.

MUSC Health Community Hospital at Nexton will be a 311,221-square-foot facility with 128 beds, to provide a range of specialized inpatient and outpatient services. Estimated at a cost of $325 million, the project is expected to be operational in three years. One of the area's newest planned communities, Nexton is located in Summerville at the crossroads of I-26 and US 17A in the path of metro Charleston's vigorous growth.

"The Nexton hospital will be a much-needed addition to our health care system," said MUSC President David J. Cole, M.D., FACS.

"Our network of MUSC hospitals, clinics and other care facilities is positioned to provide patients with the right care, at the right time and in the right location. As the only publicly assisted, comprehensive, statewide academic medical center, MUSC has a mission and responsibility unlike any other health care facility in South Carolina. We are charged with discovering, developing, teaching and delivering the most advanced health care for every patient across the state."

"We are committed to delivering top-quality care and increased access to every patient," said Patrick J. Cawley, M.D., MHM, FACHE, MUSC Health CEO and vice president for Health Affairs, University. "To achieve this goal, we must position our health care network in synchronicity with the energetic growth of the greater Charleston community."

Previously, the state health plan identified the need for 147 additional MUSC beds to serve the tri-county area (Berkeley, Charleston and Dorchester counties), based on MUSC's existing hospital occupancy and fill rates. MUSC Health Community Hospital at Nexton is designed to meet many of the increasing health care demands by bringing consistent, high quality and compassionate care to a convenient, neighborhood location.

Source: Medical University of South Carolina (2018).

Mini Case Study Questions

1. Create a SWOT analysis that might have led to University Hospital's decision to build a new facility. What must the SWOT have contained for University Hospital to reach this decision and gain state approval?
2. How would you market this new hospital?

Points to Remember

- SWOT is a good planning tool to assess an organization both internally and externally.
- Strategy selection relies on matching the community's needs with a healthcare organization's strengths or opportunities.
- Successful strategy implementation requires execution of the plan along with transparent accountability and managerial control.
- Operational (tactical) plans are one-year road maps supporting the path to strategic goals.
- Marketing is a multipronged challenge for healthcare providers.
- Patients, the public at large, physicians, and payers are all target markets for healthcare organizations.
- A consistent message in marketing is essential to creating an effective brand.

Challenge Yourself

1. What is the relationship between strategy and marketing? Is it possible to have a good strategy and poor marketing results? What about the other way around? Is it possible to have good marketing with a poorly conceived strategic plan?
2. How do you see strategic planning as helpful to the overall healthcare system?

For Your Consideration

1. Dig deeper into the Wellbe Hospital scenario from the case study. What would you look for in establishing a clinic in Shaleville? What criteria would you use to move ahead? How would you market the clinic?
2. Select a healthcare organization you know. Create a questionnaire you might use to help inform a SWOT analysis of that organization.
3. Using the same healthcare organization, perform that SWOT analysis. You might not have access to all the information you need for the strengths and weaknesses sections, so you may have to rely on reputation. You can, however, do an external assessment (covering threats and opportunities) without detailed knowledge of an organization.

References

Al Ghamdi, K. M., and N. A. Moussa. 2012. "Internet Use by the Public to Search for Health-Related Information." *Internatonal Journal of Health Informatics* 81 (6): 363–73.

American Marketing Association. 2013. "Definition of Marketing." Published July. www.ama.org/AboutAMA/Pages/Definition-of-Marketing.aspx.

Andreasen, A. R. 2006. *Social Marketing in the 21st Century*. Los Angeles: SAGE Publications.

Bonnafous-Boucher, M., and J. D. Rendtorff. 2016. *Stakeholder Theory: A Model for Strategic Management*. New York: Springer.

Boston Consulting Group (BCG). 1973. *The Experience Curve—Reviewed*. Accessed May 22, 2018. www.bcg.com/documents/file13904.pdf.

Cellucci, L. W., C. Wiggins, and T. J. Farnsworth. 2014. *Healthcare Marketing: A Case Study Approach*. Chicago: Health Administration Press.

Centers for Medicare & Medicaid Services (CMS). 2015. "Hospital HCAHPS." Last modified May 15. www.cms.gov/Research-Statistics-Data-and-Systems/Research/CAHPS/hcahps1.html.

Ford, E., T. Huerta, R. Schilhavy, N. Menachemi, and V. Wells. 2012. "Effective US Health System Websites: Establishing Benchmarks and Standards for Effective Consumer Engagement." *Journal of Healthcare Management* 57 (1): 47–74.

Ginter, P. M., W. J. Duncan, and L. E. Swayne. 2013. *Strategic Management of Health Care Organizations*, 7th ed. San Francisco: Jossey-Bass.

Hambrick, D., I. MacMillan, and D. Day. 1982. "Strategic Attributes and Performance in the BCG Matrix." *Academy of Management Journal* 25 (3): 510–31.

Harris, J. M. (ed.). *Healthcare Strategic Planning*, 4th ed. Chicago: Health Administration Press.

Humphrey, A. 2005. "SWOT Analysis for Management Consulting." *SRI Alumni Association Newsletter*. Published December. www.sri.com/sites/default/files/brochures/dec-05.pdf.

Janoff, S., and M. Weisbord. 2010. *Future Search: Getting the Whole System in the Room for Vision, Commitment, and Action*, 3rd ed. San Francisco: Barrett-Kohler.

Jurevicius, O. 2014. "GE McKinsey Matrix." *Strategic Management Insight*. Published August 19. www.strategicmanagementinsight.com/tools/ge-mckinsey-matrix.html.

Kotler, P., N. Roberto, and N. R. Lee. 2002. *Social Marketing: Improving the Quality of Life*, 2nd ed. Los Angeles: SAGE Publications.

Krentz, S., and R. Gish. 2000. "Using Scenario Analysis to Determine Managed Care Strategy." *Healthcare Financial Managment* 59 (9): 41–43.

Kruger, R. A., and M. A. Casey. 2015. *Focus Groups: A Practical Guide for Applied Research*, 5th ed. Los Angeles: SAGE Publications.

Matoff-Stepp, S., B. Applebaum, J. Pooler, and E. Kavanagh. 2014. "Women as Health Care Decision-Makers: Implications for Health Care Coverage in the United States." *Journal of Health Care for the Poor and Underserved* 25 (4): 1507–13.

Medicaid.gov. 2017. "Financial Management." Accessed July 23, 2018. www.medicaid.gov/medicaid/finance/index.html.

Medical University of South Carolina (MUSC). 2018. "MUSC Receives DHEC Approval for Certificate of Need to Build 128-Bed Hospital in Berkeley County." Press release issued July 24. http://academicdepartments.musc.edu/pr/pressrelease/2018/musc-receives-dhec-approval-for-certificate-of-need-to-build-128-bed-hospital-in-berkeley-county.htm.

MedicareResources.org. 2015. "How Does Medicare Reimbursement Work?" Accessed July 23, 2018. www.medicareresources.org/faqs/how-does-medicare-reimbursement-work/.

Porter, M. E. 1985. *Competitive Advantage: Creating and Sustaining Superior Performance*. New York: Simon & Schuster.

Quick MBA. 2010. "GE/McKinsey Matrix." Accessed May 22, 2018. www.quickmba.com/strategy/matrix/ge-mckinsey/.

Reinhardt, U. E. 2009. "Is Employer-Based Health Insurance Worth Saving?" *New York Times*. Published May 22. http:/economix.blogs.nytimes.com/2009/05/22/is-employer-based-health-insurance-worth-saving/.

Wayland, M., and W. McDonald. 2016. *Strategic Analysis for Healthcare: Concepts and Practical Applications*. Chicago: Health Administration Press.

Whitney, D., and A. Trosten-Bloom. 2010. *The Power of Appreciative Inquiry*, 2nd ed. San Francisco: Barrett-Kohler.

Ziglar, Z. 1976. *See You at the Top*. New York: Pelican.

CHAPTER 14

ASSESSING QUALITY IN HEALTH SERVICE DELIVERY AND MANAGEMENT

Important Terms

- Assessment
- Benchmarking
- Best practices
- Fishbone diagram
- Outcome
- Pay-for-performance
- Process
- Quality of care
- Risk management
- Root cause analysis
- Standards
- Structure

Learning Objectives

After reading this chapter, you will be able to do the following:

- Explain and apply a standard, three-step approach to assessment
- Discuss the importance of benchmarking and best practices
- Describe root cause analysis
- Understand program assessment tools used in both management and clinical settings

Case Study: A Longer Than Necessary Hospitalization

Stanley Londborg is a 64-year-old man with a long-standing history of a seizure disorder. He also has hypertension (high blood pressure) and chronic obstructive pulmonary disease (COPD). He is no stranger to the hospital because of his health issues. At home, he takes a number of medications, including three for his COPD and three—levetiracetam, lamotrigine, and sodium valproate—to help control his seizures.

Mr. Londborg came to the emergency room (ER) last week because he was wheezing and having trouble breathing. The physician there conducted a physical examination that yielded signs of an acute worsening of his COPD. Known as COPD exacerbation, this often is the result of a relatively mild respiratory tract infection, but could be due to something more serious, such as pneumonia.

The physician in the ER ordered a chest X-ray, which showed no signs of pneumonia, so Mr. Londborg was determined to have a relatively mild respiratory tract infection. He was admitted to the hospital for treatment. Before leaving the ER, Mr. Londborg also underwent routine blood work, which showed an elevation in his creatinine, a sign his kidneys were being forced to work harder due to his infection.

On the medical floor, the care team treated Mr. Londborg with oral steroids and inhaled bronchodilators (standard medical therapy for his condition), which resulted in a gradual improvement in his respiratory symptoms. Nurses also gave him intravenous (IV) fluids for the kidney issue, which slowly resolved. Mr. Londborg was steadily improving, so it seemed this visit to the hospital would be one of his shorter ones.

On his third morning in the hospital, however, Mr. Londborg complained to the intern, a first-year resident, on his care team about acute pain in his left leg. This symptom potentially indicated a blood clot known as deep vein thrombosis (DVT). The fear with DVT is that blood clots in the legs may dislodge and travel to the lungs and cause a pulmonary embolism, which can be deadly. The care team immediately ordered an ultrasound of Mr. Londborg's lower extremities.

The resident on the care team, who oversees the intern, then checked Mr. Londborg's medication orders and was surprised to see that the admitting doctor had not ordered prophylaxis for DVT—that is, preventive blood thinners, such as heparin or enoxaparin. The resident was surprised because, typically, all patients admitted to the hospital receive this treatment to prevent blood clots from forming while they lie in their beds. Further, nothing about Mr. Londborg's medical record suggested he should not have received this treatment as an important precautionary measure.

The ultrasound, unfortunately, confirmed the presence of a blood clot in Mr. Londborg's left calf. Due to his impaired kidney function, treatment for the blood clot required him to remain in the hospital on IV medication. Mr. Londborg's stay was going to be longer than expected. At 10 p.m. on his eighth day in the hospital, a member of the environmental services staff (also known as housekeeping) found Mr. Londborg on the floor of his room. She immediately alerted the nurses on the ward. The nurses noted seizure activity and called the overnight medical team to Mr. Londborg's bedside. The team responded quickly and gave him IV medication that stopped his seizure. Because no one witnessed his fall and seizure, Mr. Londborg underwent an emergent CT scan of his head to check for any sign of bleeding. After his mental status improved (it is common for patients to be confused for a time after a seizure), he complained of pain in his left shoulder and elbow, but X-rays of these joints showed no evidence of a traumatic fracture from his fall.

After ensuring that Mr. Londborg was stable, the overnight care team reviewed the chart and the medication history to try to determine the cause of Mr. Londborg's sudden seizure. They found that one of his seizure medications, levetiracetam, had not been given that day. There was a notation in the medication administration record from the daytime nurse indicating that the ordered dose was not available in the automatic medication dispensing system on the floor when it should have been.

Further discussions the following day with the daily care team of doctors and nurses revealed that the nurses did not notify the physicians or the pharmacy that the essential medication was not administered. The medication system did not include an automatic alert, either. Fortunately, the overnight physicians restarted Mr. Londborg on his medication, and he suffered no apparent permanent harm. Mr. Londborg was discharged after ten days in the hospital. Most hospitalizations for COPD are far shorter. In fact, many last only a couple of days.

Source: Adapted from the Institute for Healthcare Improvement (Hilliard 2013).

Introduction: Quality

In healthcare, the word ***quality*** often refers to the care provided to patients. However, patient care is not the only area where excellent quality is a goal. High-quality management processes, procedures, and techniques ensure that programs, departments, and organizations operate effectively and efficiently. By leading well-designed and appropriately implemented management processes, healthcare managers create the basis and the environment for the delivery of high-quality care.

Quality
Defined by the Institute of Medicine (2018) as "the degree to which health care services for individuals and populations increase the likelihood of desired health outcomes and are consistent with current professional knowledge."

The National Academy of Medicine defines quality as "the degree to which health care services for individuals and populations increase the likelihood of desired health outcomes and are consistent with current professional knowledge" (AHRQ 2018). In this chapter, you will read about quality of care for the patient, but also discover the role management plays in establishing an environment conducive to high-quality patient care.

While the case study you just read is clearly medical in nature, there are some aspects of it that will be of interest to administrators. (Note that quality of patient care should *always* be "of interest" to administrators. However, in this case, "of interest" refers to things administrators can do to help the clinical team improve the quality of care provided to patients like Mr. Londborg.) The challenge here is to find what went wrong with Mr. Londborg's visit to the hospital. The tempting answer is "everything," but both administrators and clinicians have the duty to ascertain specifically what went wrong in the process of care so it can be corrected and, ideally, never happen again.

This is an important question from the quality-of-patient-care perspective. It is also an important management issue, related to avoiding unnecessary costs. In this case, Mr. Londborg suffered a potentially life-threatening blood clot, a seizure that could have caused severe injury, and multiple episodes of pain. What should have been a routine matter—a mild respiratory tract infection addressed with a two- or three-day stay in the hospital—expanded into a case with multiple complications resulting in a ten-day stay with added tests such as the CT scan and ultrasound. Not only did Mr. Londborg receive poor care, but he and his insurer became responsible for much higher costs.

Simply put, the team at Mr. Londborg's hospital needs to assess the processes in this episode of care to determine the cause(s) of his extended hospital stay.

As you learned in chapter 8, quality improvement methods such as Six Sigma might help resolve the underlying problems that caused Mr. Londborg's unnecessarily long hospitalization.

Root cause analysis
The process of dissecting a positive or negative incident into its most basic segments and discovering the source of its characteristics and outcomes.

This chapter will focus on a different method of quality improvement called **root cause analysis**. Using this method, we will assess the care process at work in Mr. Londborg's case, and then strategize on how to improve and monitor it going forward.

Root Cause Analysis: Finding the Problem

On its face, we can see multiple errors in Mr. Londborg's hospital experience. Our challenge will be finding where errors in the process occurred, not for placing blame, but for reevaluating the processes and correcting the problem. In short, the challenge is to identify the root cause of the difficulties arising in Mr. Londborg's care.

Fishbone diagram
A visualization tool for categorizing the potential causes of a problem (or poor outcome) to identify its root causes. Also called a *cause-and-effect diagram*.

One of the most common tools for performing a root cause analysis is a **fishbone diagram**. The tool takes its name from its appearance, which generally looks like a collection of fish bones, with a central spine and several offshoots (exhibit 14.1). This is a tool used to help improve processes by identifying all the root causes creating the problem.

This is not a blame-seeking or blame-assigning exercise; the goal is to find out what is wrong and why, and then identify ways to fix it. An effective root cause analysis consists of data collection, investigation, determination, reporting of root causes, implementation of corrective actions, and monitoring for sustainability (Rooney and Vanden Heuvel 2004). Before we can apply that analysis to the facts of this case, a more detailed explanation of how it works is in order.

EXHIBIT 14.1
Fishbone Diagram

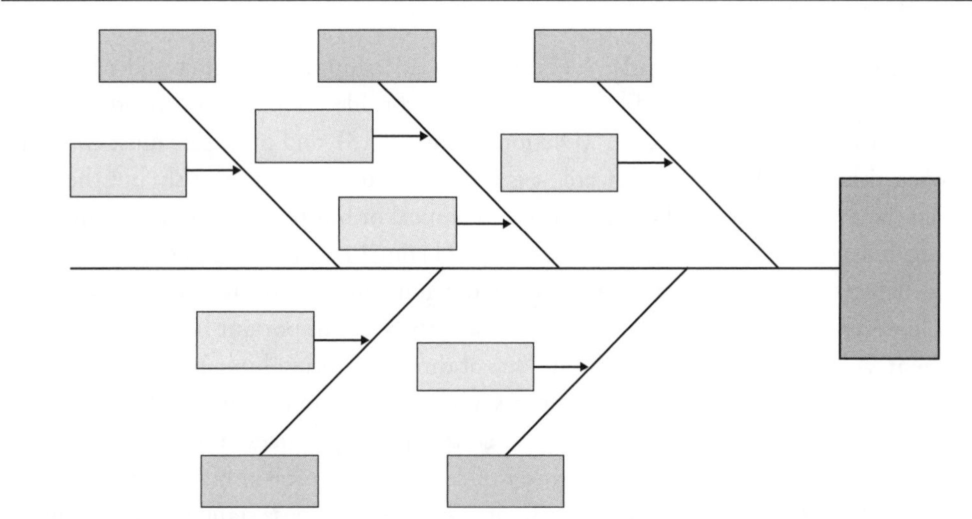

An **assessment** can take several forms. One standard assessment process looks quite simple on paper (Rue and Byars 2004):

Assessment
The act of measuring, appraising, and evaluating.

1. Set standards.
2. Monitor.
3. Take corrective action as needed.

SETTING STANDARDS

In any endeavor, how does one know how good is actually good enough? How many mistakes are acceptable? In some industries, it is very clear. For example, few people would travel on an airline that reported, on average, *only* 1 percent of its flights crashed. With some major airlines flying more than 4,000 flights each day, this rate would indicate 40 plane crashes per day (Quora 2015). And that is for only one airline! On the other hand, a student missing 1 percent of the answers on an exam would earn a grade of 99 percent, which by anyone's standards is an excellent grade. On the care-giving side of healthcare, setting **standards** is a bit more difficult. As we can see from the introductory case, each patient comes in with his own set of very individualized diagnoses, health levels, and preexisting conditions, some of which are known and some of which are unknown. In addition, each caregiver has her own set of skills and abilities. Given that the inputs (the patient and the provider) in any patient care procedure are so varied, how can standards for desired patient care **outcomes** ever be accurately set?

Standards
Customary, appropriate, and acceptable criteria or outcomes.

Outcome
The end result, product, or conclusion to a process or event.

Risk Management

In the process of setting standards, the healthcare leadership team must consider how best to manage the risk associated with the action under consideration. The word *risk* means "a possible, usually negative outcome" (Dictionary.com 2018), and managers must eliminate as much risk as possible. In healthcare, it is impossible to eliminate all risk, but the more certain the manager can be about all aspects of clinical or business performance, the lower the organization's risk will be for adverse events. Having best practice protocols, processes, and structures in place to ensure compliance with regulations and the law are good strategies to help decrease the likelihood of adverse events. These are important facets of **risk management**. Adverse events tend to fall into one of three categories: human error, equipment failure, or systems failure, either alone or in some combination (McIlwain 2006).

Risk management
Systems, processes, and structures put in place to decrease the likelihood of adverse events.

In assessing risk, leaders will want to consider best practices and benchmarks, two concepts discussed later as part of the process of developing clinical or business performance standards. In addition, certain regulatory bodies sometimes impose standards of care on the provider organization. Likewise, the payer community has begun to incentivize the provider community to adhere to certain quality standards as well.

Pay-for-performance
A financial reward system for healthcare providers in which a portion of their monetary compensation is related to improvement in patient outcomes and other indicators of improved performance.

The **pay-for-performance** model that is rapidly becoming a larger part of the healthcare reimbursement picture specifies outcomes in a variety of circumstances. The term, also known as P4P, is generally understood to be "any type of performance-based provider payment arrangements including those that target performance on cost measures" (Thomas and Caldis 2007, 1). Thus, for example, Medicare will no longer reimburse hospitals for avoidable readmissions for specific conditions (CMS 2018). The underlying premise behind this policy is that the readmission was an undesirable outcome, attributable to something that happened in the course of the patient's care and, therefore, should not be reimbursed.

Standards with regard to outcomes help define "good quality" of care. They provide the payer leverage, incentivizing providers to improve the **process** of care.

Process
Activity proximately or directly related to the delivery of care to the patient as well as the actual act of caregiving.

Monitoring

Once standards are developed, there must be a process—monitoring—in place to ensure that the organization, team, or individual is in compliance with them. The long-established framework for evaluating quality of care is the examination of structure, process, and outcomes (Donabedian 1966).

Structure
The environment and the set of conditions that exist, relating to both physical premises and qualifications of the staff. Structure is a necessary condition for quality to occur, but by itself, it is insufficient to produce quality healthcare.

Structure refers to the physical environment as well as the qualifications of the people associated with providing care. Not only does the building need to be an appropriate place to provide care, employees should be qualified and current in their competencies to provide appropriate care. In that vein, for example, the percentage of physicians who are board certified in their specialties is an important measure of structure. Likewise, this can also mean providing employees the materials and equipment they need to perform their duties. Are there enough handwashing stations in proximity to where providers see patients, for example? Are medications stored appropriately? Buildings and physical plants must meet specific safety criteria, such as fire and building codes. These are all examples of the "structure" associated with patient care.

Ensuring adequate structure and good process are necessary for quality performance, but "adequate" and "good" are only minimal standards. They are not sufficient to produce high-quality care. Best practices associated with the process of providing care must be in place. Clinicians learn **best practices** in their own patient care disciplines. These best practices evolve; what was proper and adequate in the past may no longer be acceptable as science advances. Processes need to be up-to-date, well communicated, taught, reinforced, and upheld. In the case at the beginning of the chapter, the patient presented in the emergency department with certain risk factors. Specifically, Mr. Londborg was older than age 60, dehydrated, and a critical care admission—all known risk factors for DVT prophylaxis on admission to a hospital. He should have received medication to avoid DVT (National Guideline Clearinghouse 2015).

Best practices
The actions, processes, and procedures used in a profession, discipline, or industry to achieve the best possible outcomes.

The Agency for Healthcare Research and Quality (AHRQ) as well as the National Institutes of Health's National Center for Complementary and Integrative Health have both promulgated clinical guidelines based on scientific evidence and a rigorous review process. They represent the best practices for a wide variety of medical conditions. The AHRQ guidelines help practitioners understand the appropriate preventive screens for a wide variety of illnesses (AHRQ 2014).

As the science of medicine advances and management techniques improve, it becomes imperative for both clinicians and managers to continue to understand the latest knowledge in their respective fields. Clinical guidelines change over time because the ongoing study of medicine provides new information regarding drugs, devices, and techniques that are more effective. Management changes as a result of improved technology and greater understanding of human motivation. See chapter 5 for additional information on how management theories and approaches have evolved.

Comparing how an organization stacks up against a standard or a similar organization's results is known as **benchmarking**. It applies to both clinical and administrative processes. We just made such a comparison between the process of providing care to Mr. Londborg and an established clinical guideline.

Benchmarking
The process of comparing one organization or situation to similar organizations or situations using uniform measures.

Once you have determined that the outcome was undesirable (readmission to the hospital) or that the care process fell short of best practices (missed medication), you become obligated to fix the problem. Before you can "fix the problem," however, you need to determine with a higher level of precision what, exactly, went wrong. There were multiple steps in the care provided to Mr. Londborg, several of which caused his protracted hospital stay. Sorting those events into a workable framework to help develop a solution requires a method of organizing the information into a logical sequence. The process of monitoring the events must examine the entire chain of events more closely. To this end, a root cause analysis can aid in determining where the process of care needs to be improved to achieve a better patient outcome and reduce unnecessary costs.

McDonald and Leyhane (2005) offer the following six-step process for conducting a root cause analysis specific to healthcare:

1. *Determine whether an immediate risk to patients* or providers exists, and act accordingly.
2. Clearly *define the role of leaders and facilitators*, because effective analysis requires a multidisciplinary team made up of staff at all levels closest to the event and those with decision-making authority.
3. *Determine the sequence of events*, contributing conditions, and assumptions related to the critical event.
4. *Analyze causal factors*—those that, if eliminated, would have prevented the occurrence or reduced its severity.
5. *Identify changes* and develop action plans across disciplines.
6. *Present the recommended improvements*, such as redesign or development of new systems and processes, to senior leaders for review and approval of implementation, including timelines, monitoring strategies, and reporting structures.

Returning to our case at the beginning of the chapter, note that several things did not go well during Mr. Londborg's stay. By using a team approach to obtain multiple perspectives, we can construct a fishbone diagram (shown in exhibit 14.2) that displays what might be the result from the first four steps. Steps five and six will be addressed in the next section.

As you can see, the diagram includes everything that went wrong with Mr. Londborg's visit, sorted into categories that most closely describe what kind of error occurred. This chart tells the administrator, working with clinical colleagues, where to turn to fix a host of issues associated with Mr. Londborg's misadventure.

In this case, some of the boxes have a heavier outline to delineate the true "root" of the problem. Had Mr. Londborg been administered the DVT medication, he would not have had an extended stay in the hospital and most likely would have been discharged on day 3. Recall that it was on day 3 that he complained of pain in his leg and the care team diagnosed a DVT, necessitating a longer stay. It was in the subsequent days (day 8) that his care team failed to provide his antiseizure medication, leading to a seizure, his fall, and the need to extend his stay even further. Had he been given the DVT medication in the first place, the ensuing events would not have occurred. As we know, however, he did not receive the DVT prophylaxis and all the ensuing events did occur. After identifying the

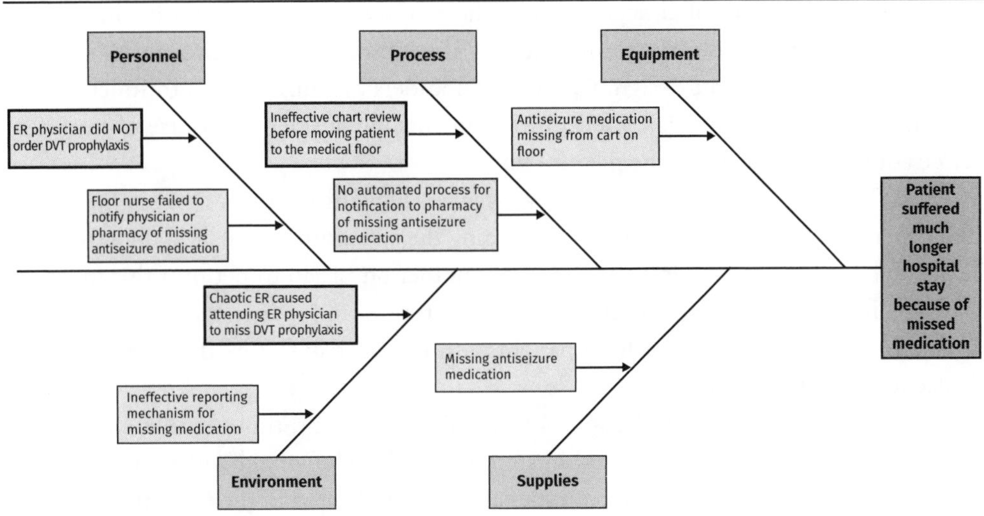

Exhibit 14.2 Root Cause Analysis of Events in Mr. Londborg's Hospitalization

root cause(s) of what went wrong, administrators and clinicians alike can and must now go about the business of taking corrective action.

Taking Corrective Action as Needed

By definition, healthcare requires intense levels of interactions among staff members, so when things go wrong, it is human nature to assign blame. However, root cause analysis, one of the most powerful tools of risk management, dissects the problem into its most basic segments in an attempt to discover the true source of the problems.

Steps four and five from the McDonald and Leyhane (2005) framework come into play here as the team doing the analysis would prepare for step six. For the sake of brevity, we will examine only the heavier-weight boxes of exhibit 14.2 as we consider step five, "Identify changes":

a. ER physician did not order DVT prophylaxis (Personnel)

b. Chaotic ER distracted attending ER physician (Environment)

c. Ineffective chart review before moving patient to medical floor (Process)

Items "a" and "b" are closely related. By their nature, emergency departments are sometimes chaotic places. With an obligation to treat all patients, they see everything from dog bites and emergency childbirths to heart attacks, car accident injuries, gunshot wounds, and much more. Nothing can prevent events in the outside world that result in patients who need multiple kinds of emergency care. These events sometimes occur in clusters that defy prediction. As a result, the team reviewing this episode of care may want to consider the emergency department design. Can hospital leaders organize the ER to function in a way that provides the physician a few quiet moments to consider the course of treatment before admitting a patient to the medical floor?

As for item "c," that same team may consider changing the process of care to include an independent review of the chart before sending the patient to the medical floor. It would be possible for a nurse, physician assistant, or another physician to perform this function. Having a fresh set of eyes on the chart at this juncture would reduce the risk of failing to order an important medication for a patient with known risk factors that indicate a particular course of treatment.

Regardless, these potential solutions require review and thoughtful consideration by a multidisciplinary team, as noted in step two of the McDonald and Leyhane (2005) framework. Cost and human resource issues are both implicated in the potential solutions.

Process Evaluation in a Business Setting

One of management's important functions is to create an environment conducive to clinicians providing the best possible healthcare services. Managers accomplish this through the allocation of resources in efficient and effective ways and in taking steps to ensure the organization complies with all applicable laws and regulations. To that end, managers can employ many of the same tools used in the clinical setting to assess the effectiveness of management functions.

In short, all the steps previously described can also apply to most business processes. While it may be more challenging to find information related to "best practices," it is still possible—and desirable—to improve management effectiveness using the same tools and processes discussed earlier.

Now, let us consider a second case.

An Unwelcome Surprise

If there was anything Jamal Bell didn't like, it was surprises at work—particularly surprises with bad news. How in the world had this happened? How could he possibly not have seen it coming?

Jamal had earned his bachelor's degree in health administration three years earlier, and after completing his one-year administrator-in-training program for long-term care (LTC) administration, he had passed the nursing home administrator's exam in his state with flying colors. He then accepted the position of assistant administrator at West Wind

Manor, a small, 20-bed skilled nursing facility that was one of 11 facilities in the region owned by Healthy Elderly, Inc.

Jamal's immediate boss, West Wind's administrator, also had duties at the three other Healthy Elderly facilities in the county and was only at West Wind about one day each week. This meant that, as the administrator on site, Jamal was responsible for day-to-day operations and direct supervision of all the department heads and managers. With such a broad span of control, he knew he would have to rely heavily on the department heads and managers underneath him. Luckily, they had all been at West Wind longer than he, and they all seemed to know their areas well.

One of the things Jamal was proudest of was that everyone at West Wind genuinely liked him—managers, staff, and clients alike. He knew everyone by name and had an easygoing, friendly, open-door management style. He held monthly management meetings where each manager gave a verbal report of her area and was free to bring up any concerns or problems that had arisen. These meetings usually went smoothly, and Jamal and his management team often had time at the end to discuss new ideas for programs and for the care West Wind provided.

LTC facilities must meet a vast number of criteria to maintain Medicare and Medicaid eligibility. In the past, site visits by inspectors to ensure quality of care and compliance with regulations had been regularly scheduled, but they were now conducted on an unannounced, random basis. West Wind had not had a site visit in the two years Jamal had been there. That is, until the previous week, when the inspectors had simply shown up.

Jamal, of course, knew his facility would eventually go through a site inspection, but he had not really been concerned, as things seemed to be running so well. West Wind's financials were strong, there was relatively low turnover among staff, and client complaints were few and far between. The facility was clean, the food was good, and the recreation events were well designed and well attended. So Jamal was shocked when the site visit team reported a large number of major and minor infractions. Jamal was given a short time in which to respond to the site team's report and to create a correction plan for each of the following infractions the team found:

1. The refrigeration unit failed to keep foods chilled to an appropriate temperature. At the time of the site visit, foods containing mayonnaise were perilously close to becoming tainted.
2. Food service workers failed to wear appropriate protective gloves and failed to wash their hands before and after handling raw meat.
3. One of the medication carts was unattended and unlocked.
4. The community/activity room was uncleaned and had traces of food in multiple places.

5. Several residents had pressure ulcers (bedsores).
6. Review of financial records revealed that West Wind was behind in paying its bills, with accounts receivables exceeding the industry average.

Jamal sat down at his desk with the site team's report and sighed. The surprise bad news frustrated him because he did not understand how this could have happened. How should he address the concerns raised in the report?

Jamal decided that the tool he should use to review the infractions was root cause analysis. He and his team would take the list of infractions, break them into appropriate categories, and examine what happened (or did not happen) in each circumstance to begin considering possible corrective action. In this instance, a root cause analysis could help determine the reasons for important shortcomings, which in turn could lead to more effective monitoring.

Using the six steps described earlier would facilitate the determination of not only what went wrong (the list of infractions provides that), but why. Again, here is a synopsis of the McDonald and Leyhane (2005) framework:

1. *Determine whether an immediate risk to patients* or providers exists.
2. Clearly *define the role of leaders and facilitators.*
3. *Determine the sequence of events.*
4. *Analyze causal factors.*
5. *Identify changes and develop action plans across disciplines.*
6. *Present the recommended improvements to senior leaders* and implement.

Exhibit 14.3 is a possible outcome of the process Jamal and his team used to analyze the regulatory site team's findings. As you can see, the violations show up in all five categories. Note also that the category labeled "Supplies" in exhibit 14.2 has been changed to "Finances" here. The point is there is nothing magical about the categories. Each can be adapted to fit the circumstances to help determine what went wrong. There is nothing about "Supplies" in the review team's list of infractions, so Jamal and his colleagues can change it to "Finances" to be consistent with the review team's findings of poor handling of accounts payable. Conversely, the categories otherwise used in exhibit 14.2 for Mr. Londborg's case all apply here, so the West Wind team can use them for assessing business and management processes as well. Were there violations stemming from other areas, these categories, too, could be changed. In addition, it would be acceptable to add or subtract categories if necessary. The danger in adding categories is that the process loses its meaning if there are too many.

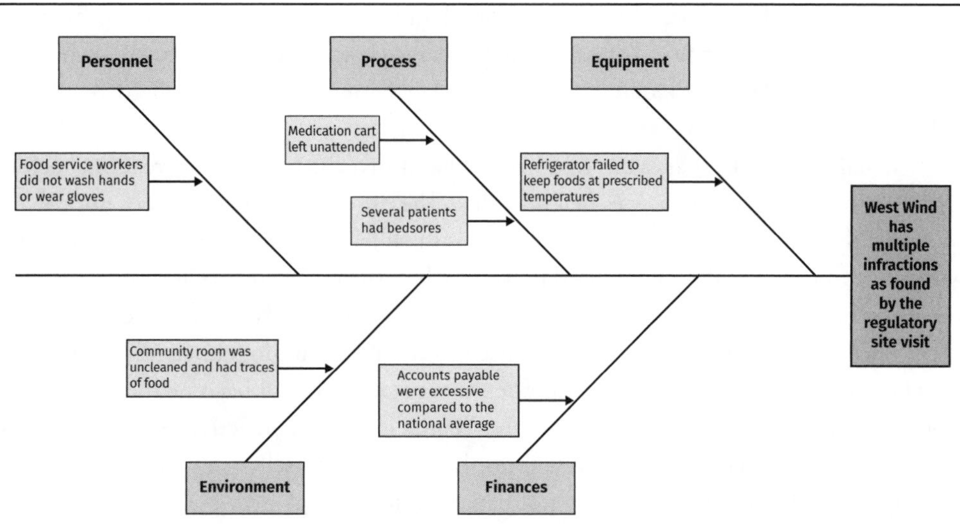

Exhibit 14.3 Root Cause Analysis of West Wind Violations

In examining what went wrong, the management team must consider how to avoid making these mistakes again. The case remarks, "How could he possibly not have seen this coming?" Conducting the root cause analysis to understand what went wrong will only work to prevent it from happening again, if Jamal and his team understand that part of the underlying problem here is a systemic failure to monitor operations effectively.

Monitoring the Improvements

One glaring red flag in Jamal's "Unwelcome Surprise" case is that the management team provided only verbal reports at monthly meetings. The root cause analysis will show areas for improvement. In those areas and others, written reports should become part of the routine monitoring process in the aftermath of the assessment and improvement recommendations. The most common way of presenting information as part of the monitoring function is in a written report. Verbal reports, such as those presented at Jamal's monthly meetings, do not provide actual documentation. They could easily be incomplete, overlooking an important detail. Written reports may be in the form of spreadsheets for finances and summaries of various activities.

For example, Jamal believed West Wind's financials were strong. Perhaps they are, but the accounts receivable function is not. What was the basis for Jamal's belief? A verbal report is insufficient for the detail required. Perhaps Jamal heard only what he wanted to hear; perhaps the financial officer glossed over the facts about accounts receivables in her verbal report.

On a more basic level, how would Jamal and his team go about setting financial goals? To ensure that West Wind's financial performance is adequate, Jamal needs to compare West Wind to similar LTC facilities on several financial measures—benchmarks—and set realistic standards.

Jamal also thinks that West Wind is clean and that the food and recreational activities are good. But, again, how does he know this? The use of verbal reports does not convey appropriately or fully the complete picture and is the likely culprit. Jamal and his top management team need to take a long, hard look at each of the review team's areas of inspection and, using benchmarking, set reasonable and achievable standards for each area.

The leadership team should be actively engaged in determining the standards so everyone will understand and embrace them. Then those standards will become the baseline for written reports for effectively monitoring West Wind's management activities going forward.

Using these techniques, Jamal will not have to ask himself again, "How could this have happened? How could I possibly not have seen it coming?"

Conclusion

This chapter addressed the issue of quality from both clinical and management perspectives. Many evaluative methods of assessing quality apply to both. The root cause analysis is a primary example. In setting standards of care, or of conducting business, an organization should consider benchmarking its process against others, or engage in additional research to discover best practices. Once it has adopted standards, its leadership team needs to monitor performance to ensure those standards are being met (the control step). Finally, the idea of monitoring with an eye toward continuous improvement is imperative. Using risk-management tools such as a root cause analysis can help detect opportunities for improvement. The delivery of high-quality care depends, in part, on the environment administrators create through the implementation of high-quality standards in the practice of management.

Mini Case Study: What Disney Can Teach Walter Reed

The US Army is paying Walt Disney Inc. $800,000 in consultant fees to serve as a benchmark for its treatment of veterans. Walter Reed Army Medical Center has received unfavorable reviews from veterans frustrated by receiving the "runaround," not getting their questions answered, being constantly faced with an impersonal bureaucracy, and being cared for in a shabby, if not unhealthy, environment (Vogel 2008).

Disney will help Walter Reed Army Medical Center by sharing best practices regarding customer service. Walter Reed staff members hope they can put the "care" back into "healthcare" for the veterans.

Mini Case Study Questions

1. What common ground do you think Disney shares with Walter Reed?
2. How would you recommend that Walter Reed Army Medical Center evaluate the program's outcomes for the treatment of veterans?

Points to Remember

- The structure of providing care—the physical facilities as well as the training and competence of the staff—is an underlying component of quality of care.
- The process of care is also critically important in achieving a high quality of care.
- The outcome is likewise a part of considering the quality of care.
- Benchmarking—the process of comparing one organization to another or to a well-established standard—is an important consideration in improving both care and management operations.
- Risk management is an organization's way to minimize the uncertainty associated with a particular process and to minimize the possibility of an adverse outcome.
- The root cause analysis is an important tool in developing improvements in both care and managerial settings.
- Multiple perspectives are necessary for the development of a thorough root cause analysis.

Challenge Yourself

Assume that the infractions the site review team found at West Wind include three items:

1. Noncompliance with fire safety standards—specifically, an insufficient number of fire extinguishers, inaccessible fire extinguishers, and insufficient testing of fire extinguishers
2. Inadequate activities for the residents, activities not sufficiently stimulating, and not enough of them
3. Insufficient monitoring of medications provided to patients, resulting in improper dosages being provided to patients at the wrong time

Develop a root cause analysis and propose a correction plan of standards, monitoring, and corrective action.

For Your Consideration

1. Provide a healthcare management example of benchmarking. Where could the benchmarking information be found for your example?
2. The beginning of this chapter states that although the standard assessment process might look simple on paper, it is complex and often hard to implement in healthcare settings. What specific factors might make assessment more challenging in healthcare than in other industries?
3. Provide an example of best practices. Where could "best practice" information be found for your example?

References

Agency for Healthcare Research and Quality (AHRQ). 2018. "Quality." Accessed May 2. www.ahrq.gov/topics/quality.html.

———. 2014. "Guide to Clinical Preventive Services, 2014: Recommendations of the US Preventive Services Task Force." Reviewed June. www.ahrq.gov/professionals/clinicians-providers/guidelines-recommendations/guide/index.html.

Centers for Medicare & Medicaid Services (CMS). 2018. "Readmissions Reduction Program." Accessed April 26. www.cms.gov/medicare/medicare-fee-for-service-payment/acuteinpatientpps/readmissions-reduction-program.html.

Dictionary.com. 2018. "Risk." Accessed August 25. www.dictionary.com/browse/risk.

Donabedian, A. 1966. "Evaluating the Quality of Medical Care." *Milbank Memorial Fund Quarterly* 44 (3): 166–202.

Hilliard, R. 2013. "Case Study: An Extended Stay." Institute for Healthcare Improvement. Accessed June 16, 2016. www.ihi.org/education/IHIOpenSchool/resources/Pages/Activities/CaseStudyAnExtendedStay.aspx.

Institute of Medicine (IOM). 2018. "Crossing the Quality Chasm: The IOM Health Care Quality Initiative." Accessed November 26. www.nationalacademies.org/hmd/Global/News%20Announcements/Crossing-the-Quality-Chasm-The-IOM-Health-Care-Quality-Initiative.aspx.

McDonald, A., and T. Leyhane. 2005. "Drill Down with Root Cause Analysis: Know the Source of the Spark While Protecting Yourself from Fire." *Nursing Management* 36 (10): 26–31.

McIlwain, J. 2006. "A Review: A Decade of Clinical Risk Management and Risk Tools." *Clinician in Management* 14 (4): 189–99.

National Guideline Clearinghouse. 2015. "Venous Thromboembolism in Adults Admitted to Hospital: Reducing the Risk." Accessed June 16, 2018. www.guideline.gov/summaries/summary/49437/venous-thromboembolism-in-adults-admitted-to-hospital-reducing-the-risk?q=prophylaxis+DVT.

Quora. 2015. "How Many Flights Are There a Day Per Airline?" Accessed June 16, 2018. www.quora.com/How-many-flights-per-day-are-there-per-airline.

Rooney, J., and L. Vanden Heuvel. 2004. "Root Cause Analysis for Beginners." *Quality Progress* 37 (7): 45–53.

Rue, L., and L. Byars. 2004. *Supervision: Key Link to Productivity*. Boston: McGraw-Hill Irwin.

Thomas, F., and T. Caldis. 2007. "Emerging Issues of Pay-for-Performance in Health Care." *Health Care Financing Review* 29 (1): 1–4.

Vogel, S. 2008. "Trying Some Disney Attitude to Help Cure Walter Reed." *Washington Post*. Published February 25. www.washingtonpost.com/wp-dyn/content/article/2008/02/24/AR2008022401993.html.

CHAPTER 15

HEALTH INFORMATICS

Important Terms

- Accounts receivable
- American Recovery and Reinvestment Act (ARRA)
- Average days in accounts receivable
- Clinical decision support systems
- Computerized physician order entry (CPOE)
- Electronic health record (EHR)
- Health informatics
- Health Information Technology for Economic and Clinical Health (HITECH) Act
- Health Insurance Portability and Accountability Act (HIPAA)
- HIPAA Privacy Rule
- Institute of Medicine
- Meaningful use
- Medical Identity Fraud Alliance (MIFA)
- Medical identity theft
- Medicare Access and CHIP Reauthorization Act (MACRA)
- Office of the National Coordinator for Health Information Technology (ONC)
- Patient portal
- Protected health information (PHI)

Learning Objectives

After reading this chapter, you will be able to do the following:

- ➤ Describe health informatics
- ➤ Explain the history of health information technology (HIT) adoption in the United States
- ➤ Define the electronic health record (EHR)

- Evaluate the benefits and issues surrounding health information technologies
- Describe the Health Insurance Portability and Accountability Act (HIPAA)
- Define protected health information (PHI)
- Explain how information technology supports organizational goals

Case Study: HIPAA and Memorial Hermann Health System

In September 2015, a patient was asked to show her identification when she arrived for an appointment at the Memorial Hermann Health System (MHHS) gynecologic clinic. She was scheduled for an annual visit that would include her doctor following up on an abdominal cyst that had been identified at her 2014 annual appointment (Maruca 2015). She never got to see the doctor.

The patient had given the staff member her photo identification upon request when she arrived for her appointment. The staff member thought the photo identification looked like a fake Texas driver's license and asked the patient to produce another form of photo identification, which she could not do (Kuyers 2017). The staff member phoned the Texas Department of Public Safety to find out if they could help determine if the driver's license was authentic, and the Texas Department of Public Safety advised the staff to contact law enforcement, which they did. Law enforcement determined the driver's license was false and arrested the patient (Kline 2017). She was charged with one felony count of tampering with a government record because deputies discovered a fake Social Security card when they searched her purse (Barajas 2015).

It was later revealed the patient had lived in Texas for more than ten years on an expired visa, and the incident at MHHS spurred discussion and protest about the role of hospitals that refuse medical care to illegal immigrants. Moreover, there was public concern that immigrants would become afraid to seek medical care for fear of being arrested. The incident became the focus of debate on healthcare and undocumented workers in the United States (Schiller 2015). In response to protesters at Memorial Hermann, the hospital issued to 15 media outlets press releases in which they reported the patient's name, explaining she was not being denied medical care. Rather, they said the issue had been about the patient identification at check-in and MHHS ensuring the patient was indeed who she said she was (Morse 2017). MHHS also published the patient's name on its website and mentioned it during meetings with an advocacy group, state representatives, and a state senator (US Department of Health and Human Services 2017a)—a clear violation of the **HIPAA Privacy Rule**.

Health Insurance Portability and Accountability Act (HIPAA) Privacy Rule
The part of HIPAA that establishes safeguards to protect confidentiality and privacy and specifically identifies protected health information.

Financial donations were given to help the family post the patient's $35,000 bond, and after two weeks in the Harris County jail, she was released and allowed to return home. Six months after the incident, she pleaded guilty to having a false driver's license and was sentenced to 40 hours of community service and a $200 fine (Hixenbaugh 2017).

In May 2017, MHHS agreed to settle the alleged HIPAA disclosure violation regarding protected health information (PHI). MHHS agreed to adopt a corrective action plan and pay the US Department of Health and Human Services' Office for Civil Rights (OCR) $2.4 million. The fine and corrective plan were in response to MHHS's publishing the patient's name and using it during meetings with the advocacy group, state representatives, and state senator. The agreed-upon corrective action plan included MHHS's promise to update its policies and procedures regarding PHI and to conduct training so MHHS staff are educated about PHI and allowable uses and disclosures. OCR Director Severino stated the following (US Department of Health and Human Services 2017b):

> Senior management should have known that disclosing a patient's name on the title of a press release was a clear HIPAA Privacy violation that would induce a swift OCR response. . . . This case reminds us that organizations can readily cooperate with law enforcement without violating HIPAA, but that they must nevertheless continue to protect patient privacy when making statements to the public and elsewhere.

Introduction

We saw in the case study the failure of management to understand the law regarding **protected health information (PHI)**. You were introduced to the **Health Insurance Portability and Accountability Act** (**HIPAA**) in chapter 10, and after reading this case, you may surmise why the law is important enough to be discussed again in this chapter on **health informatics**, a term that describes the "field that is concerned with the optimal use of information, often aided by the use of technology, to improve individual health, health care, public health, and biomedical research" (Hersh 2009).

Protected health information (PHI)
Information from which a specific person or patient can be identified and that relates to physical or mental health, the provision of healthcare, or the payment for healthcare.

Health Insurance Portability and Accountability Act (HIPAA)
A law that took effect in 2003 and established a baseline of acceptable protection for patient privacy and confidentiality.

Health informatics
The study of the creation and implementation of information technology–based innovation to advance health services.

Healthcare managers use data every day to assess costs, generate budgets, evaluate patient care quality, and bill for services rendered. However, while using the data, it is equally important to safeguard that data, particularly any data that might infringe upon patient confidentiality. Thus, healthcare managers have responsibilities to all stakeholders to have a working knowledge of health information technology (HIT) used in the healthcare workplace, as well as the policies, procedures, and laws that govern our access to and use of data.

In the last chapter, we saw how critical it is for managers to create an environment conducive to delivering high-quality care. In this chapter, you will see that it is equally vital for healthcare managers to know how to leverage technology to yield better information, which leads to both better care and better organizational performance. Moreover, managers must be aware of the issues of privacy and security surrounding HIT. You will learn about these issues and see how HIT helps to bring about patient-centered care.

Health Informatics and the Origins of Health Information Technology in the US Healthcare Delivery System

Healthcare was slower to adopt information technology (IT) than other industries, such as retail and banking. For example, the growth of IT at Walmart, the largest discount retailer in the world, helped the company create efficiencies in its practices, grow its businesses, and increase profits (Wailgum 2007). Walmart opened its first store in 1962. By 1975, it had more than 125 stores generating $340.3 million in sales, and Walmart had leased a computer to help with inventory control (Wailgum 2007). By 1977, the company had built a computer network for ordering merchandise from its suppliers, and by 1987, it had a barcode labeling system in its more than 880 stores (Wailgum 2007). The barcode system tracked sales and identified when products sold and at what price. It gave Walmart a competitive advantage because this technology enabled precise inventory management so managers and suppliers knew when to restock merchandise (Lewallen 2004). Customers could expect Walmart to always have the products they wanted in stock when they wanted them. All because of IT management.

In the banking industry, automated teller machines (ATMs) changed the way customers interfaced with their banks. Instead of only banking on weekdays during business hours, ATMs allowed customers to walk up to a machine, insert an encrypted card, and conduct bank transactions any day of the week, at any time. The first ATM is credited to a Barclays branch in England in 1967 (McRobbie 2015). The ATM card was encoded with a unique card number, expiration date, and personal identification number (PIN). A customer only had to insert a card into the ATM and verify the PIN. The machine then communicated with the bank's host processors to complete the transaction. Suddenly, rather than waiting in line at a branch, customers could expect their bank to conduct certain transactions, such as withdrawal of cash, whenever they wanted. All because of IT management.

Now, compare these examples with a patient's healthcare encounter. In the 1960s and 1970s, when Walmart and banks were employing IT to conduct business better, patients in physician offices were still dealing with paperwork. If during an appointment a physician prescribed medication, the physician handwrote that prescription on a piece of paper from a prescription pad. The physician then gave that piece of paper to the patient, who hand-delivered it to a pharmacy. The pharmacist deciphered the handwritten prescription and filled the drug order—a process that was slow, inconvenient, and presented risk for error. In the 1960s and 1970s, all prescriptions were handwritten. (In fact, most clinician orders were handwritten until after 2009, a change we will discuss later.) Patients could not expect prescriptions to be ready when they arrived at the pharmacy, and there was always the chance that pharmacists might misread a physician's writing and dispense the wrong drug. All because of the lack of IT management.

Despite this slow adoption of technology on the clinical side of healthcare, the industry *did* invest during the 1960s and 1970s in IT related to administrative and financial functions. For example, hospitals began developing IT applications in response to health insurance companies' use of IT to track and adjust premium prices based on costs (Neumann, Parente, and Paramore 1996). The outcome was a computerized billing system for hospitals. Physician practices followed suit with "super-bill" programs, which allowed them to bill different insurers "while working from a single data entry screen" (Neumann, Parente, and Paramore 1996, 426). These new IT systems also enabled hospitals and physicians to speed up certain activities, including payer and patient billing.

Institute of Medicine (IOM)
A nonprofit, nongovernment organization established in 1970 that focuses on evidence-based research for public health and science policy.

Electronic health record (EHR)
A digital record of the care provided to a patient by a healthcare organization, including the patient's up-to-date, real-time health-related information. When the record can be shared among multiple providers, it is said to have *interoperability*. Also called *electronic medical record*.

Office of the National Coordinator for Health Information Technology (ONC)
Created by President George W. Bush's executive order in 2004 to promote a national health information technology infrastructure. The 2009 HITECH Act gave ONC leadership authority for EHR implementation efforts.

The application of IT to improve patient care only came later. During the 1990s, the growth of technology as a whole spurred serious interest and investment in healthcare IT for patients. The World Wide Web was introduced in 1991 (World Wide Web Foundation 2018), and e-mail became popular shortly thereafter when Microsoft released Hotmail, its Internet-based e-mail application, in 1996 (Left 2002). Users became familiar with the ability to access and exchange information in real time, or close to it.

Also during this time, the **Institute of Medicine (IOM)** issued its support for the establishment of computer-based patient records (Dick and Steen 1991). And, in 1999, it published its groundbreaking report regarding patient deaths due to medical errors, *To Err Is Human: Building a Safer Health System*. IOM estimated that 44,000 to 98,000 people died annually from medication errors and "found that the majority of medical errors do not result from individual recklessness but because of systemic flaws in the way the health system is organized" (Havens and Boroughs 2000, 77).

The report cited several studies to illustrate its point about systemic flaws. We offer one here for illustration.

Researchers reviewed all the admissions to 22 medical and surgical units at two Boston tertiary care hospitals, Brigham and Women's and Massachusetts General, over a six-month period in 1993 (Leape et al. 1995). They identified 334 adverse drug events, which they attributed to two main causes: lack of knowledge about the drug and lack of information about the patient (Leape et al. 1995). Had a better information system been in place, the clinicians could have learned immediately about—and prevented—potential interactions that might occur between a potential drug and a patient's current prescriptions. In addition, the patient's medical history would have been complete and readily available for review by anyone involved in his or her care, including physicians, other providers, pharmacies, and laboratories.

This critical information—drug interactions and patient history—are components of a comprehensive **electronic health record (EHR)**, which is a digitalized record that documents the patient's medical history, previous diagnoses, medications, allergies, and other health-related information (HealthIT.gov 2018). Despite its importance to patient safety, however, the introduction and adoption of EHRs did not come until later, after support from President George W. Bush's 2004 executive order to establish the **Office of the National Coordinator for Health Information Technology (ONC)**, which led to efforts to develop and incentivize a national HIT strategy.

The same year the ONC was established, IOM issued another seminal report: *Patient Safety: Achieving a New Standard for Care*, which called for a commitment to patient safety and a national health information infrastructure. Then, five years later, Congress passed the 2009 **American Recovery and Reinvestment Act (ARRA)**, which included the 2009 **Health Information Technology for Economic and Clinical Health (HITECH) Act**. HITECH provided governmental endorsement and financial incentives for the adoption and implementation of EHRs, as well as their **meaningful use**. The overall goal was for healthcare providers to have access to the right data, at the right time, and in the right place. EHRs and meaningful use were further legislated in 2015, with the passage of the **Medicare Access and CHIP Reauthorization Act (MACRA)**. As it established new reimbursement rules for providers of Medicare patients, MACRA folded meaningful use into the new Merit-Based Incentive Payment System (MIPS), which examines patient outcomes and EHRs (Network for Regional Healthcare Improvement 2018).

Thus, to meet the rules as well as provide quality patient care measured by patient outcomes, healthcare providers now needed to rely on quality data that identified best practices in quality patient care. To share data, access data, and evaluate best practices, providers turned to comprehensive EHRs and other data sets related to patient protocols. The result of the political, economic, and healthcare delivery goals regarding quality patient care was the increased adoption and implementation of EHRs.

By 2012, 42 percent of hospitals had implemented an EHR system (DesRoches et al. 2013). By 2015, the Centers for Disease Control and Prevention (CDC) reported that about 87 percent of office-based physicians used an EHR (CDC 2015). And by 2016, the ONC reported that 96 percent of non-federal acute care hospitals had adopted EHRs, and more than 80 percent of other types of hospitals (small, rural, critical access) had done so (Henry et al. 2016).

American Recovery and Reinvestment Act (ARRA)
An economic stimulus bill passed by the US Congress in 2009 in response to the country's economic downturn. Included the 2009 HITECH Act.

Health Information Technology for Economic and Clinical Health (HITECH) Act
Legislation passed in 2009 to promote the adoption and meaningful use of health information technology. Also addressed privacy and security concerns associated with the use of HIT.

Meaningful use
US government standards for healthcare providers' use of electronic health records for capturing and sharing data with other providers, insurers, and patients.

Medicare Access and CHIP Reauthorization Act (MACRA)
Legislation passed in 2015 that based Medicare payments on patient outcomes; streamlined quality programs such as meaningful use into the Merit-based Incentive Payment System; and provided payments for provider participation in alternative payment models.

Health Information Technology, Meaningful Use, and the Merit-Based Incentive Payment System

Financial incentives for healthcare entities that provide care for Medicare and Medicaid patients were key for the increased adoption and implementation of EHRs. As mentioned earlier, the 2009 HITECH Act and the 2015 MACRA legislation connected financial reimbursement and EHR use—specifically influenced by providers' meeting meaningful use requirements of EHR usage that became one of the four components of the new MIPS under MACRA.

Meaningful use was divided into three stages for provider adoption. Stage one focused on electronic data capture and sharing, and stage two expanded on stage one and advanced clinical processes (CMS 2018a). Stage three was designed to improve outcomes and implement actions that lead to improved health for patients on a large scale, including improving the quality of health information exchanged and establishing a more collated information

Computerized physician order entry (CPOE)
A system in which a healthcare provider enters a medication order via electronic entry, which is sent directly to a pharmacy in real time. Replaces handwritten paper prescriptions.

network (CMS 2018b). Exhibit 15.1 explores the requirements for the stages of meaningful use involving **computerized physician order entry (CPOE)**.

To reiterate, with the introduction of MACRA in 2015, meaningful use became one of the four components of the new MIPS, which is part of the MACRA legislation. Today, providers no longer participate in a formal meaningful use program. However, adopting meaningful use actions has helped them meet the quality reporting measures defined in MIPS that provide financial incentives to use certified EHR technology. Exhibit 15.2 illustrates meaningful use and the shift to MIPS.

Exhibit 15.1 Stages of Meaningful Use of Computerized Physician Order Entry

Stage 1	Providers were to use CPOE for medication orders directly entered by any licensed healthcare professional who could enter orders into the medical record per state, local, and professional guidelines.
Stage 2	Providers were to use CPOE for medication, laboratory, and radiology orders directly entered by any licensed healthcare professional who can enter orders into the medical record per state, local, and professional guidelines.
Stage 3	Providers were to use CPOE for medication, laboratory, and diagnostic imaging orders directly entered by any licensed healthcare professional, credentialed medical assistant, or medical staff member credentialed to perform the equivalent duties of a credentialed medical assistant, who can enter orders into the medical record per state, local, and professional guidelines.

Sources: CMS (2012, 2016, 2018b).

Exhibit 15.2 Meaningful Use and the Shift to MIPS

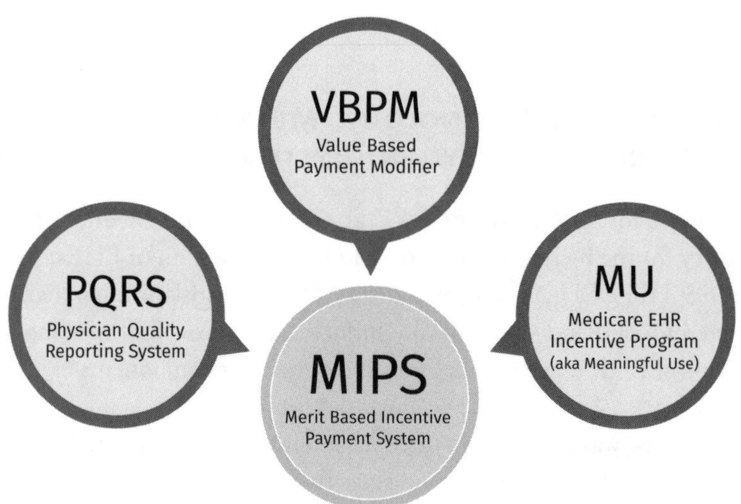

Source: Adapted from HealthIT.gov (2017).

Benefits of Health Information Technology

The expansion of health IT and providers' increased adoption and implementation of EHRs has brought benefits across the healthcare system. It has benefited public health and research, as access to de-identified data now lets researchers study past treatment protocols and determine which ones provide better outcomes. It also, as we will see, improves patient safety during emergencies, offers billing and other administrative advantages, helps clinicians make treatment decisions and prevent medication errors, and lets patients participate more actively in their care with patient portals.

Patient Safety During Emergencies

Consider, for example, the aftermath of Hurricane Katrina, a Category 5 storm that struck New Orleans in August 2005, causing flood waters as high as 13 feet in some areas and leaving 80 percent of the city submerged (Robertson and Fausset 2015). At Charity Hospital, Louisiana's largest healthcare facility, the backup generators installed for emergency use were located on the first floor; after the hurricane, they were under water and useless. For five days, in 100-degree heat, the hospital's remaining occupants endured a loss of electricity and a shortage of food, water, and medication. In these conditions, clinicians had to care for 250 patients while waiting for help to arrive (Freemantle 2005). One of the challenges they faced was a lack of access to patients' PHI (Franco et al. 2006). They did not know about patients' diagnoses or potential drug interactions. When patients could finally be evacuated to safe facilities, providers had to make sure their medical records traveled with them—by taping brief paper notes to their bodies (Franco et al. 2006).

Medical facilities were flooded throughout the area, and patient records across the region were a problem after Katrina. In a small fishing village on the Gulf Coast, for example, the practice of primary care provider Regina Benjamin had used paper records for 23 years before the storm. Benjamin explained she had not pursued implementing an EHR because of the cost: "Money was tight, as it was for many small practices throughout the country, and it eventually came down to a choice: I could either install an EHR system or pay the electricity bill" (Benjamin 2010, 505).

But after her clinic was flooded by Katrina, and she and her staff tried to salvage paper medical records by drying them in the sun, Benjamin said that "whereas I had previously decided against installing an EHR system because I couldn't afford one, I now realized I couldn't afford *not* to have one" (Benjamin 2010, 506).

Fast-forward to 2012. When a tornado landed in Harrisburg, Illinois, the emergency department at Harrisburg Hospital had to care for 53 patients in six hours; on average, they see about 20 patients in a 24-hour time frame (Abir et al. 2012). The presence of an EHR let staff register patients efficiently and provided access to their stored medical information. If patients had to be transferred to another facility, there was no need to tape their records to their bodies, as at Charity Hospital in Louisiana; rather, with a click, the information was sent digitally to the receiving institution. This smooth information sharing was because the hospital belonged to a regional health information organization (RHIO). Organizations that join RHIOs agree to share patient healthcare–related information electronically. Thus, at Harrisburg Hospital, technology improved both administrative tasks and clinical access to patient information, leading to better care, even during an emergency.

Administrative Benefits of HIT

Information technology also provides administrative benefits to hospitals and other healthcare facilities, as we will see in an example featuring a physician practice and the issue of accounts receivable benchmarks.

Accounts receivable
Dollar amounts that have been billed to patients and third-party payers but have not yet been paid.

Average days in accounts receivable
Calculation of the average number of days from date of service to payment received. Typically, the equation reads total accounts receivable ÷ (gross charges ÷ days in period).

The term **accounts receivable** refers to an important financial indicator for any business, and days in accounts receivable means the average number of days from the time service is provided until payment is received (MGMA 2009). In a 2011 case, an internal medicine clinic was experiencing **average days in accounts receivable** of 200 days, and the physician-owners had hired Amelia, a new business manager, to help improve clinic operations as well as patient and insurance billing practices (Cellucci, Benson, and Farnsworth 2011). The goal was to first reduce the average days in accounts receivable to fewer than 50 days, and then to fewer than 30 days. However, to accomplish this, Amelia had to identify the problem, examine alternative solutions to the problem, identify the best alternative, and implement it. (She engaged in the rational decision-making model we discussed in chapter 9.)

Amelia determined the problem was that the clinic's former biller (who no longer worked there) should have been submitting 500 statements per month, but had been submitting only 15 (Cellucci, Benson, and Farnsworth 2011). Moreover, the practice had recently invested in an EHR, but the former biller was not competent with the system. Amelia knew that effective performance required both the presence of an EHR and a staff that was trained and skilled in using it. She formed a team of experienced billers from the clinic's consultant group and helped the new clinic biller learn the EHR system. As a result, the clinic reduced the average days in accounts receivable to fewer than 30. However, as we saw in our discussion of effective teams in chapter 8, it took a team of dedicated employees to help the clinic accomplish this goal.

Clinical Decision Support Systems

Health information technology also offers clinical benefits, as we saw in our discussion of computerized physician order entry. With CPOE, prescribing providers can type a prescription on a computer or mobile device, reducing potential errors caused by illegible handwriting and transcription mistakes. Indeed, research has found that CPOE reduces by 70 percent the odds of making a medication error when compared to paper prescriptions (Devine et al. 2010). In addition, CPOE systems support **clinical decision support systems (CDSSs)**, so if a prescriber enters an order for a drug that interacts negatively with another medication the patient is taking, the prescriber is alerted to this drug–drug interaction. Further, comprehensive EHR systems incorporate CDSS tools that can remind caregivers about a patient's health maintenance needs, drug allergies, drug interactions, and drug guidelines (Wright et al. 2011).

Clinical decision support system (CDSS)
Computer software that presents clinicians with knowledge-based information to help provide better specialized patient care.

Patient Portals

Another benefit of health information technology is the **patient portal**, which lets patients view their data, lab test results, and care notes online so they may participate more actively in their care. However, while a systematic literature review examining patient attitudes about the use of portals for managing chronic illnesses indicated that patients were positive about the patient–provider communication portals provided (Kruse, Bolton, and Freriks 2015), patients also were concerned about the safety of secure messaging (Kruse, Bolton, and Freriks 2015). Other research also indicated a concern about security to ensure the privacy of patients' health information (Clark et al. 2015; Miller et al. 2016).

Patient portal
Secure website that allows patients access to their personal health information.

Overall, research suggests patient portals are underutilized. A national survey of US veterans in 2010 found that only about 22 percent of veterans who had utilized healthcare services at the Veterans Health Administration accessed their patient portal (Tsai and Rosenheck 2012). A 2014–2015 study on patient engagement at a not-for-profit healthcare system in Virginia found that about 21 percent of patients activated their "MyChart" patient portal accounts (Mook et al. 2018). And, another 2014 study examining patient use of the patient portal at the University of North Carolina Health Care System within 30 days after discharge found that about 16 percent of patients had used the system (Griffin et al. 2016). Thus, research indicates that the majority of patients are not using the technology.

A systematic review of publications about patient portals from 1990 to 2013 found disparities regarding who accessed their patient portals and who did not (Goldzweig et al. 2013). Factors that affected usage included race, as whites were more likely to engage in the technology (Goldzweig et al. 2013; Griffin et al. 2016; Mook et al. 2018; Tsai and Rosenheck 2012). Educational attainment also influenced usage, as persons with some college education or higher were more likely to use their patient portal (Goldzweig et al. 2013; Tsai and Rosenheck 2012). In addition, severity of illness was positively associated with use: Griffin et al. (2016) found that 34 percent of patient portal users were readmitted to the hospital within 30 days. Thus, patient portal users were more likely to be white, higher educated, and sicker. They also were satisfied with the improved patient–provider communication portals provide, but were concerned about the security of their health information.

Issues of Concern Regarding Health Information Technologies

While the benefits are many regarding the use of technology in healthcare, there also are potential negative issues worthy of consideration by healthcare managers. Let us examine an outcome of the lack of privacy and security of data—the issue of **medical identity theft**.

Medical identity theft
The stealing of another's personal health insurance information in order to submit fraudulent claims for healthcare services rendered or healthcare products purchased.

In 2014, Kathleen Meiners received a follow-up communication from Centerpoint Medical Center in Independence, Missouri, regarding their appreciation of her son's visit (Armour 2015). Meiners lived in Kansas City with her husband and son, a 39-year-old with Down's syndrome. Her son had never been to Centerpoint Medical Center (Armour 2015). Meiners contacted Centerpoint to explain this, and to prove that her son had not been a patient there, she drove him to the medical center to show the staff he had not suffered the injury they claimed nor had he received treatment for that injury there. Nonetheless, Centerpoint continued to bill Meiners throughout 2014, as did the emergency room physicians and radiologists (Armour 2015). The radiologists even sent the bill to a collection agency. The Meiners family were victims of medical identity theft.

Medical identity theft not only damages a victim's credit; it also affects the information stored in their health records. A woman in Florida was billed for a leg amputation she did not receive, and she discovered that her health records included the faulty information that she was diabetic. She said, "The person had their leg amputated because of diabetes. . . . I am not a diabetic" (Minor 2016). In another case, a retired postal worker from Texas had her wallet stolen in 2008. Two years later, she was arrested, fingerprinted, and had her mugshot taken for allegedly purchasing more than 1,700 prescription opioid pills from numerous pharmacies (Andrews 2016).

Medical Identity Fraud Alliance (MIFA)
A coalition created in 2013 to identify best practices for combating patient identity theft.

The **Medical Identity Fraud Alliance (MIFA)**, a US public–private coalition, was formed in response to the rise in medical identity theft. Charter members included Blue Cross/Blue Shield Association, AARP, Kaiser Permanente, and the US Department of Veterans Affairs. MIFA's members "provide leadership to mobilize the healthcare ecosystem; cooperate to leverage collective power; research to adequately understand the problem and guide solution building; educate consumers, industry, legislators and regulators; and empower individuals to be the first line of defense in protecting their Protected Health Information" (MIFA 2015).

MIFA, together with Kaiser Permanente, ID Experts, Experian Data Breach Resolution, and Identity Finder, sponsors the Ponemon Institute's annual study of medical identity theft. In 2014, Ponemon surveyed a stratified, random sample of adults from all regions in the United States, with a final sample of more than 1,000 respondents (Ponemon Institute 2015). The findings indicated that medical identity theft was increasing, and that it cost consumers money, time, and, potentially, reputation. Of particular interest to healthcare managers, 79 percent of the survey respondents indicated they believed it was important for healthcare providers to ensure the privacy of their health records, while 40 percent reported that prompt notification of a data breach was important (Ponemon Institute 2015).

The issue of maintaining the confidentiality of patient information is not new to healthcare. Even before EHRs, an unethical person could access paper records to obtain information, and he could view handfuls of files. However, with EHRs, the same unethical person may have access to *thousands* of digital files. To illustrate, the US Department of Health and Human Services' Office for Civil Rights (OCR) publishes a list of PHI breaches affecting 500 or more people (OCR 2018). The list is updated frequently at https://ocrportal.hhs.gov/ocr/breach/breach_report.jsf. In 2017 and 2018, cases included employee theft of identifying information on about 11,000 patients (OCR 2018; Spitzer 2018); an employee error that e-mailed Social Security numbers for more than 30,000 patients (OCR 2018); and a phishing scam that resulted in access to PHI for more than 35,000 patients (*HIPAA Journal* 2018b; OCR 2018).

The advent of technology may make patient confidentiality harder to protect, but it is also incumbent upon healthcare managers to hire ethical employees and enforce their good behavior to minimize the risk that unethical staff members will steal patient data. Managers may want to encourage employees' involvement in their respective professional development organization (e.g., American College of Healthcare Executives, Medical Group Management Association, American Health Information Management Association), which will reinforce their ethical codes of conduct. Moreover, an organization's IT professionals can institute "hard stops" in the EHR system to hide portions of the medical records from persons who do not need access to that information. For instance, one health system developed "a system of 'nesting' sensitive information so that . . . psychiatric records can be shielded from nonpsychiatric providers" (Shenoy and Appel 2017, 340). In addition, the following strategies may help reduce data breaches: nesting (i.e., shielding) personal identifying information, encrypting records, auditing access to health records, requiring all employees to sign agreements not to disclose PHI, training regarding the use of passwords, increasing knowledge of phishing schemes, and maintaining an organizational culture that promotes ethical awareness.

Still, a director of development and community relations in Vermont conceded that even though the hospital encrypted its records, audited access to health records, required employees to sign agreements not to disclose PHI, and trained employees about hospital procedures regarding PHI confidentiality, the hospital had to report two breaches within a year (Ollove 2014). The director concluded that the hospital had to rely on the honor system (Ollove 2014). Even with appropriate training, policies, and procedures, you may still find an unethical employee. And, when you do, you can refer back to chapter 12 on how to ethically terminate her employment at your facility.

Conclusion

At the beginning of this chapter, we met the managers at Memorial Hermann Health System, who publicly revealed the name of a patient. What began with a fraudulent identification card turned into a larger problem: The hospital managers were responsible for protecting the patient's information, and they did not. The outcome was a fine of $2.4 million, with an agreement to implement a corrective plan of action.

Throughout this chapter, we saw how vital it is for healthcare managers to understand the impact of health information technology on administrative tasks and patient care. We presented a brief history of IT in healthcare and discussed its benefits as well as issues that accompany its use. It is not enough for healthcare managers to know what is legally right according to HIPAA legislation regarding privacy, security, and enforcement rules. Healthcare managers also need to foster an organizational culture that promotes ethical awareness and behavior so that competent, ethical employees who have been trained to use EHR systems effectively and understand its inherent security and privacy issues can provide quality healthcare. All the promised benefits of EHRs are only possible if healthcare managers create an environment in which healthcare providers can do their jobs well and patients have confidence in the security of their medical records.

Mini Case Study: Patient Deception

In 2009, Sharon Holmes had a routine mammogram at Perry Hospital in Georgia and was told the results were negative: She did not have cancer. But only two months later, she felt a lump in her breast and underwent another mammogram. The results of this new test said she had aggressive breast cancer, and the disease had spread to her lymph nodes (Brumback 2014; Newsome and McLaughlin 2014).

Holmes was determined to be one of about 1,300 women who had received falsified mammogram readings at Perry Hospital. This was discovered after another patient, who had also received a negative reading for her mammogram taken at Perry, received a positive diagnosis following a second mammogram at a different facility three months later. An investigation at Perry into these discrepancies uncovered the 1,300 cases, in which women had not had their mammograms read by a radiologist. Ten of the patients had been given false negatives, and two women later died from breast cancer. When investigators discovered that one of the radiologists who had supposedly read one of the mammograms on a particular date was not working at the hospital on that date, the lead radiological technologist confessed. She said that personal issues had caused her to fall behind in her work, so over the course of 18 months she had regularly logged into the hospital's computer system, assumed the identities of the radiologists, and signed off on the mammograms as negative (Brumback 2014).

The technologist pleaded guilty in 2010 and was sentenced to up to six months in prison, ten years' probation, and a $12,500 fine. Moreover, she is not allowed to work in the healthcare field for ten years.

Mini Case Study Questions

1. Identify the security breach in this mini case. Consider the issue of the radiological technologist's access to the radiologists' passwords in your response.

2. Assume you are a healthcare manager at Perry. What corrective plan would you introduce to ensure an event like this does not occur again?
3. The falsified mammogram actions were discovered by chance. How could an in-house audit have identified the radiologic technologist's actions sooner? How might the radiologists have noticed they were not reading the mammograms?

Points to Remember

- HIPAA is important legislation regarding protection for patient privacy and confidentiality.
- Privacy and security regarding health information matters should be the concern of all healthcare administrators and providers.
- The increased use of EHRs is directly related to the political environment, which introduced financial incentives for EHR adoption and implementation.
- Health information technology has both benefits and issues associated with its use.
- Medical identity theft not only may affect reimbursement of services provided, but also may result in faulty patient health information being recorded.
- Healthcare managers have a responsibility to safeguard proper use of health information technology by establishing appropriate training and professional development opportunities for employees.
- Healthcare managers also have a responsibility to safeguard proper use of health information technology by establishing an ethical culture that promotes the use of technology to support the organization's goals of providing quality patient care.

Challenge Yourself

1. The case study at the beginning of this chapter introduced a patient who was asked to show identification at Memorial Hermann Health System, and she produced a fake driver's license. Criticism and debate about immigrants' access to healthcare, and MHHS' subsequent press releases and conversations, resulted in the health system agreeing to pay $2.4 million to the US Department of Health and Human Services' Office for Civil Rights and to implement a corrective action plan to ensure compliance regarding PHI. After reading the section on medical identity theft, why do you think MHHS asks patients for identification when they arrive at their facility? What would you recommend as the proper course of action?
2. Contact your local hospital or healthcare center and ask to interview personnel associated with its disaster plan. How have they prepared to protect patient health

information during a disaster? How have they prepared to share patient data with other hospitals and healthcare centers in case of patient transfer during a disaster?

3. Reflect on the comment made by the director of development and community relations in Vermont regarding the hospital's need to rely on the honor system for PHI confidentiality. List three actions healthcare managers could take so they do not have to rely on an honor system. Consider training, professional development, and corrective action plans in your response.

For Your Consideration

1. This chapter's discussion of patient portals noted that research shows the majority of patients are not using this technology. Suggest two possible reasons they are not doing so.
2. Offer one example to illustrate how information technology supports organizational goals for administrative tasks and another example for patient care.

Exercise 15.1 Ethics and Subsequent Use of Electronic Health Record Data

We discussed in this chapter the role of ethics regarding privacy and security of health information. Consider the role of ethics regarding employee interactions with EHRs, including the importance of entering accurate data, maintaining confidentiality, and taking actions to avoid data breaches. If your library has access to the following article, review the three recommendations of Lee (2017) to minimize risk and maximize benefit and the role of both technological innovation in ethics integration. The full reference is: Lee, L. 2017. "Ethics and Subsequent Use of Electronic Health Record Data." *Journal of Biomedical Informatics* 71: 143–46.

If your library does not have access to this journal, Lee's (2017) three recommendations are as follows:

1. Researchers and healthcare administrators working with EHR management should evaluate EHR validity.
2. Healthcare managers should provide ethical training regarding data management and the importance of protecting health data.
3. Healthcare managers should hold employees accountable for data breaches.

Exercise 15.1 Question

1. Offer examples to illustrate how Lee's recommendations could be put into action.

Exercise 15.2 Snooping into Patient Records

Cleveland-based University Hospitals informed about 700 patients that one of its employees had been snooping into their medical records, which by law should be confidential (McCann 2014). Upon investigation, University Hospitals learned the employee had been accessing patient financial and health information for more than three years. The employee was terminated.

In Massachusetts, an employee was hired in 2010 at Tufts Health Plan. Between 2010 and 2014, she sent personal data on more than 8,700 plan members to an individual in Florida with whom her brother used the information to file false income tax returns. The employee was arrested and charged with stealing personal identifying information, including names, birth dates, and Social Security numbers (US Department of Justice 2017). The employee pleaded guilty and was sentenced to three months in prison and three years of supervised release, and to pay $52,000 in restitution. One man was sentenced to two years in prison, the other to a term of one year and one day.

These are just two examples of snooping, an action in violation of HIPAA. By law, only employees whose job it is to access patient information may do so. Still, HIPAA breaches continue. A review of the 39 PHI breaches reported in February 2018 alone found that 16 of them (41 percent) were the result of employee actions (*HIPAA Journal* 2018a).

Exercise 15.2 Questions

1. With reference to the information provided in the chapter, discuss examples of how snooping may be addressed. Describe, for example, what you as a healthcare manager could do regarding policies and procedures for nesting personal identifying information, encrypting records, auditing access to health records, requiring all employees to sign agreements not to disclose PHI, training on the use of passwords, and increasing knowledge of phishing schemes.
2. Conduct an Internet search with the terms "HIPAA" and "snooping." Read in detail about one case you find. What do you think healthcare managers in that case might have done to prevent the breach from occurring?

References

Abir, M., F. Mostashari, P. Atwal, and N. Lurie. 2012. "Electronic Health Records Critical in the Aftermath of Disasters." *Prehospital and Disaster Medicine* 27 (6): 620–22.

Andrews, M. 2016. "The Rise of Medical Identity Theft." *Consumer Reports*. Published August 25. www.consumerreports.org/medical-identity-theft/medical-identity-theft/.

Armour, S. 2015. "How Identity Theft Sticks You with Hospital Bills." *Wall Street Journal*. Published August 7. www.wsj.com/articles/how-identity-theft-sticks-you-with-hospital-bills-1438966007.

Barajas, M. 2015. "Woman Arrested at Gynecologist Appointment Could Face Deportation." *Houston Press*. Published September 11. www.houstonpress.com/news/woman-arrested-at-gynecologist-appointment-could-face-deportation-7754827.

Benjamin, R. 2010. "Finding My Way to Electronic Health Records." *New England Journal of Medicine* 363 (6): 505–6.

Brumback, K. 2014. "Ex-Technician Falsified Mammograms." *Atlanta Journal-Constitution*. Published April 28. www.pressreader.com/usa/the-atlanta-journal-constitution/20140428/281891591278738.

Cellucci, L., K. Benson, and T. Farnsworth. 2011. "Health Information Technology, Patient Flow, and the New Manager: Evaluation of Three Clinics." *Annual Advances in Business Cases* 30: 82–89.

Centers for Disease Control and Prevention (CDC). 2015. "National Electronic Health Records Survey: 2015 State and National Electronic Health Record Adoption Summary Tables." Accessed August 15, 2018. www.cdc.gov/nchs/data/ahcd/nehrs/2015_nehrs_web_table.pdf.

Centers for Medicare & Medicaid Services (CMS). 2018a. "Promoting Interoperability (PI)." Updated July 31. www.cms.gov/Regulations-and-Guidance/Legislation/EHRIncentivePrograms/index.html.

———. 2018b. "Stage 3 Program Requirements for Providers Attesting to Their State's Medicaid Promoting Interoperability (PI) Programs." Updated April 25. www.cms.gov/Regulations-and-Guidance/Legislation/EHRIncentivePrograms/Stage3Medicaid_Require.html.

———. 2016. *Stage 2 – Modified Stage 2 – Stage 3 Comparison of Eligible Professional Measures and Objectives*. Published November. http://dhs.pa.gov/cs/groups/webcontent/documents/document/c_253196.pdf.

———. 2012. "Stage 1 vs. Stage 2 Comparison Table for Eligible Professionals." Updated August. www.cms.gov/Regulations-and-Guidance/Legislation/EHRIncentivePrograms/Downloads/Stage1vsStage2CompTablesforEP.pdf.

Clark, S., L. Costello, A. Gebremariam, and K. Dombkowski. 2015. "A National Survey of Parent Perspectives on Use of Patient Portals for Their Children's Health Care." *Applied Clinical Informatics* 6 (1): 110–19.

DesRoches, C., D. Charles, M. Furukawa, M. Joshi, P. Kralovec, F. Mostashari, C. Worzala, and A. Jha. 2013. "Adoption of Electronic Health Records Grows Rapidly, but Fewer Than Half of US Hospitals Had at Least a Basic System in 2012." *Health Affairs* 32 (8): 1478–85.

Devine, E., E. Williams, D. Martin, D. Sittig, P. Tarczy-Hornoch, T. Payne, and S. Sullivan. 2010. "Prescriber and Staff Perceptions of an Electronic Prescribing System in Primary Care: A Qualitative Assessment." *BMC Medical Informatics and Decision Making* 10: 72.

Dick, R., and E. Steen. 1991. *The Computer-Based Patient Record: An Essential Technology for Health Care*. Washington, DC: National Academies Press.

Franco, C., E. Toner, R. Waldhorn, B. Maldin, T. O'Toole, and T. Inglesby. 2006. "Systemic Collapse: Medical Care in the Aftermath of Hurricane Katrina." *Biosecurity and Bioterrorism: Biodefense Strategy, Practice, and Science* 4 (2): 135–46.

Freemantle, T. 2005. "Trapped Hospital Workers Kept Most Patients Alive." Published September 18. www.chron.com/news/hurricanes/article/Trapped-hospital-workers-kept-most-patients-alive-1502571.php.

Goldzweig, C., G. Orshansky, A. Towfigh, D. Haggstrom, I. Miake-Lye, J. Beroes, and P. Shekelle. 2013. "Electronic Patient Portals: Evidence on Health Outcomes, Satisfaction, Efficiency, and Attitudes: A Systematic Review." *Annals of Internal Medicine* 159 (10): 677–87.

Griffin, A., A. Skinner, J. Thornhill, and M. Weinberger. 2016. "Patient Portals: Who Uses Them? What Features Do They Use? And Do They Reduce Hospital Readmissions?" *Applied Clinical Informatics* 7 (2): 489–501.

Havens, D., and L. Boroughs. 2000. "'To Err Is Human': A Report from the Institute of Medicine." *Journal of Pediatric Health Care* 14 (2): 77–80.

HealthIT.gov. 2018. "What Is an Electronic Health Record (EHR)?" Reviewed March 21. www.healthit.gov/faq/what-electronic-health-record-ehr.

———. 2017. "Meaningful Use." Reviewed September 5. www.healthit.gov/topic/federal-incentive-programs/meaningful-use.

Henry, J., Y. Pylypchuk, T. Searcy, and V. Patel. 2016. "Adoption of Electronic Health Record Systems Among U.S. Non-Federal Acute Care Hospitals: 2008–2015." ONC Data Brief 35. Published May. https://dashboard.healthit.gov/evaluations/data-briefs/non-federal-acute-care-hospital-ehr-adoption-2008-2015.php.

Hersh, W. 2009. "A Stimulus to Define Informatics and Health Information Technology." *BMC Medical Informatics and Decision Making*. Published May 15. https://doi.org/10.1186/1472-6947-9-24.

HIPAA Journal. 2018a. "Analysis of February 2018 Healthcare Data Breaches." Published March 19. www.hipaajournal.com/february-2018-healthcare-data-breaches/.

———. 2018b. "ATI Physical Therapy Data Breach Impacts 35,000 Patients." Published March 22. www.hipaajournal.com/ati-physical-therapy-data-breach-impacts-35000-patients/.

Hixenbaugh, M. 2017. "Memorial Hermann to Pay $2.4M After Sharing Patient Name in Press Release." *Houston Chronicle*. Published May 10. www.houstonchronicle.com/news/article/Memorial-Hermann-to-pay-2-4M-after-sharing-11137038.php.

Institute of Medicine (IOM). 2004. *Patient Safety: Achieving a New Standard for Care*. Washington, DC: National Academies Press.

———. 1999. *To Err Is Human: Building a Safer Health System*. Washington, DC: National Academies Press.

Kline, M. 2017. "6 Takeaways from Memorial Hermann HIPAA Settlement: Press Releases Lead to $2.4 Million Payout." *HIPAA & Health Information Technology* blog. Posted May 14. https://hipaahealthlaw.foxrothschild.com/2017/05/articles/privacy/6-takeaways-memorial-hermann-hipaa-settlement-press-releases-lead-2-4-million-payout/.

Kruse, C., K. Bolton, and G. Freriks. 2015. "The Effect of Patient Portals on Quality Outcomes and Its Implications to Meaningful Use: A Systematic Review." *Journal of Medical Internet Research* 17 (2): e44.

Kuyers, S. B. S. 2017. "Memorial Hermann's Use of Patient Name in Press Release Leads to $2.4 Million HIPAA Settlement." *Health Law & Policy Matters* blog. Posted May 18. www.healthlawpolicymatters.com/2017/05/18/memorial-hermanns-use-of-patient-name-in-press-release-leads-to-2-4-million-hipaa-settlement/.

Leape, L., D. Bates, D. Cullen, J. Cooper, H. Demonaco, T. Gallivan, R. Hallisey, J. Ives, N. Laird, G. Laffel, R. Nemeskal, L. Petersen, K. Porter, D. Servi, B. Shea, S. Small, B. Sweitzer, T. Thompson, and

M. Vliet. 1995. "Systems Analysis of Adverse Drug Events." *Journal of the American Medical Association* 274 (1): 35–43.

Lee, L. 2017. "Ethics and Subsequent Use of Electronic Health Record Data." *Journal of Biomedical Informatics* 71: 143–46.

Left, S. 2002. "Email Timeline." *The Guardian*. Published March 13. www.theguardian.com/technology/2002/mar/13/internetnews.

Lewallen, B. 2004. "Wal-Mart & the Bar Code." *Frontline*. Published November 16. www.pbs.org/wgbh/pages/frontline/shows/walmart/secrets/barcode.html.

Maruca, W. 2015. "Did Practice Violate HIPAA by Tipping off Immigration Authorities?" *HIPAA & Health Information Technology* blog. Posted September 25. https://hipaahealthlaw.foxrothschild.com/2015/09/articles/articles/did-practice-violate-hipaa-by-tipping-off-immigration-authorities/.

McCann, E. 2014. "Employee Sacked After Snooping Patient EMR Records." *Healthcare IT News*. Published December 2. www.healthcareitnews.com/news/employee-sacked-after-snooping-patient-emr-records.

McRobbie, L. 2015. "The ATM Is Dead. Long Live the ATM!" Smithsonian.com. Published January 8. www.smithsonianmag.com/history/atm-dead-long-live-atm-180953838/.

Medical Group Management Association (MGMA). 2009. "Revenue Cycle and Accounts Receivable Management." In *Medical Practice Management Body of Knowledge Review: Financial Management, Vol. 2*, 2nd ed., 75–96. Englewood, CO: MGMA.

Medical Identity Fraud Alliance (MIFA). 2015. "New Medical Identity Fraud Alliance Research Reveals More Than Two Million Victims Affected by Medical Identity Theft in 2014." Published February 23. www.prnewswire.com/news-releases/new-medical-identity-fraud-alliance-research-reveals-more-than-two-million-victims-affected-by-medical-identity-theft-in-2014-300039152.html.

Miller, D., C. Latulipe, K. Melius, S. Quandt, and T. Arcury. 2016. "Primary Care Providers' Views of Patient Portals: Interview Study of Perceived Benefits and Consequences." *Journal of Medical Internet Research* 18 (1): e8.

Minor, T. 2016. "Could You Fall Victim to Medical Identity Theft?" *News4Jax*. Posted February 11. www.news4jax.com/news/investigations/local-woman-a-victim-of-medical-identity-theft.

Mook, P. J., A. W. Trickey, K. E. Krakowski, S. Majors, M. A. Theiss, C. Fant, and M. A. Friesen. 2018. "Exploration of Portal Activation by Patients in a Healthcare System." *Computers, Informatics, Nursing* 36 (1): 18–26.

Morse, S. 2017. "Memorial Hermann Ordered to Pay $2.4 Million over Immigrant Incident." *Healthcare IT News*. Published May 10. www.healthcareitnews.com/news/memorial-hermann-ordered-pay-24-million-over-immigrant-incident.

Network for Regional Healthcare Improvement. 2018. "What Is MACRA." Accessed August 15. www.nrhi.org/work/what-is-macra/what-is-macra/.

Neumann, P., S. Parente, and L. Paramore. 1996. "Potential Savings from Using Information Technology Applications in Health Care in the United States." *International Journal of Technology Assessment in Health Care* 12 (3): 425–35.

Newsome, J., and E. McLaughlin. 2014. "Former Hospital Technician Behind Bogus Mammogram Results Gets Jail Time." CNN. Published April 16. www.cnn.com/2014/04/16/health/georgia-false-mammogram-cancer-sentencing/index.html.

Office for Civil Rights (OCR). 2018. "Cases Currently Under Investigation." Accessed May 28. https://ocrportal.hhs.gov/ocr/breach/breach_report.jsf.

Ollove, M. 2014. "Nearly Half of Identity Thefts in U.S. Are Medical Info." *USA Today*. Published February 7. www.usatoday.com/story/news/nation/2014/02/07/stateline-identity-thefts-medical-information/5279351/.

Ponemon Institute. 2015. *Fifth Annual Study on Medical Theft*. Published February. https://static.nationwide.com/static/2014_Medical_ID_Theft_Study.pdf.

Robertson, C., and R. Fausset. 2015. "10 Years After Katrina." *New York Times*. Published August 26. www.nytimes.com/interactive/2015/08/26/us/ten-years-after-katrina.html.

Schiller, D. 2015. "Immigrant Mother Arrested at Gynecologist's Office Draws National Attention." *Houston Chronicle*. Published September 17. www.houstonchronicle.com/news/houston-texas/houston/article/Immigrant-mother-arrested-at-gynecologist-s-6512587.php.

Shenoy, A., and J. Appel. 2017. "Safeguarding Confidentiality in Electronic Health Records." *Cambridge Quarterly of Healthcare Ethics* 26 (2): 337–41.

Spitzer, J. 2018. "Employee at Carolina Digestive Health Associates Steals PHI." *Becker's Health IT & CIO Report*. Published April 19. www.beckershospitalreview.com/cybersecurity/employee-at-carolina-digestive-health-associates-steals-phi.html.

Tsai, J., and R. Rosenheck. 2012. "Use of the Internet and an Online Personal Health Record System by US Veterans: Comparison of Veterans Affairs Mental Health Service Users and Other Veterans Nationally." *Journal of the American Medical Informatics Association* 19 (6): 1089–94.

US Department of Health and Human Services. 2017a. "Memorial Hermann Health System Resolution Plan Agreement and Corrective Action Plan." Accessed August 15, 2018. www.hhs.gov/sites/default/files/mhhs_ra_cap.pdf.

———. 2017b. "Texas Health System Settles Potential HIPAA Disclosure Violations." Press release published May 10. www.hhs.gov/about/news/2017/05/10/texas-health-system-settles-potential-hipaa-disclosure-violations.html.

US Department of Justice. 2017. "Former Tufts Health Plan Employee Sentenced for Disclosing Personal Patient Information." Press release published May 31. www.justice.gov/usao-ma/pr/former-tufts-health-plan-employee-sentenced-disclosing-personal-patient-information.

Wailgum, T. 2007. "45 Years of Wal-Mart History: A Technology Time Line." *CIO*. Published August 17. www.cio.com/article/2437873/infrastructure/45-years-of-wal-mart-history--a-technology-time-line.html.

World Wide Web Foundation. 2018. "History of the Web." Accessed August 15. https://webfoundation.org/about/vision/history-of-the-web/.

Wright, A., D. Sittig, J. Ash, J. Feblowitz, S. Meltzer, C. McMullen, and B. Middleton. 2011. "Development and Evaluation of a Comprehensive Clinical Decision Support Taxonomy: Comparison of Front-End Tools in Commercial and Internally Developed Electronic Health Record Systems." *Journal of the American Medical Informatics Association* 18 (3): 232–42.

GLOSSARY

Academic health center (AHC): A teaching hospital that provides healthcare services to the community, trains physicians, and engages in medical research.

Accommodating style: A conflict style involving low concern for one's own position and high concern for that of others.

Accountable care organization (ACO): A form of health services delivery organization that includes multiple kinds of providers who work together to improve care delivery to the individual patient as well as to improve the health status of a particular population, such as a group of employees or Medicare enrollees. The providers work as a team because of a reimbursement mechanism that incentivizes improvement in patient outcomes.

Accounts receivable: Dollar amounts that have been billed to patients and third-party payers but have not yet been paid.

Active listening: The process of paying close attention to a message so that it is received accurately.

Activities of daily living (ADL): Functions that are generally done for oneself, such as eating, bathing, dressing, grooming, and taking care of bodily functions.

Activity-based budgeting: Creating a financial plan that focuses on the manager's allocating costs to each activity performed on behalf of the unit's responsibilities (e.g., patient care).

Acute care: Short-term care for patients who have a relatively severe illness.

Adjourning stage: The final stage of teamwork, during which team members review outcomes and successes and individuals disengage from the team.

Administrative rule: Language written by an agency that explains a piece of legislation in active terms to carry out the law's mandate. It may also be something that describes the agency's process or procedures. This seldom-featured part of the policymaking process is as important as the legislative process that enacted the law.

Adverse selection: The phenomenon that occurs when there is a disproportionate percentage of patients with greater-than-average need for medical and hospital care enrolling in an insurance plan.

Affordable Care Act (ACA): Also known as the Patient Protection and Affordable Care Act, legislation that was promulgated by the Obama administration to bring the United States one step closer to "universal coverage," or insurance that covers everyone in the country.

Age Discrimination in Employment Act, 1967: Act prohibiting age discrimination in employment for those 40 years or older.

Aggressiveness: Behavior that is hostile and combative.

Ambulatory surgery center (ASC): A facility capable of performing surgery on an outpatient basis, with a patient's arrival and departure on the same day.

American College of Healthcare Executives (ACHE): An international professional society of 48,000 healthcare executives who lead hospitals, healthcare systems, and other healthcare organizations. ACHE has 78 chapters that provide access to networking, education, and career development at the local level. ACHE publishes *Healthcare Executive, Journal of Healthcare Management*, and *Frontiers of Health Services Management.* It also has its own publishing division, Health Administration Press, which published this book.

American Recovery and Reinvestment Act (ARRA): An economic stimulus bill passed by the US Congress in 2009 in response to the country's economic downturn. Included the 2009 HITECH Act.

Americans with Disabilities Act, 1990: Act prohibiting discrimination in employment, public services, accommodations, and telecommunications for those with disabilities.

Ancillary services: Services provided by a hospital that are incidental to patient care, such as imaging and laboratory services. Clinicians use these services for both inpatients and outpatients.

Assertiveness: Behavior that is positive and self-confident.

Assessment: The act of measuring, appraising, and evaluating.

Assisted living facility: A living arrangement for older adults who can live independently but require some nonnursing support with some activities of daily living in order to do so.

Association of University Programs in Health Administration (AUPHA): An international association of more than 400 colleges and universities dedicated to improving health by promoting excellence in healthcare management education. AUPHA provides opportunities for member programs to learn from each other by influencing practice and by promoting the value of healthcare management education. AUPHA publishes *Journal of Health Administration Education.*

Authoritarian: A leadership style in which power is concentrated in the leader.

Autonomy: The state of being self-governing. The liberty to rule one's self, free of the controlling influence of others.

Average days in accounts receivable: Calculation of the average number of days from date of service to payment received. Typically, the equation reads total accounts receivable ÷ (gross charges ÷ days in period).

Avoidance style: A conflict style involving low concern for self and low concern for others; often presents itself as withdrawal or lack of cooperation.

Benchmarking: The process of comparing one organization or situation to similar organizations or situations using uniform measures.

Beneficence: An obligation to help and provide benefits to others.

Best practices: The actions, processes, and procedures used in a profession, discipline, or industry to achieve the best possible outcomes.

Bias: A tendency to apply a negative or positive bent to a situation because of prejudicial thought.

Bribe: Money or favor given or promised in order to influence the judgment or conduct of a person in a position of trust.

Budget: A statement that indicates financial administration for a set period of time. This is basically a guide to the organization's priorities.

Bundled payment: Payment to providers based on expected costs for clinically defined episodes of care.

Centers for Medicare & Medicaid Services (CMS): The federal government agency that administers the Medicare program and the federal portion of the Medicaid and CHIP programs. CMS is part of the US Department of Health and Human Services. Note that even though the "centers" portion of the name is plural, the CMS acronym is singular.

Change participants: The staff members whose work behaviors may be affected by any implemented changes.

Change process: The process whereby managed change is envisioned and implemented (successfully or unsuccessfully) in an organization.

Charity write-off: The cost of providing service to people who cannot pay, requiring the provider to take a financial loss.

Civil Rights Act, 1991: Act containing provisions regarding the right to a trial and the receipt of damages in cases of intentional discrimination.

Civil Rights Act, Title VII, 1964: Act prohibiting discrimination in employment on the basis of sex, race, color, national origin, and religion. Applies to organizations with 15 or more employees.

Civility: Positive interpersonal behavior that includes kind, courteous treatment of others.

Clinical decision support system (CDSS): Computer software that presents clinicians with knowledge-based information to help provide better specialized patient care.

Clinical ethics: The overarching framework of morals and principles underscoring the provision of medical care to patients.

Clinical integration: The coordinated delivery of patient care by a team across conditions, providers, settings, and time to achieve high-quality care. Best effectuated by a common (electronic) health record to keep all providers informed.

Collaboration: Working together to achieve designated goals.

Community health center (CHC): One of a network of clinics designed to provide patient care in a designated area.

Community hospital: Hospitals, ranging from large teaching hospitals to small inpatient facilities, that provide medical services to their communities.

Community rating: The process of establishing insurance premiums based on the average healthcare demands of an entire community or population without regard to any risk factors, resulting in identical premiums for every plan member regardless of age, gender, or other health risk.

Competencies: A set of professional and personal skills, knowledge, values, and traits that guide a leader's performance, behavior, interactions, and decisions.

Competitive advantage: A set of attributes that puts a company in a favorable or superior business position.

Compromising style: A conflict style involving a reasonable level of concern for self and for others; aims to keep both sides equal and actively searches for the middle ground, ensuring that one side does not give in more than the other.

Computerized physician order entry (CPOE): A system in which a healthcare provider enters a medication order via electronic entry, which is sent directly to a pharmacy in real time. Replaces handwritten paper prescriptions.

Confidentiality: Holding information as secret and private.

Contractual allowance: The amount a provider discounts from the cost of service in exchange for treating a higher volume of patients.

Control: To guide or check; the act of accountability.

Coordination of care: Deliberate communication and organization of healthcare actions between two or more providers and the patient to ensure better health outcomes.

Copay: A fixed amount paid by the patient out of pocket, usually at the time a healthcare service is provided. The copayment is required by the insurance company as a condition of the insured receiving service.

Corporate citizenship: The social responsibility of both not-for-profit organizations and for-profit businesses, and the extent to which they meet legal, ethical, and economic responsibilities, as expected by stakeholders.

Covered lives: The number of people and dependents enrolled in a particular health plan. There is no standard term for such a person, as they may be referred to as beneficiary, member, insured, subscriber, or the like.

Criticality: The ultimate importance of an issue and its material effect on the individuals and time pressure involved in resolving the conflict.

Cultural adaptability: The willingness and ability to understand cultural differences and act upon that understanding to yield cooperative outcomes.

Cultural relativism: Understanding another culture based on its own standards, beliefs, and traditions.

Decision-making process: The thought and action that lead one to choose from a set of options.

Deductible: The aggregate amount an insured must pay before the insurance begins to pay for the insured's care. For example, a $2,000 deductible means the patient must pay $2,000 before full coverage will begin.

Delegation: Assigning tasks to others; the ability to get work done through others.

Democratic: A leadership approach in which team members share governance.

Direct costs: Expenses associated with a specific activity provided by a unit.

Discrimination: Prejudice or unjust treatment of people based on group characteristics rather than individual merit.

Disease prevention: The result of education and other health-promotion efforts designed to help people become healthier and stay healthy.

Diversity: A list of characteristics, including gender, race, ethnicity, educational level, socioeconomic status, culture, language, religion, disabilities, sexual orientation, and age, that indicates an individual's background.

Dominating style: A conflict style involving high concern for self and low concern for others; demanding and imposing one's will on others with little or no concern about the impact on the other party.

Downward communication: Communication that is primarily informational and initiated by the superior in the organization.

Dustbin delegation: Delegating only unpleasant, boring tasks that the manager does not want to do.

Effective: Having a definite or desired effect.

Effective communication: Communication in which the receiver receives and understands the message as the sender intended it.

Efficient: Productive, with minimum waste or effort.

Electronic health record (EHR): A digital record of the care provided to a patient by a healthcare organization, including the patient's up-to-date, real-time health-related information. When the record can be shared among multiple providers, it is said to have *interoperability*. Also called *electronic medical record.*

Emergency Medical Treatment and Labor Act of 1986 (EMTALA): Legislation created to address the perceived problem of "patient dumping"—the refusal to treat uninsured patients, who are instead transferred to charitable hospitals without being seen by a clinician or receiving care. EMTALA requires hospitals and their affiliated physicians to screen and to continue to treat emergency patients until they are stabilized or transferred.

Emotional intelligence: The ability to identify and manage your own emotions and the emotions of others.

Employer-sponsored insurance (ESI): Insurance plans for which the employer pays part of the premium for the benefit of the employees and sometimes their family members. The primary way Americans obtain health insurance.

Equal Employment Opportunity Act, 1972: Legislation containing the provision that the Equal Employment Opportunity Commission may sue in federal courts if there is reasonable cause to believe employment discrimination occurred based on race, color, religion, sex, or national origin.

Equal Employment Opportunity Commission (EEOC): The US government agency that enforces federal employment discrimination laws.

Ethics: An internalized understanding of how one should behave.

Ethnocentrism: The tendency to judge aspects of other cultures based upon the standards, beliefs, and traditions of one's own culture.

Excess of revenue over expenses: In a nonprofit organization, the remaining cash after revenues minus expenses.

Expense: Costs incurred by a unit's actions (associated with services provided) or overhead costs not directly related to generating revenue.

Explanation of benefits (EOB): A statement sent by a health insurance company to covered individuals explaining what medical treatments and services were paid for on their behalf.

Federal poverty level (FPL): An economic measure used by the federal government to determine the eligibility for certain federal programs intended to assist people living in poverty. The FPL varies with family size and is lower for smaller families and higher for larger families.

Federally qualified health center (FQHC): A clinic designated to serve an underserved area or population, offering a sliding fee scale and comprehensive healthcare services.

Feedback: Critical assessment of information or action.

Fee-for-service: A method of paying physicians for services in which each service carries a fee.

Fidelity: The quality of being faithful, accurate, and steadfast to an ideal, obligation, trust, or duty.

Fishbone diagram: A visualization tool for categorizing the potential causes of a problem (or poor outcome) to identify its root causes. Also called a *cause-and-effect diagram.*

Fixed costs: Expenses that will be incurred regardless of volume of activity or usage.

Forming stage: The first stage of teamwork, during which members are given their charge or the purpose of the team.

Four Rights approach: Delegating by identifying the right task, the right person, the right communication, and the right feedback.

Functions of management: The basic responsibilities of a manager, which include planning, organizing, leading, and controlling.

Germ theory: The theory stating that invisible microorganisms invade the body to cause disease.

Good stewardship of resources: The careful and responsible management of something entrusted to one's care.

Graduate medical education: Formal education in residency programs available to physicians who have graduated from medical school.

Gross domestic product (GDP): The monetary value of all finished goods and services produced in a country by individuals and companies for a specified period of time, usually one year. In 2016, the GDP for the United States was $18.57 trillion. By comparison, the GDP for the second-largest economy in the world, China, was $11.2 trillion.

Groupthink: Conformity to group values and ethics that can lead to negative outcomes.

HCAHPS scores: Results on the Hospital Consumer Assessment of Healthcare Providers and Systems survey, the first national, standardized, publicly reported survey of patients' perspectives on hospital care.

Health informatics: The study of the creation and implementation of information technology–based innovation to advance health services.

Health Information Technology for Economic and Clinical Health (HITECH) Act: Legislation passed in 2009 to promote the adoption and meaningful use of health information technology. Also addressed privacy and security concerns associated with the use of HIT.

Health Insurance Portability and Accountability Act (HIPAA): A law that took effect in 2003 and established a baseline of acceptable protection for patient privacy and confidentiality.

Health Insurance Portability and Accountability Act (HIPAA) Privacy Rule: The part of HIPAA that establishes safeguards to protect confidentiality and privacy and specifically identifies protected health information.

Health literacy: The degree to which one has and understands health information essential to making informed health decisions.

Health maintenance organization (HMO): A healthcare-providing organization that generally has a closed panel (limited number) of physicians (and other providers, including hospitals) that agrees to provide all the medical and hospital care an individual may need, for a fixed, predetermined fee.

Health promotion: Activities designed to influence individual behaviors that affect personal health.

Health Resources and Services Administration (HRSA): The federal agency that deals with issues relating to access, equity, quality, and cost of care. It is part of the Department of Health and Human Services.

Hill-Burton Act: Bipartisan legislation aimed at funding the growth of community hospitals in the United States.

Home health agency: An organization that provides medical and other health services in the patient's home.

Hospice: A program that assists with the physical, emotional, spiritual, psychological, social, and financial needs of a dying patient and the patient's family. This service may be provided in the patient's home or in a facility.

Hospital outpatient department: A part of a hospital designated for the treatment of outpatients: people with health problems who visit the hospital for diagnosis or treatment, but who do not need to be admitted for overnight care.

Human resource management: The management of activities related to healthcare employees.

Incremental budgeting: Creating a financial plan that is increased or decreased according to previous expenditures for a set period of time.

Indirect costs: Expenses that are not associated with a specific unit activity.

Industrial revolution: The shift from an agrarian economy to an industrial economy in Western countries in the eighteenth and nineteenth centuries. This shift resulted in changes to social and economic organization.

Informed consent: A legal document in all 50 states that constitutes an agreement for a proposed medical treatment, nontreatment, or invasive procedure. It requires physicians to disclose the benefits, risks, and alternatives to the proposed treatment, nontreatment, or procedure. It is the method by which fully informed, rational persons may be involved in choices about their healthcare.

Institute of Medicine (IOM): A nonprofit, nongovernment organization established in 1970 that focuses on evidence-based research for public health and science policy.

Instrumental activities of daily living (IADL): Essential activities of daily living, as well as more specialized activities such as shopping, preparing meals, handling money, doing housework and laundry, and driving or using public transportation.

Integrity: Firm adherence to a code of ethics or to a moral code of behavior.

Internalize: To incorporate values, beliefs, or norms as self-guiding principles.

Interprofessionalism: An interdisciplinary healthcare team comprising members from different health professions.

Interprofessional team: A team that forms when two or more professionals from different disciplines collaborate to enable better patient outcomes.

Iron triangle: The interlocking relationships among the cost of care, its quality, and access to it.

Job description: A document that clearly defines the tasks, duties, responsibilities, and performance standards associated with a position.

Joint Commission: A not-for-profit accrediting agency that assesses an organizations' ability to meet standards of performance in key healthcare operations.

Justice: Fairness. Ensuring that everyone is treated equitably.

Kickback: A form of bribery; the offering, giving, receiving, or soliciting of any item of value to influence the actions of another as a result of the recipient's activity to provide illicit value to the giver.

Laissez-faire: A "hands-off" leadership approach.

Lateral communication: Communication between staff members of the same status.

Lead: To be in charge of or responsible for people or tasks.

Leadership: The act of engaging a group of people, often within an organization, to set and achieve goals.

Level of authority: An employee's empowerment to carry out delegated tasks. Levels include the authority to search for information, the authority to provide recommendations, and the authority to fully implement a task.

Liability: Being in a position to likely incur an undesirable responsibility or obligation, usually monetary.

Licensed practical nurse (LPN): A person licensed by the state to carry out specified nursing duties under the direction of a registered nurse.

Litigious: Contentious and prone to become involved in lawsuits.

Long-term care facility (LTC): A facility that provides rehabilitative, restorative, or ongoing skilled nursing care to patients or residents requiring assistance with activities of daily living.

Malpractice: Injury or harm to a patient or customer directly caused by negligence, intentional tort, or breach of contract by a professional.

Managed care organization (MCO): A general term applied to a variety of organizations that provide services intended to reduce healthcare costs by managing access to care.

Managerial ethics: A set of principles and rules that define what is right and what is wrong in an organization. It is the guideline that helps direct a lower manager's decisions in the scope of his or her job when presented with a conflict of values.

Meaningful use: US government standards for healthcare providers' use of electronic health records for capturing and sharing data with other providers, insurers, and patients.

Medicaid: A joint federal–state program that provides insurance coverage for those who cannot afford it. The federal government funds 50 to 75 percent of the costs and controls the broad parameters of the program, which is otherwise administered by the states. The formula that allocates the federal funds is inverse to the relative wealth of the state, meaning that poorer states receive more while richer states receive less.

Medical Group Management Association (MGMA): A professional association of medical group practice professionals with more than 40,000 members who lead and manage more than 12,500 organizations. Members includes administrators, CEOs, physicians in management, board members, and office managers.

Medical Identity Fraud Alliance (MIFA): A coalition created in 2013 to identify best practices for combating patient identity theft.

Medical identity theft: The stealing of another's personal health insurance information in order to submit fraudulent claims for healthcare services rendered or healthcare products purchased.

Medical staff privileges: Permission to practice in the hospital granted to physicians who pass the hospital's credentialing process. Physicians already granted privileges at the hospital frequently oversee this process; it is a form of peer review and acceptance.

Medicare: The federal program that provides health insurance coverage for people older than 65. Medicare Part A covers hospital costs; Part B covers part of the cost of ambulatory care; Part C is a managed care alternative; and Part D provides a benefit for the partial expense of prescription drugs.

Medicare Access and CHIP Reauthorization Act (MACRA): Legislation passed in 2015 that based Medicare payments on patient outcomes; streamlined quality programs such as meaningful use into the Merit-based Incentive Payment System; and provided payments for provider participation in alternative payment models.

Mission statement: An enduring statement of purpose defining what an organization does, whom it serves, and how it does it.

Moving forward: Implementing the managed change.

Multitasking: Doing more than one thing at a time.

National health expenditures (NHE): An economic indicator showing the aggregate amount the United States spends on healthcare each year, frequently expressed as a percentage of the gross domestic product.

Nonmaleficence: The quality of causing no injury or harm and committing no misconduct or wrongdoing.

Nonprogrammed decision: A decision for which there is no set procedure in place and that must be resolved via rational thinking and action.

Nonverbal cues: In communication theory, the behaviors of persons who are interacting with one another. Body language, posture, and facial expressions may elaborate the message that is being sent or received.

Norming stage: The third stage of teamwork, during which team members agree upon working styles, conflict is reduced, and group cohesiveness emerges.

Nurse practitioner (NP): A registered nurse who has completed additional educational requirements (a master's degree or higher) and has qualifications that permit conducting an extended evaluation of the patient with a focus on primary care and patient education.

Occupational Safety and Health Act, 1970: Act mandating worksite safety for employees.

Office of the National Coordinator for Health Information Technology (ONC): Created by President George W. Bush's executive order in 2004 to promote a national health information technology infrastructure. The 2009 HITECH Act gave ONC leadership authority for EHR implementation efforts.

Open door management: Always working with your office door open to show you are available to everyone all the time.

Organizational culture: The shared values, beliefs, and taken-for-granted assumptions of an organization's employees.

Organizational ethics: The ethics of an organization; how an organization responds to an internal or external stimulus.

Organizational fit: An employment candidate's qualification for the position advertised and ability to work well with others in the specific work environment.

Organizational politics: Informal, unofficial, and sometimes behind-the-scenes efforts to sell ideas, influence an organization, increase power, or achieve other targeted objectives.

Organize: To coordinate and carry out tasks.

Outcome: The end result, product, or conclusion to a process or event.

Patient-centered medical home (PCMH): A healthcare delivery model in which the primary care provider ensures the patient receives the right treatment at the right time by the right provider in a way they can understand and that helps them be an active participant in their care.

Patient portal: Secure website that allows patients access to their personal health information.

Patient's role on the healthcare team: Patients' responsibilities to be proactive regarding becoming healthier, staying healthy, and actively engaging with their healthcare team when appropriate.

Pay-for-performance: A financial reward system for healthcare providers in which a portion of their monetary compensation is related to improvement in patient outcomes and other indicators of improved performance.

Per capita expenditure: The total amount spent on healthcare—that is, the national health expenditures (NHE)—divided by the population.

Performance evaluation: The process of reviewing employees' work behavior and efforts.

Performing stage: The fourth stage of teamwork, during which team members are engaged in the work and purpose of the team.

Pharmacy benefit manager (PBM): A company used by managed care providers and insurers to improve the efficiency of providing patients the drugs covered by their plan.

Physician assistant (PA): A healthcare professional with advanced training who is licensed to practice medicine under the supervision of a physician.

Plan: To devise or create a way to accomplish a defined task.

Population health: The health outcomes of a designated population, including the distribution of such outcomes within this population.

Positive duty: The duty of commission. The requirement to engage in an action actively and intentionally.

Post-acute care facility (PAC): A facility that offers a continuum of care depending on patient or resident need.

Power: The ability to enact one's own will based on status, rank, knowledge, level of education, reputation, or a combination of these and other factors.

Pregnancy Discrimination Act, 1978: Act prohibiting discrimination in employment based on pregnancy.

Problem-solving style: A conflict style involving high concern for self and high concern for others; searches for more than the middle ground and actively works toward finding the best possible outcome for all parties.

Process: Activity proximately or directly related to the delivery of care to the patient as well as the actual act of caregiving.

Profession: A body of knowledge shared by people who have received specialized education and training and share common values.

Professional: A person who has received specialized education and training and has qualified to serve in a specific occupation.

Professionalism: Knowledge and understanding of beliefs and behaviors expected of a professional.

Profit: In a for-profit organization, total income or cash flow minus expenditures.

Protected health information (PHI): Information from which a specific person or patient can be identified and that relates to physical or mental health, the provision of healthcare, or the payment for healthcare.

Provider network: A list of hospitals, doctors, and other providers with whom a health plan has contracted and who, therefore, are contractually obligated to provide care for the covered lives in the health plan at a negotiated payment rate.

Public hospital: Publicly owned medical facility found mostly in major metropolitan areas, though sometimes in rural counties as well; frequently treats uninsured patients or those insured through Medicaid.

Quadruple Aim: The goals of improving the patient experience, the health of a population, *and* the provider's experience while reducing healthcare costs.

Quality: Defined by the Institute of Medicine (2018) as "the degree to which health services for individuals and populations increase the likelihood of desired health outcomes and are consistent with current professional knowledge." See chapter 14.

Quality improvement: A systematic, formal approach to analyzing performance and efforts to improve service.

Rational decision-making process: Steps that assist when one is determining what course of action to take.

Receiver: One who is given the message produced by the sender.

Refreezing: Stabilizing the forces that have brought about a newly implemented change so they become part of the organization.

Registered nurse (RN): A healthcare professional who, having graduated from formal training, has been licensed by the state to ensure a specific level of competence in rendering nursing care.

Rehabilitation: Therapies that help restore someone to normal or close-to-normal life.

Rehabilitation hospital: A hospital devoted to the rehabilitation of patients with various neurological, musculoskeletal, orthopedic, and other medical conditions following stabilization of their acute medical issue with a goal of restoring all or most of their pre–acute care functioning.

Relationship conflict: Disagreement and antagonism unrelated to the specific situation and interpersonal in nature.

Relationship management: The connections between you and your workplace with stakeholders. These connections depend on how you and the stakeholders treat each other in the context of work. Acting with integrity and treating each other with civility helps lead to positive relationship management.

Residential care community: A facility that provides room, board, housekeeping, supervision, and personal care assistance with basic activities such as personal hygiene, dressing, eating, and walking for people generally older than age 60.

Resistance to change: Change participants' hesitation or refusal to comply with the vision for the future of operations and management's attempts at carrying out that vision.

Retail clinic: A "walk-in" clinic usually located in a drugstore or other retail store, most often staffed by a nurse practitioner who can provide a variety of primary care services and diagnoses.

Retention: The keeping of employees at an organization.

Revenue: Income produced from providing goods or services.

Risk: A possible, usually negative, outcome. Managers must eliminate as much risk as possible, although in healthcare it is impossible to eliminate all risk.

Risk management: Systems, processes, and structures put in place to decrease the likelihood of adverse events.

Rolling budgeting: A financial plan that is reviewed and updated on a regular, ongoing basis, such as every month or quarter, to reflect recent activities.

Root cause analysis: The process of dissecting a positive or negative incident into its most basic segments and discovering the source of its characteristics and outcomes.

Running a morning dash: Spending an hour on the most important thing on your to-do list first thing each morning, even before checking your messages or e-mail.

Scenario planning: A planning tool that provides a structured way to think about the future and how things might unfold that could affect an organization's well-being.

Scientific management: The study of management activities based on theory and research.

Scientific method of inquiry: The formal process of research. Steps include observation and description, hypothesis formulation, data gathering, data analysis, discussion of the findings, and conclusion.

Sender: The producer of a message.

Sexual harassment: The illegal practice of unwelcome sexual behavior in the workplace.

Shared savings program: A payment strategy that incentivizes healthcare providers to reduce spending for a defined patient population by offering them a percentage of any net savings realized because of their efforts.

Situationally appropriate: In a conflict, taking into account the power and criticality of the issue and each party's willingness to confront the other.

Social determinants of health: The conditions in which people live and work that affect their access to appropriate healthcare and their ability to be an effective and responsible patient.

Social insurance: A system of compulsory payments made by everyone to the government to provide assistance to a designated subset of the population for a specific service or set of services. Medicare Part A is a good example: Every employee and employer contributes to the Medicare Trust Fund through a taxing mechanism. Those funds are used to provide hospitalization benefits to everyone older than age 65.

Socialization process: The process whereby people learn values, beliefs, and norms.

Social marketing: The creation, communication, and delivery of information, events, and programs to influence individual behavior for the benefit of both the individual and the community as a whole.

Social Security Act of 1935: Massive legislation that created direct federal benefits for American citizens in the form of cash payments to the elderly. The act also provided for unemployment insurance and worker's compensation for injured workers.

Special interest group: A collection of organizations and individuals dedicated to a particular cause or profession acting in the policymaking arena with the intent of advancing their point of view and seeking an advantage with respect to policy outcomes.

SSLL dilemma: The basic conflict between "smaller-sooner" (short-term, more immediate costs and benefits) and "larger-longer" (long-term, and perhaps riskier, future payoffs).

Stakeholder: An individual, group, or entity that has an interest in organizational success.

Standards: Customary, appropriate, and acceptable criteria or outcomes.

Statement of operations: A statement that shows the revenues, expenses, and net income of an organization.

Storming stage: The second stage of teamwork, during which team members learn about one another. This stage is characterized by conflict and emotional issues that may inhibit a team's progress.

Strategy development: The part of the planning process in which the organization assesses its internal and external environments and begins to match capability with opportunity to lay the foundation for a strategic plan.

Strategy implementation: The part of the planning cycle in which the organization attempts to operationalize the strategic plan to meet its strategic goals.

Structure: The environment and the set of conditions that exist, relating to both physical premises and qualifications of the staff. Structure is a necessary condition for quality to occur, but by itself, it is insufficient to produce quality healthcare.

SWOT: Stands for strengths, weaknesses, opportunities, and threats. A basic tool of internal and external assessment that any organization can use as part of its strategic planning.

Tactical (operating) plan: Shorter-term, smaller-scale, specific plan intended to carry out the larger goals of the strategic plan. Departments or divisions develop these plans focused on annual objectives. Examples include an operating plan, marketing plan, and fund-raising plan.

Task conflict: Disagreement about tasks, goals, methods, or desired outcomes.

Teaching hospital: A hospital that provides care for the citizens of its local community and residency training programs for medical school graduates preparing to enter a specialty.

Team: A group of people who work toward a shared task and hold themselves mutually accountable for effective performance.

Teamwork climate: How well healthcare team members perceive they work together to provide patient care.

Termination: End of an employee's contract with a company.

360 evaluation: A review process in which the supervisor, the employee, and staff members who work with the employee assess the work behavior and efforts of an employee.

Time inventory log: A tool that illustrates how time is used by briefly noting activities at regular intervals, such as each hour or half hour, during the workday.

Time management: The practice of using time effectively to achieve professional and personal goals.

Tort: An intentional wrong that results in injury or harm. Breach of contract is a category of tort.

Triple Aim: The goals of improving the patient experience and health of the population while reducing healthcare costs.

Trust: Assured reliance on character, ability, strength, or truth. Putting confidence in a person, place, or thing.

Truth telling: A positive duty to provide accurate, complete, and honest information at all times as part of the respect for other persons.

Unfreezing: Reducing the forces that are keeping an organization in its current state.

Uniformed Services Employment and Reemployment Rights Act, 1994: Act prohibiting discrimination of veterans in civilian employment, protecting their seniority, status, and salary.

Upward communication: Communication that allows supervisors to know about staff members' concerns, issues, or recommendations.

Values statement: A statement defining an organization's culture. It expresses values that are important and that guide the organization's work and its interactions with patients, the community, and employees.

Variable costs: Expenses that will change as the volume of activity changes.

Verbal cues: In communication theory, the tone and manner of the message sent and received.

Vision statement: A statement identifying a specific desired future state of an organization; usually an inspiring goal for the organization many years into the future.

Worker's compensation: Insurance overseen by the state for employees who are injured while performing work or work-related activities.

Working memory: Part of short-term memory associated with storing and managing information for learning, reasoning, and comprehension.

Zero-based budgeting: Creating a financial plan for a set period of time that requires each budget item to be justified according to the unit's goals.

INDEX

Note: Italicized page locators refer to exhibits.